Thoracic Surgery Atlas

Thoracic Surgery Atlas

Mark K. Ferguson, MD

Professor, Department of Surgery
Director, Thoracic Surgery Service
The University of Chicago
Chicago, Illinois

Illustrator: Jill Rhead

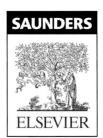

SAUNDERS
ELSEVIER

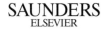

SAUNDERS
ELSEVIER

1600 John F. Kennedy Blvd.
Ste 1800
Philadelphia, PA 19103-2899

**WF
17
F353t
2007**

THORACIC SURGERY ATLAS   ISBN: 978-0-7216-0325-4

Copyright © 2007 by W. B. Saunders, Inc., an affiliate of Elsevier

---

Notice

Library of Congress Cataloging-in-Publication Data
Ferguson, Mark K.
   Thoracic surgery atlas / Mark K. Ferguson ; artist, Jill Rhead.—1st ed.
      p.   ;   cm.
   Includes bibliographical references and index.
   ISBN 978-0-7216-0325-4 (alk. paper)
   1. Chest—Surgery—Atlases. I. Title.
   [DNLM: 1. Thoracic Surgical Procedures—methods—Atlases.   WF 17 F353t 2008]
RD536.F462 2008
617.5'4059—dc22

                                                        2007019409

Publishing Director: Judith Fletcher
Developmental Editor: Joanie Milnes
Project Manager: David Saltzberg
Design Direction: Ellen Zanolle

Printed in China

Last digit is the print number: 9 8 7 6 5 4 3 2 1

To Phyllis, who illuminates all that she encounters.

Preface

Writing a surgical atlas is an undertaking that, from its inception, is doomed to failure. Surgical science, including anatomy, physiology, and pathophysiology, is a field that is subject to hypothesis testing leading to objective information. Controversies, when they exist, are usually resolved through clinical or laboratory research. Surgical practice, particularly with regard to surgical techniques, is quite a different matter. The range of possible approaches to a single problem is endless, including choice of instruments, selection of incisions, methods of dissection, and the order in which accepted steps are carried out, to name but a few. That surgeons have, for more than a century, agreed to disagree on many of these points underscores the difficulty of producing an atlas that most readers will feel resonates with their own surgical practices. In addition, surgery is perforce a dynamic field. Many of the techniques illustrated herein did not exist at the time when I was in training. Undoubtedly, additional new techniques will arise before the ink on these pages has dried. Finally, trying to teach the active physical process of surgical technique through images and the written word is bound to lead to dissatisfaction on a number of levels.

Then why was this atlas produced? Thoracic surgery is performed all or in part by a variety of surgical specialists, including general surgeons, dedicated thoracic surgeons, cardiothoracic surgeons, and sometime head and neck surgeons. It is estimated that, in the United States, over 50% of thoracic surgical procedures are performed by specialists other than board certified thoracic surgeons. After reviewing products available from other publishers, it was evident that a concise atlas covering all basic aspects of modern day thoracic surgery was lacking, leaving the individuals performing thoracic surgery to seek out information from a variety of other sources. This atlas was created to fill that void.

At the time of its conception, this project was estimated to take about a year to complete; in fact, its gestational period far exceeded that of a pachyderm. Fortunately, progress in thoracic surgical technique has not proceeded so rapidly as to render this atlas outmoded at the time of publication. The procedures and approaches included were selected with the objective of providing information that was as timely and timeless as possible. Hopefully the reader will find the information useful for many years to come. The key to producing a beautiful and useful surgical atlas is to identify an expert medical illustrator. I was extremely fortunate to work on this project with Jill Rhead, who has extensive experience illustrating cardiothoracic surgical procedures. The illustrations were created initially in digital format based on ideas I presented to Jill. I then suggested changes, often on several occasions, and Jill digitally revised the files until the final images were agreed upon. Any inaccuracies in the images are the responsibility of the author; the beauty of the images is entirely the work of Jill Rhead.

The orientation of the illustrations in this work is at variance with what is typically seen in an atlas or textbook of thoracic surgery. Abdominal surgical atlases usually orient their images vertically on the page. In contrast, thoracic surgery atlases traditionally picture the surgical patient in a lateral decubitus position, and the images are portrayed from the perspective of the surgeon who is standing at the back of the patient. There were several reasons for breaking with tradition and orienting the images vertically in this atlas. First, the transition from the anatomic images at the beginning of the chapters to the procedural images later in the chapters is made more fluid if the images are maintained in the same orientation. Second, those of us who take surgeons-in-training through thoracic operations often stand on the "wrong" side of the table during the operation, facing the patient, providing a very different perspective than what is traditionally presented. Third, the gradual transition from open thoracic procedures to thoracoscopic operations has necessitated the adoption of new ways to view hilar and mediastinal structures, often from anterior rather than posterior. Finally, since it is never clear what direction this challenging specialty of ours will take next, providing images unbiased by traditional orientation permits us to view all future possibilities with an open mind.

The average reader, and this is certainly true of this author, has no understanding of the intricacies of the medical publishing business. That my estimates for completing portions of this atlas were years rather than months off target was usually accepted with good humor by the wonderful professionals with whom I worked. I am certain that these delays raised all sorts of havoc with their schedules, yet producing a top quality text was the ultimate goal that we all shared. I am particularly grateful to Joe Rusko, the Acquisitions Editor who initially suggested the possibility of a thoracic surgical atlas; Judith Fletcher, the Publishing Director who has overseen the last few years of production; and Joanie Milnes, the Associate Development Editor who has shouldered the detail work necessary to get this atlas through the production phase. The vast experience of the Elsevier publishing group has left an indelible mark on the final product.

The question that has been in the back of my mind during the writing of this atlas is: what will my trainees want to know as they are learning each procedure? I have been fortunate, as have many in academic surgery, to work with a large number of outstanding surgical residents. They are the brightest, most enthusiastic, and hardest working people I have ever met. Their needs are what inspired this text. I can only hope that it in some small way repays them for their dedication to furthering the art and science of surgery.

Mark K. Ferguson, MD

Contents

Thoracic Surgery Atlas

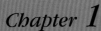

Incisions

1-1   Anatomy

The organs of the thorax are contained within a relatively rigid enclosure formed by the spine, sternum, and ribs. Unlike the abdomen, a single incision in the chest, no matter how long, does not provide adequate access to every region of interest. In addition, in contrast to most intraabdominal organs, intrathoracic organs are in a relatively fixed position. Therefore, a detailed knowledge of the anatomy of the chest wall is important in selecting the appropriate location and extent of incisions.

A lateral approach is typical for exposure of the lungs and mediastinum, but the use of posterior, anterior, subcostal, and supraclavicular incisions is not uncommon. The appropriate incision is one that provides optimal exposure to the region of the thorax that will entail the greatest technical difficulty during the operation. For example, for most major lung resections, adequate exposure of the pulmonary hilum is necessary, whereas for resection of a superior sulcus tumor, exposure of the brachial plexus and first rib is mandatory. Aside from adequate exposure, incisions should be selected that minimize pain and postoperative dysfunction. Finally, the cosmetic appearance of an incision, while not important during the conduct of an operation, may form the most lasting impression of the surgeon's skill for both the patient and the referring physician. Incisions should not disfigure breast tissues, especially in women, and preferably should not be visible when casual clothing is worn.

Incisions are characterized by their location, orientation, and the muscles that must be divided during their creation. The naming of incisions is sometimes arbitrary. What one surgeon means by a posterolateral thoracotomy may be entirely different from what another surgeon perceives it to be. The terms used in this text, while somewhat random, are also descriptive; in most instances, the use of eponymous terms has been avoided.

To understand the elements that are necessary for opening and closing an incision, a thorough knowledge of the regional anatomy is vital. With the patient in a true lateral position the muscles of the lateral chest wall are well exposed (Fig. 1-1A). The muscles of the lateral chest wall of greatest interest are the latissimus dorsi and the serratus anterior. The broadest muscle of the back, the latissimus dorsi, originates from the spinous processes of the lower thoracic and upper lumbar vertebrae, the sacrum, and the iliac crest, and inserts on the upper humerus. It is innervated by the thoracodorsal nerve, and adducts, extends, and rotates the arm medially. The serratus anterior arises from the anterolateral portions of ribs 1–9 and inserts on the scapula. It interdigitates with insertions of the oblique major muscles of the abdominal wall. The serratus anterior muscle is innervated by the long thoracic nerve and both rotates the scapula forward and elevates the ribs. Superior to the latissimus dorsi is the teres major, which normally is not involved in thoracic incisions. It extends from the scapula to the humerus, and assists in rotating, extending, and abducting the arm. The trapezius overlaps portions of the teres major and latissimus dorsi posteriorly. A triangular gap between these muscles, which is evident posterolaterally—the auscultatory triangle—provides direct access to the chest wall.

The serratus anterior is also visible from an anterior perspective, although the pectoralis muscles and rectus abdominus are more prominent (Fig. 1-1B). The pectoralis major originates from the medial clavicle, manubrium, sternum, rib cartilages 1–6, and the aponeurosis of the external obliques. It inserts on the greater tubercle of the humerus, is innervated by the anterior thoracic nerve, and serves to adduct and medially rotate the arm. Pectoralis minor originates from the costochondral junctions of the upper ribs and inserts on the scapula. It is also innervated by the anterior thoracic nerve, and its actions are to rotate the scapula down and/or elevate the ribs. The lower rib cage is stabilized by the external abdominal obliques, which originate from the anterior and lateral surfaces of ribs 5–12 and insert in the iliac crest, inguinal ligament, and anterior surface of the rectus sheath. The obliques are innervated by the lower thoracic nerves.

The most important muscles of the posterior chest wall include the trapezius, the rhomboids, and the paraspinous muscles (Fig. 1-1C). The trapezius origins

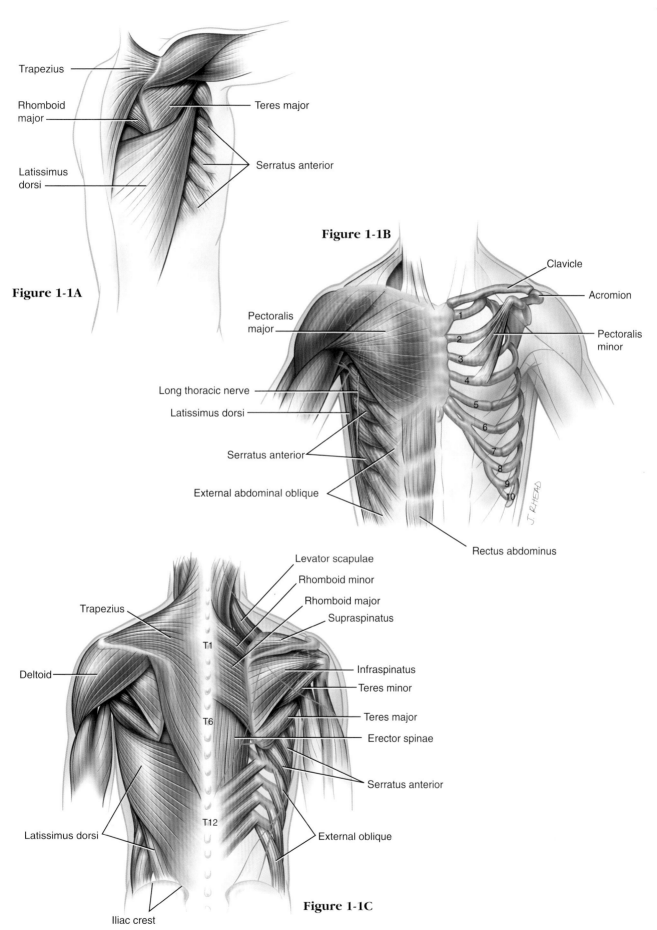

Figure 1-1A

- Trapezius
- Rhomboid major
- Latissimus dorsi
- Teres major
- Serratus anterior

Figure 1-1B

- Clavicle
- Acromion
- Pectoralis major
- Pectoralis minor
- Long thoracic nerve
- Latissimus dorsi
- Serratus anterior
- External abdominal oblique
- 1
- 2
- 3
- 4
- 5
- 6
- 7
- 8
- 9
- 10
- Rectus abdominus

J. RHEAD

Figure 1-1C

- Levator scapulae
- Rhomboid minor
- Rhomboid major
- Supraspinatus
- Trapezius
- Deltoid
- Infraspinatus
- Teres minor
- Teres major
- Erector spinae
- Serratus anterior
- Latissimus dorsi
- External oblique
- Iliac crest
- T1
- T6
- T12

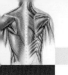

extend from the occiput, along the nuchal ridge, and down the thoracic vertebrae and associated ligaments. Its insertions are the lateral clavicle, the acromion, and the spine of the scapula. It is innervated by the accessory nerve, and its function is to rotate the scapula and tilt the head. The rhomboid major and minor originate from thoracic vertebrae 1 through 4 and cervical vertebrae 6 and 7, respectively, and insert on the medial margin of the scapula, below and above its spine, respectively. They are innervated by the dorsal nerve of the scapula, and draw the scapula medially and slightly upward. The paraspinous muscles, or erector spinae muscles, lie deep to the thoracolumbar fascia, and are innervated by dorsal branches of the thoracic and lumbar nerves.

Some special incisions require a thorough knowledge of the bony anatomy of the thoracic inlet, including trapdoor incisions, first rib resection, partial sternotomy, partial sternal resection, and partial claviculectomy. The clavicles are separated from the manubrium by articular discs (Fig. 1-1D). They are attached to the first ribs by costoclavicular ligaments, and are joined at the superior aspect of the manubrium by the interclavicular ligament. This results in a semi-rigid structure in which the heads of the clavicles are located anterosuperior to the junction of the first rib and the manubrium.

Chest wall resections that include portions of the vertebral bodies; management of dumbbell tumors that extend into the neural foramina; and spine surgery for primary tumors, metastatic disease, and degenerative diseases all require a thorough knowledge of spinal anatomy. Vertebrae are interconnected by intertranverse ligaments joining the transverse processes, and by the anterior longitudinal ligament. The rib heads each interface with the vertebral bodies at inferior (on the superior vertebral body) and superior (on the inferior vertebral body) facets. The ribs are attached to the transverse processes by superior, lateral, and medial costotransverse ligaments, to the vertebral bodies by radiate ligaments, and to the discs by interarticular ligaments (Fig. 1-1E). A cross-sectional view of the interface between the ribs and the vertebral bodies helps to delineate these complex relationships (Fig. 1-1F). The ribs can easily be disarticulated from the vertebrae; alternatively, sharp dissection across the articular surface with en bloc removal of the transverse process is routinely performed. Less commonly, partial vertebrectomy is possible by using an osteotome to remove a portion of the vertebral body along with the attached rib head.

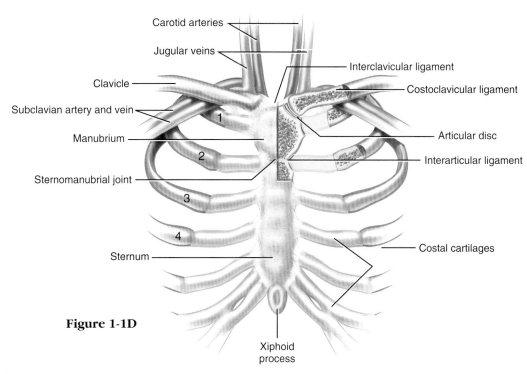

Carotid arteries

Jugular veins

Clavicle

Subclavian artery and vein

Manubrium

Sternomanubrial joint

Sternum

Interclavicular ligament

Costoclavicular ligament

Articular disc

Interarticular ligament

Costal cartilages

1

2

3

4

Figure 1-1D

Xiphoid process

Figure 1-1E

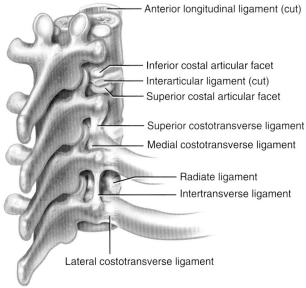

Anterior longitudinal ligament (cut)

Inferior costal articular facet

Interarticular ligament (cut)

Superior costal articular facet

Superior costotransverse ligament

Medial costotransverse ligament

Radiate ligament

Intertransverse ligament

Lateral costotransverse ligament

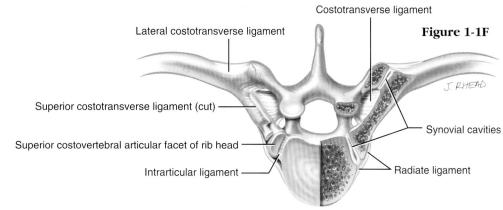

Costotransverse ligament

Lateral costotransverse ligament

Figure 1-1F

Superior costotransverse ligament (cut)

Superior costovertebral articular facet of rib head

Intrarticular ligament

J. RHEAD

Synovial cavities

Radiate ligament

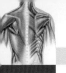

1-2 Lateral Thoracotomy

The lateral thoracotomy and its variations are the most commonly used incisions in general thoracic surgery. They provide access to all structures in the ipsilateral hemithorax and to much of the mediastinum. Incisions vary depending on their length and which muscles are divided. During a lateral thoracotomy, the latissimus dorsi is divided and the serratus anterior is preserved.

The patient is placed in a true lateral position, ensuring that the upper arm is rotated slightly cephalad and extended anteriorly (Fig. 1-2A). This rotates the scapula forward, providing access to the paraspinal region. The lower leg is flexed and the upper leg is straight, which permits the weight of the upper leg to widen the intercostal spaces if the patient is placed in mild reverse Trendelenberg position. This also helps to move the patient's hip a little lower. A small pad or bag of intravenous fluid is placed under the chest wall immediately inferior to the axilla to prevent pressure on the brachial plexus. The head is supported so that the cervical spine is in a neutral position.

The incision extends from the angle of the ribs posteriorly to just anterior to the anterior margin of the latissimus dorsi. The latissimus dorsi is divided without separating the muscle from the surrounding soft tissues, thus avoiding the creation of dead space (Fig. 1-2B). Care is taken to ligate or cauterize the neurovascular bundles, which are identified as thick white bundles that lie across the incision in the muscle.

The serratus anterior is evident just deep to the latissimus dorsi. Under most circumstances, this muscle is preserved and can easily be retracted anteriorly after appropriate mobilization. Its posterior margin runs obliquely across the incision, and the soft tissues just posterior to this margin are divided to the level of the ribs. The muscle is elevated with a finger, and the inferolateral free margin is divided from its soft tissue attachments (Fig. 1-2C). The origins of the muscle on the ribs are encountered anteriorly, and small communicating arterial branches are often evident. These attachments are divided with electrocautery to ensure adequate hemostasis.

The scapula is elevated with a retractor, and the fascia posterior to the serratus anterior is divided. The ribs are counted from above (usually the second rib is the highest rib that can be palpated) and the level for the intercostal incision is identified. Under most circumstances the thoracic cavity is opened without resecting a rib. The intercostal muscles are divided from posterior to anterior on the surface of the rib lying at the inferior margin of the interspace, thus avoiding injury to the neurovascular bundle. The intercostal muscle division extends as far as necessary to permit spreading the ribs to the extent desired to perform the operation.

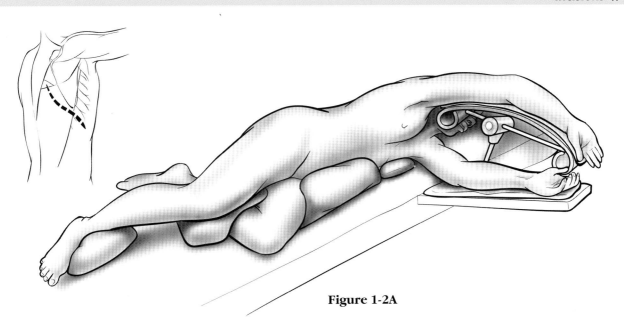

Figure 1-2A

Figure 1-2C

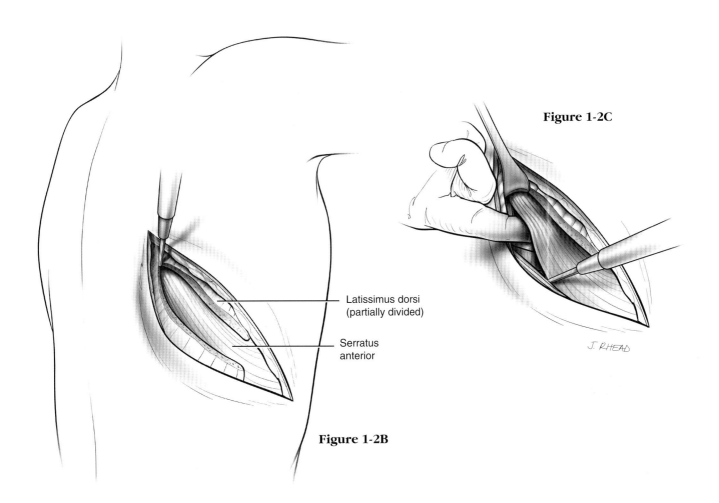

Latissimus dorsi
(partially divided)

Serratus
anterior

J. RHEAD

Figure 1-2B

If substantial rib spreading is necessary, the intercostal incision is extended from just anterior to the sympathetic chain to just lateral to the internal thoracic vessels. Extending the intercostal incision reduces the risk of rib fracture and, compared to a smaller intercostal incision, produces little additional discomfort and no additional dysfunction. If even greater access is needed, a 1-cm segment of either rib bordering the incision is excised from beneath the paraspinous muscles. Resecting the rib in this location permits maximum distraction of the ribs and provides excellent muscle and fascial coverage of the cut ends of the ribs. In patients in whom additional exposure is needed, particularly when there are extensive pleural adhesions resulting from prior inflammation or surgery, one of the ribs bordering the incision is removed subperiosteally.

Chest retractors are placed at right angles to separate the ribs and fully distract the soft tissues anteriorly and posteriorly (Fig. 1-2D). Closure of the incision is accomplished after drainage tubes are placed. The ribs are reapproximated with one or two sturdy figure-of-eight sutures placed through the intercostal space superior to the upper rib and between the neurovascular bundle and the lower rib (Fig. 1-2E). If a rib has been fractured by the chest retractor one of the sutures is placed so that it straddles the fracture. The use of absorbable suture material and exclusion of the neurovascular bundle help eliminate post-thoracotomy pain.

The serratus anterior is placed back in its normal position and the free margin is sutured to the connective tissue from which it was originally divided. The edge of the latissimus dorsi is closed in separate anterior and posterior layers to help eliminate the possibility of dehiscence while limiting the amount of muscle necrosis caused by full thickness sutures (Fig. 1-2F). The skin is closed in a standard fashion.

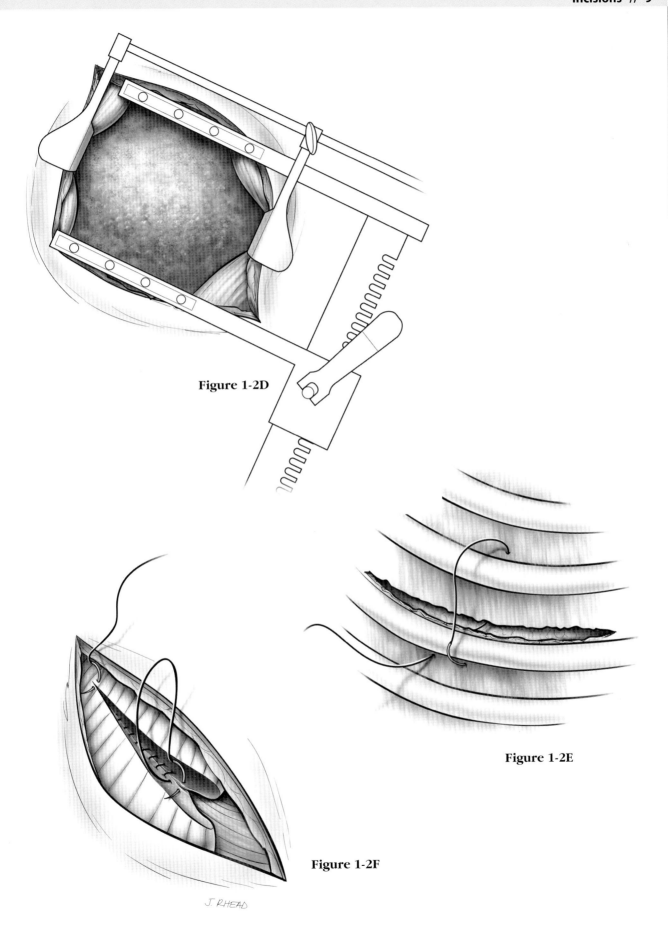

Figure 1-2D

Figure 1-2E

Figure 1-2F

J. RHEAD

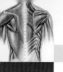

1-3   Lateral Muscle Sparing Thoracotomy

A lateral muscle sparing thoracotomy is useful for almost all the same purposes for which a lateral thoracotomy is appropriate. Exposure is somewhat more limited, but the additional time that is sometimes spent during the intrathoracic portion of the operation is usually more than compensated for by the rapidity with which the incision is opened and closed. Advantages to the use of this incision include improved cosmesis and improved function of shoulder girdle muscles. In addition, preservation of the latissimus dorsi helps when complications arise after general thoracic procedures that require soft tissue flaps for management.

The patient is placed in a true lateral position. A variety of locations may be used for the incision. A vertical incision may be placed just anterior to the latissimus dorsi, or an angled incision may be placed parallel to the fibers of the serratus anterior. A useful option is to make an 8-to-10-cm incision that constitutes the anterior portion of a standard lateral thoracotomy. Its posterior extent is just posterior and inferior to the tip of the scapula, and it extends parallel to the underlying intercostal spaces to a point that is just anterior to the anterior border of the latissimus dorsi (Fig. 1-3A).

The incision is developed to the level of the latissimus dorsi fascia, and suprafascial flaps are raised superiorly and inferiorly, concentrating on the anterior extent of the flaps to permit adequate mobilization of this edge of the muscle. Extending the flaps too far posteriorly, superiorly, or inferiorly increases the likelihood that a seroma will collect postoperatively. The anterior edge of the latissimus dorsi is grasped. A vertical incision is made along it, and the plane between the latissimus and serratus anterior is incised (Fig. 1-3B). This plane is developed bluntly. The latissimus is retracted posteriorly. The posterolateral edge of the serratus anterior is palpated and the connective tissue along it is incised. The edge of the muscle is elevated with a finger and is developed (Fig. 1-3C).

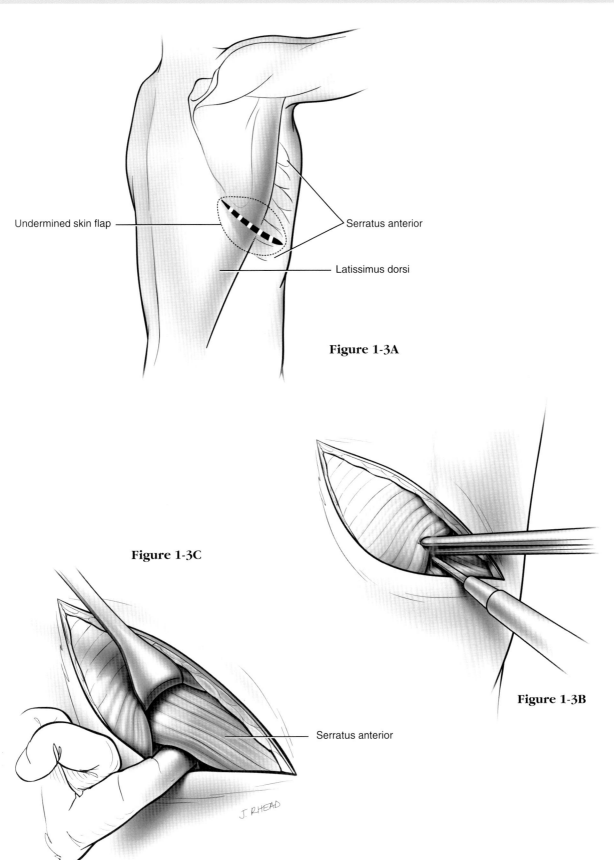

Undermined skin flap

Serratus anterior

Latissimus dorsi

Figure 1-3A

Figure 1-3C

Figure 1-3B

Serratus anterior

J. RHEAD

A retractor is placed under both muscles, exposing the ribs and intercostal muscles. The ribs are counted from below because the incision at this point is too small to permit placing a hand superiorly to count the ribs from above. The fourth interspace cannot be accessed from this incision, but access to the fifth, sixth, and seventh interspaces is feasible. The intercostal muscles of the desired interspace are incised from posterior to anterior, providing sufficient room for a Tuffier retractor. After gentle spreading, the intercostal muscles are further divided anteriorly and posteriorly from inside the thorax. A second Tuffier retractor is placed at right angles to the first, permitting distraction of the latissimus dorsi and the serratus anterior (Fig. 1-3D).

Closure is accomplished after placement of a thoracostomy tube. The ribs are reapproximated with a single figure-of-eight absorbable suture, excluding the neurovascular bundle. The anterior portion of the serratus is sometimes slightly avulsed from its connective tissue, and this junction is closed with a running suture (Fig. 1-3E). The latissimus dorsi is placed back in its normal anatomic position, but does not need to be sutured in place. Because little or no suturing of the muscle layers is required, Scarpa's fascia is closed with a running suture to ensure the incision has an airtight boundary (Fig. 1-3F). The skin is closed using a standard technique.

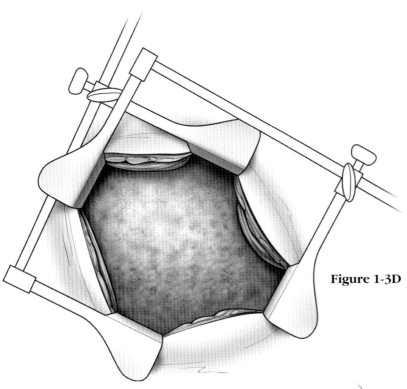

Figure 1-3D

Figure 1-3E

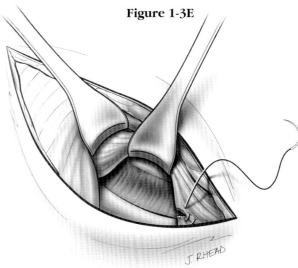

J. RHEAD

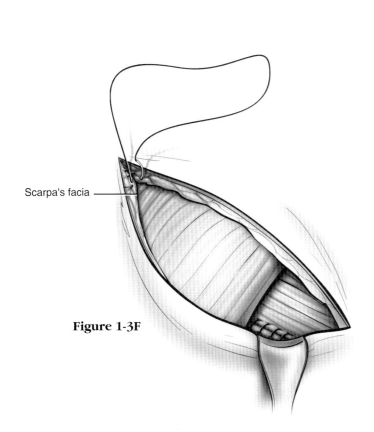

Scarpa's facia

Figure 1-3F

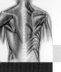
1-4 Posterolateral Thoracotomy

The posterolateral thoracotomy, which decades ago was the standard thoracotomy incision for most procedures, is now used less commonly than smaller incisions because of the greater amount of postoperative pain and functional disability associated with it. The incision provides maximal exposure for almost all intrathoracic procedures, and is particularly advantageous for reoperations and more complex procedures.

The patient is placed in a true lateral position, possibly with slight rotation anteriorly. It is important that the surgical field includes the region adjacent to and sometimes overlying the spine. The incision is similar to the standard lateral thoracotomy except that the posterior portion of the incision is extended superiorly, medial to the scapula, to facilitate division of the rhomboid major and possibly a portion of the trapezius (Fig. 1-4A).

After division of the latissimus dorsi, the serratus is reflected anteriorly or may be divided, depending on how much anterior exposure is required. The plane deep to the rhomboids is developed bluntly, and the rhomboid major is divided in a superior direction. If additional exposure is needed, the trapezius may be divided through a small part of its width (Fig. 1-4B).

The interspace for the thoracotomy is opened and the paraspinous muscles are elevated off of the ribs bordering this interspace. It is best to use electrocautery for this dissection because of the presence of numerous, small perforating vessels, injury to which can create annoying bleeding (Fig. 1-4C). Typically, a segment of only one rib is removed; short segments of both ribs can be removed, depending on the amount of rib distraction required for the procedure. The rib to be divided is cleared of the overlying periosteum with a periosteal elevator and is dissected circumferentially with a Doyen, preserving the intercostal vessels and nerve. The area of dissection is limited to the region of the rib underlying the paraspinous muscles so that the cut ends of the rib do not impinge directly on the patient's skin after the incision is closed. A rib cutter is used to excise a 1-cm segment of rib so that the cut ends do not rub together once the incision is closed (Fig. 1-4D).

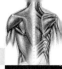

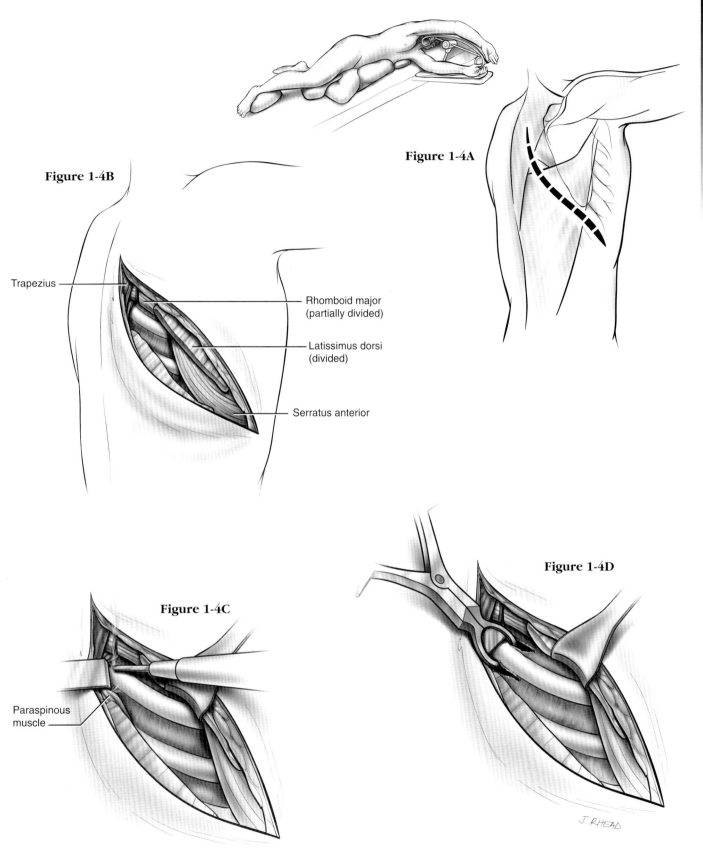

Figure 1-4A

Figure 1-4B

Trapezius

Rhomboid major
(partially divided)

Latissimus dorsi
(divided)

Serratus anterior

Figure 1-4C

Paraspinous
muscle

Figure 1-4D

J. RHEAD

A rib spreader is placed, and a second chest retractor may be used at right angles to it to achieve maximum exposure (Fig. 1-4E). After chest drains are placed at the conclusion of the operation, the ribs are reapproximated with figure-of-eight sutures, taking care to exclude the neurovascular bundle of the inferior rib by placing the suture between the rib and its neurovascular bundle.

The trapezius and rhomboid major are reapproximated with separate running sutures (Fig. 1-4F). The serratus is repaired with a running suture if it was divided. The latissimus is closed in two layers, taking adequate bites of the posterior and anterior fascia with each respective running suture (Fig. 1-4G).

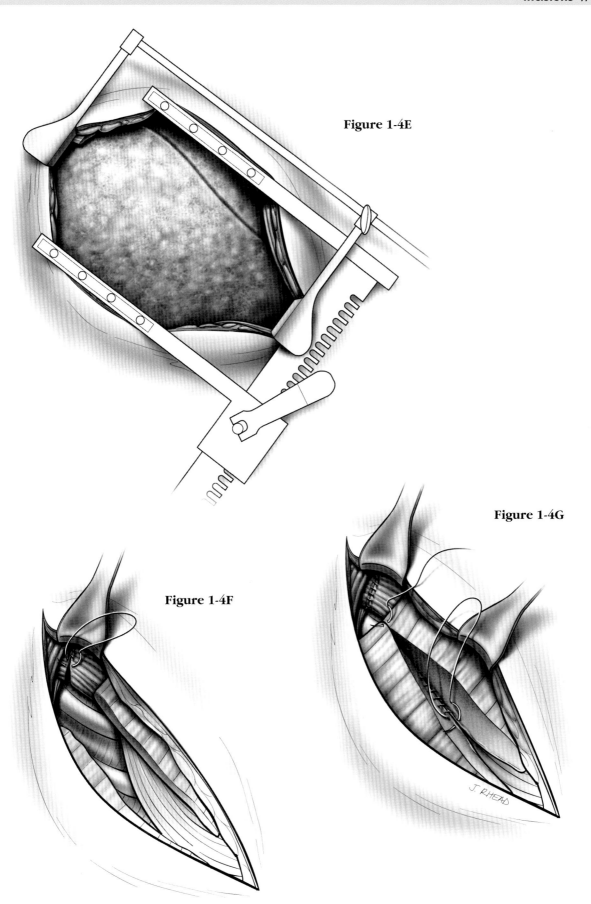

Figure 1-4E

Figure 1-4G

Figure 1-4F

J. R. HEAD

1-5 Anterolateral Thoracotomy

Anterolateral thoracotomies are used by some surgeons as the incision of choice for most pulmonary procedures. The potential advantages are better access to the anterior hilum and a wider interspace within which to work. There is also no need to place the patient in a true lateral position. These factors are especially advantageous for management of patients who are victims of penetrating chest trauma. Placing patients in a lateral position is time-consuming, potentially threatens cardiovascular stability, and limits exposure to the opposite hemithorax. The potential disadvantages include poor visualization of the posterior mediastinum, inadequate access to the apex of the hemithorax, and inability to access posterior ribs if chest wall resection is contemplated. The patient is placed supine or semirecumbent with a roll under the side of the incision. The ipsilateral arm may be placed along the patient's side, positioned over the face, or extended lateral to the head (Fig. 1-5A).

The incision is made in or near the inframammary crease. The surgeon should take care not to incise the breast tissues, especially in women, because of the devastating, long-term aesthetic consequences such a scar produces. If a random open lung biopsy is the indication for surgery, a 5-cm incision is sufficient. The breast tissue is elevated in the plane superficial to the pectoralis fascia, the muscles of the pectoralis are split, and the sixth or fifth interspace is opened. A rib spreader is not required. For more extensive procedures, a 10-to-15-cm incision is used, extending postersuperiorly around the breast tissue and towards the axilla (see Fig. 1-5A).

The upper edge of the incision is elevated with skin hooks or rake retractors and the breast tissue is elevated in a suprafascial plane until the interspace designated for the incision is accessible (Fig. 1-5B). Limiting the flap dissection to the area necessary for adequate exposure reduces the likelihood of a seroma developing postoperatively. The pectoralis muscle is divided anteriorly over the interspace selected for the incision; the fifth interspace is accessed for most pulmonary surgery and trauma, whereas the fourth interspace is used most commonly for mediastinal and cardiac procedures (Fig. 1-5C). As the pectoralis incision is extended laterally, it is curved to run parallel to the pectoralis fibers, which are then separated along their length rather than being divided. The intercostal muscles are divided in the selected interspace, taking care to preserve the internal mammary vessels. If additional exposure is necessary, one or both costal cartilages may be divided with an angled rib cutter after controlling the internal mammary vessels.

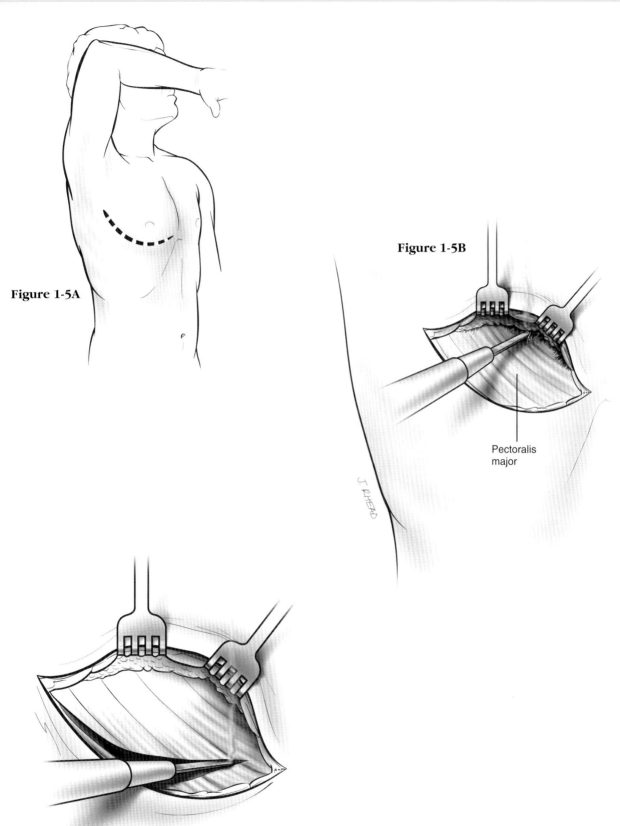

Figure 1-5A

Figure 1-5B

Pectoralis
major

Figure 1-5C

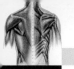

At the conclusion of the operation a chest drain is placed and the ribs are reapproximated with a figure-of-eight suture that excludes the intercostal neurovascular bundle inferiorly. The pectoralis muscle is closed with a running suture, emphasizing the importance of developing a suprafascial plane during the initial dissection (Fig. 1-5D). A flat suction drain is positioned beneath the skin flap if a large area has been dissected to help reduce the risk of seroma formation. Scarpa's fascia is reapproximated with a running suture, and the skin is closed in a standard manner (Fig. 1-5E).

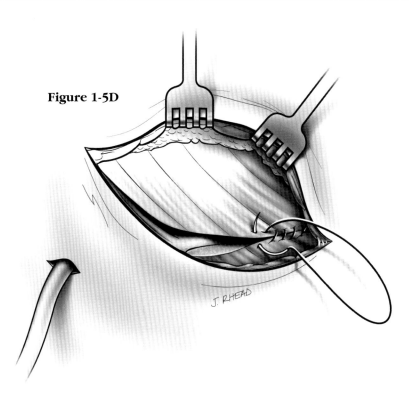

Figure 1-5D

J. R HEAD

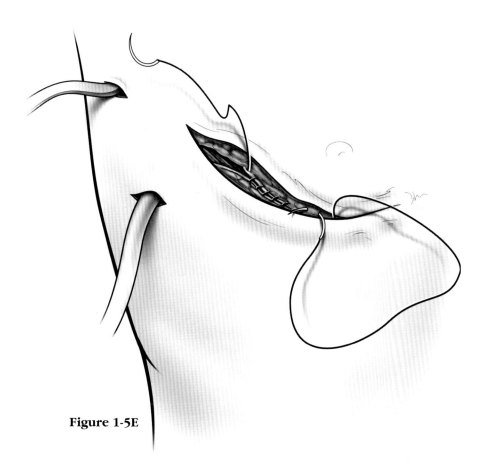

Figure 1-5E

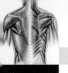

1-6   Axillary Thoracotomy

There are many variations to the axillary thoracotomy, which range from a very limited incision for apical bleb or first rib resection to a larger thoracotomy that is used routinely by some surgeons for major lung resection. This atlas will focus on the more limited options. So-called axillary thoracotomies that are used for standard lung resection operations are really variations of muscle sparing incisions that were summarized above. The primary advantages of a true axillary thoracotomy are preservation of shoulder girdle muscles that are routinely divided during anterolateral, lateral, and posterolateral thoracotomies (pectoralis major, latissimus dorsi, serratus anterior); improved exposure to the apex of the hemithorax; and ease of closure. Potential disadvantages include limited exposure of the majority of the hemithorax should there be unexpected findings requiring more extensive surgery, and limited exposure if bleeding complications occur during chest wall procedures, such as first rib resection.

The patient is positioned in a true lateral or a semi-lateral position (Fig. 1-6A). The ipsilateral arm is elevated off of the chest wall to permit access to the axilla. Among the various ways to accomplish this, one is to pad the arm carefully and then suspend it from a bracket mounted at the head of the table. Care must be taken not to over-extend the arm, which can cause injury to the brachial plexus, and adequate padding ensures that no pressure injury will occur. It is usually not necessary to shave the axillary hair. Its presence provides a good guideline for positioning the incision, which is located just inferior to the hairline.

An incision 5 to 6 cm long is sufficient for most operations. The incision extends from the posterior margin of the pectoralis major to the anterior margin of the latissimus dorsi. The incision is deepened to the chest wall as the aforementioned muscles are retracted (Fig. 1-6B). Care is taken to preserve the long thoracic nerve and artery, which course over the ribs through the region of the incision, typically more in the posterior aspect of the field. The third rib is identified by palpation. Options at this point include making an incision through the intercostal muscles or resecting a 5-to-6-cm segment of the third rib; the latter is typically necessary to permit adequate exposure to the apex of the lung (Fig. 1-6C). If the incision is used for other reasons, such as first rib resection, blunt dissection is used to develop the plane onto the first rib. In this situation care is taken to avoid injury to the intercostobrachial nerve.

When the procedure is completed, a chest drain is placed if the pleural space has been entered and there is concern about pulmonary air leak or excess pleural fluid accumulation. In situations in which the pleural space has been entered but no pulmonary procedure has been performed and thus there is no concern about pleural fluid accumulation, air is evacuated from the pleural space by sustained positive pressure ventilation during wound closure. The retracted chest wall muscles are allowed to fall back into place. No fixation of these muscles is usually necessary. The Scarpa's fascia layer is closed with a running suture (Fig. 1-6D) and the skin is closed in a standard fashion. In patients in whom no pleural drain is placed, a small pneumothorax evident on the postoperative chest radiograph is usually well tolerated and requires no specific intervention, assuming there is no concern about ongoing air leakage into the pleural space.

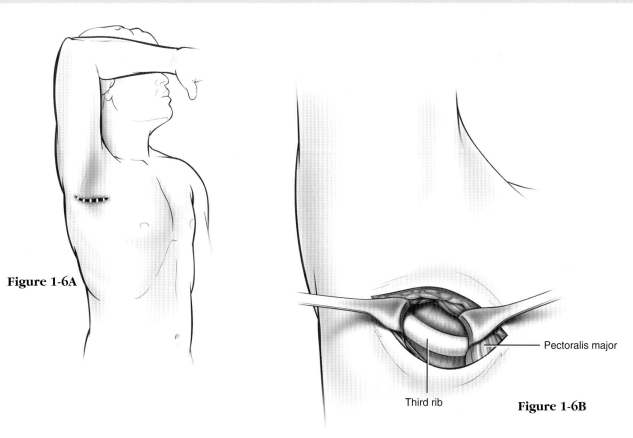

Figure 1-6A

Pectoralis major

Third rib

Figure 1-6B

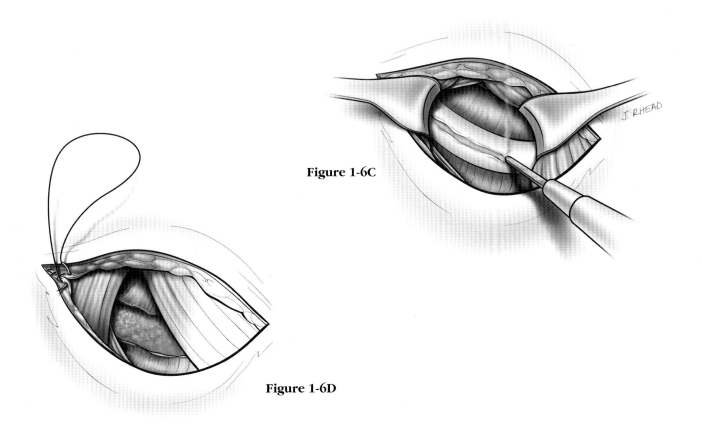

Figure 1-6C

J. RHEAD

Figure 1-6D

1-7 Sternotomy and Its Variations

The definitive sternotomy incision has been the mainstay for surgical approaches to the pericardium, heart, and great vessels for decades. The classic incision provides excellent exposure suitable to most cardiac procedures for acquired disease, as well as for operations on the thymus and intrathoracic trachea; on occasion, it is the incision of choice for elective pulmonary surgery. Because of its midline location, the postoperative pain associated with sternotomy is less than for standard thoracotomy incisions. The main drawback to routine use of a sternotomy incision is the risk of sternal malunion, which usually is associated with a postoperative infection. The recent growing interest in reducing the "invasiveness" of surgery has engendered a variety of partial sternotomy approaches to the mediastinal contents, which permit the use of smaller skin incisions. In addition to this cosmetic advantage, leaving more of the sternum intact may help reduce the incidence of sternal wound infection by helping to maintain the rigidity of the chest wall.

The patient is placed in a supine position and a folded sheet with the electrocautery grounding pad on its surface is placed along the spine, slightly arching the back. The arms are usually tucked at the patient's side.

The length of the incision varies according to what type of exposure is necessary. A complete sternotomy can be achieved by an 8-to-10-cm incision centered between the sternal notch and the xiphoid process if cosmesis is important. Under special circumstances, particularly in young women, it is possible to perform a bilateral submammary incision, raising flaps cephalad to permit a complete sternotomy and further improve on the cosmetic results of the incision. The typical incision, however, extends from near the sternal notch to the level of the xiphoid process (Fig. 1-7A). After dividing the subcutaneous tissues, the pectoralis fascia overlying the sternum is divided with cautery. Careful palpation of the edges of the sternum is invaluable in accurately centering the incision. Cautery is used superior to the manubrium to divide the interclavicular ligament (Fig. 1-7B), and the retrosternal space is then bluntly dissected from above with a finger. After scoring the sternal periosteum, an oscillating bone saw is centered at the top of the manubrium. Ventilation is suspended, and the saw is drawn in a caudad direction (Fig. 1-7C). Reversing the course of the saw for a distance of several centimeters at the level of the manubriosternal junction and then resuming the caudad direction of movement may help prevent entry into the right pleural space. The division is completed to or through the xiphoid process, the saw

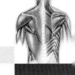

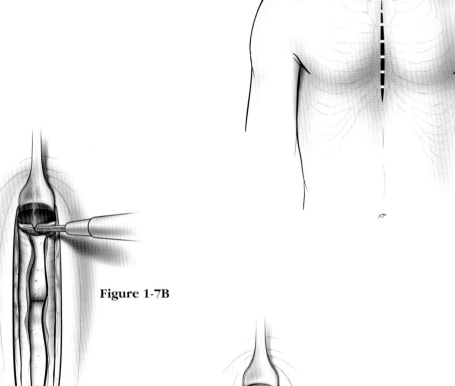

Figure 1-7A

Figure 1-7B

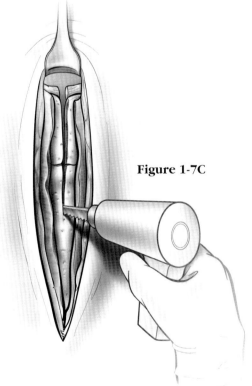

Figure 1-7C

is withdrawn, and ventilation is resumed. Bleeding is controlled from the superficial and deep sternal periosteal surfaces with electrocautery.

Next, a sternal retractor is placed (Fig. 1-7D). Positioning the retractor as inferiorly as possible (commensurate with adequate exposure) helps reduce injury to the first and second ribs as well as the brachial plexus. The pleural reflections, particularly on the right side, may be swept laterally with a sponge to better expose the pericardium. If substantial sternal spreading is anticipated, the connective tissue overlying the innominate vein must be dissected to avoid trauma to the vein as the sternal margins are distracted.

At the conclusion of the procedure a mediastinal drain is placed; pleural drains are placed if the pleural space was entered and either visceral air leak or fluid accumulation is anticipated. There are a variety of methods for closing the sternum, the most common being sternal wire placement. Simple through-and-through wires are as effective as figure-of-eight techniques, unless there is a transverse fracture of the sternum, which is better stabilized with the latter method. Alternatively, if instability is anticipated, the sternum can be closed with plates and screws. The problem with this technique is the inability to reenter the mediastinum emergently should acute postoperative complications develop. Sternal wires are placed in sufficient number to completely stabilize the edges, including two wires in the manubrium and at least four more wires inferior to this (Fig. 1-7E). If the sternum is wide enough the wires are placed through the bone. In situations in which the sternum is narrow (a common finding in women) or the sternal division is positioned off the midline, the wires are placed around the sternum, taking care to avoid injury to the internal mammary vessels. The pectoralis fascia is closed so that the sternal wires are not visible (Fig. 1-7F). The subcutaneous tissues and skin are closed in a standard fashion.

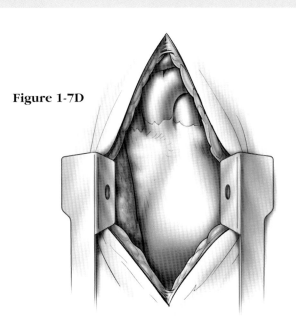

Figure 1-7D

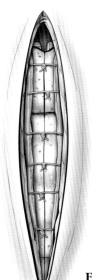

Figure 1-7E

Figure 1-7F

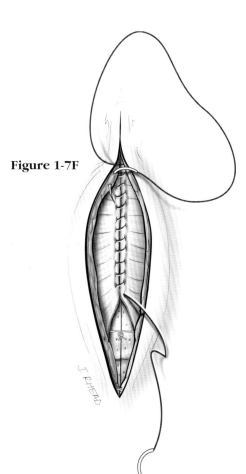

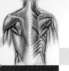

A partial sternotomy is useful for limited additional access to the anterosuperior mediastinum. The skin incision extends from the sternal notch to just below the manubrial-sternal junction; it is often combined with a collar incision initially performed for tracheal, thymic, thyroid, or parathyroid surgery (Fig. 1-7G). The tissues overlying the sternum are divided as described above. The sternal saw is used to divide the sternum to the level of the manubrial-sternal junction or just below it. A small (Tuffier) rib spreader is positioned between the halves of the divided sternum to accomplish gentle spreading of the sternum (Fig. 1-7H). If excessive spreading is performed, the sternum will inevitably fracture transversely in an uncontrolled manner near the inferior margin of the sternal incision. It is sometimes possible to obtain additional exposure on one side of the chest or the other by angling the retractor as the sternum is spread so that the bone opens in a clamshell fashion. There is no need to drain the mediastinum unless the pleura space has been entered or undue drainage is anticipated. Closure of the sternum is accomplished with wires as described above.

Partial sternotomy can be performed by electively dividing the sternum transversely at the end of the vertical sternal division (Fig. 1-7I). This is usually performed with a partial division of the upper sternum but is also possible to perform when dividing the lower sternum only. Dividing the sternum transversely avoids the uncontrolled fracture that often occurs with a partial sternotomy only, and permits improved visualization of the mediastinum. The transverse division may be performed by angling the sternal saw across the sternum but can also be accomplished in a more delicate manner using a Lebsche sternal knife and mallet (Fig. 1-7J). Usually the internal mammary vessels are not injured during this procedure unless there is undue distraction of the ends of the transversely divided sternal edge. After placement of drains (if deemed necessary), closure of the sternum is accomplished with wires as described above.

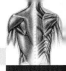

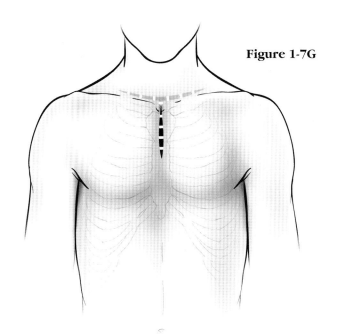

Figure 1-7G

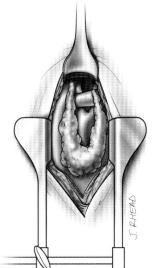

Figure 1-7H

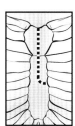

Figure 1-7I

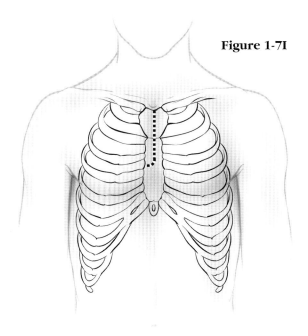

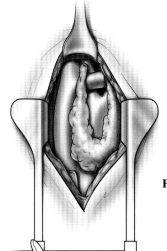

Figure 1-7J

The sternotomy may be extended in a supraclavicular direction, usually on the right side, for improved exposure of the innominate and subclavian vessels as well as the right carotid artery (Fig. 1-7K). The skin incision is extended superior to the clavicle for a distance of 8 to 10 cm, and the strap muscles are divided from their attachments to the sternum. It is not usually necessary to divide the anterior scalene muscle for additional exposure. Placing the sternal retractor somewhat higher than usual enables adequate distraction of the sternal edges, permitting control of the aforementioned vessels (Fig. 1-7L).

A partial sternotomy may also be used as the basis of a trapdoor incision, which gives access to the superior mediastinum and the superior sulcus region, most commonly on the right side (Fig. 1-7M). This operation combines a partial J-type sternotomy through the second or third interspace with the supraclavicular extension of a standard sternotomy, both described above. The major necessary addition to complete the trapdoor incision is extension of the inferior lateral arm of the incision into the breast tissue and through the pectoralis major muscle. Once the transverse division of the sternum is accomplished, the internal mammary vessels are ligated and the intercostal incision is extended laterally. A rib-spreading retractor (Tuffier) is placed to elevate the trapdoor section of the chest wall in clamshell fashion (Fig. 1-7N). For additional exposure of the mediastinum in its middle and cephalad portions, the transverse incision can be positioned at the fourth or fifth interspace, and is then sometimes referred to as a hemiclamshell incision. This provides ideal exposure for large anterior mediastinal masses, such as thymomas and germ cell tumors.

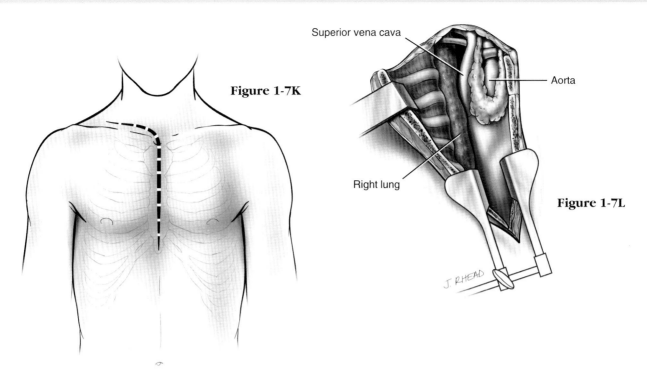

Figure 1-7K

Superior vena cava

Aorta

Right lung

Figure 1-7L

J. R. HEAD

Figure 1-7M

Figure 1-7N

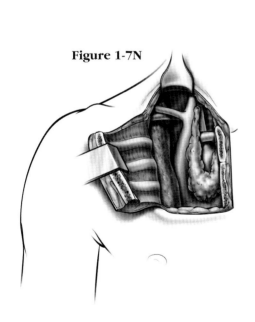

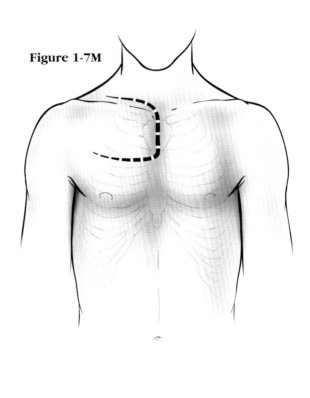

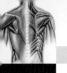

1-8 Transverse Sternothoracotomy

The transverse sternothoracotomy is selected when additional exposure to the mediastinum as well as the lungs is necessary. This incision was used routinely in the early days of cardiac surgery, particularly for pericardiectomy, but was quickly replaced by median sternotomy when procedures on the heart itself became common. This incision has experienced a resurgence in popularity for carefully selected indications, including excision of large mediastinal masses, double lung transplantation, and excision of bilateral pulmonary metastases. A version of this incision is sometimes employed by trauma surgeons as an extension of an emergency anterior thoracotomy performed to resuscitate a patient who is in extremis. Enthusiasm regarding this incision should be tempered by factors such as increased postoperative pain, possibly increased chest wall dysfunction, and the risk of malunion of the sternum.

The patient is positioned supine with the arms at the sides, abducted laterally on arm boards, or positioned alongside the head on arm boards, taking care not to place undue tension on the brachial plexus. One of the latter two positions for the arms is selected if posterolateral extension of the incision is anticipated for access to the pulmonary hila. The skin incision is performed along the inframammary crease, curving upwards in the midline to provide access to the level at which the sternotomy will be performed (Fig. 1-8A). Dermal flaps are raised in a suprafascial manner to give access to the appropriate intercostal space, usually the fourth or fifth. Injury to the pectoralis fascia during creation of the flaps hinders adequate subsequent closure of the incision. The pectoralis muscle is divided at the level of the chosen interspace. As the incision is extended laterally, following the curve of the underlying interspace brings the incision in the pectoralis muscle parallel to its fibers. The muscle can then be separated along the direction of its fibers superiorly, avoiding additional destruction of the muscle (Fig. 1-8B). After the pleural spaces are opened bilaterally, the internal mammary vessels are divided. The retrosternal space is bluntly dissected with a finger, and the sternum is divided with an oscillating sternal saw, a Gigli saw, or a Lebsche sternal knife (Fig. 1-8C). Bilateral rib retractors are placed to provide exposure to the mediastinum and lungs (Fig. 1-8D).

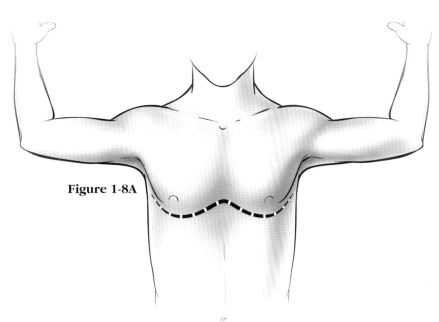

Figure 1-8A

Figure 1-8B

Figure 1-8C

Fourth rib

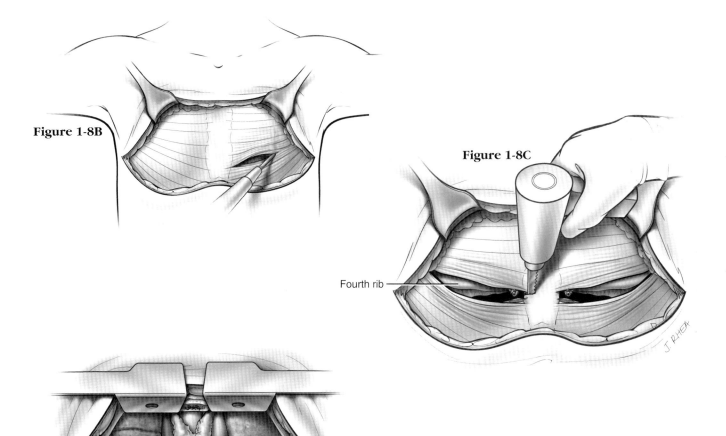

Figure 1-8D

At the conclusion of the operation pleural drains are placed. The sternum is reapproximated with two or three sternal wires (Fig. 1-8E). It is sometimes helpful to place Steinmann pins or a K wire to prevent sternal override. The ribs are reapproximated with a pericostal suture on each side. The pectoralis muscle is closed with a running suture and the fascia is closed over the sternum to completely cover the sternal wires (Fig. 1-8F). Drains are placed beneath the skin flaps and the skin incision is closed in layers in a standard fashion (Fig. 1-8G).

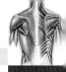

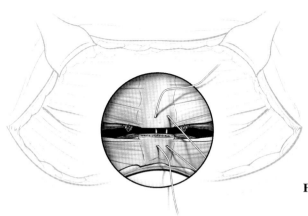

Figure 1-8E

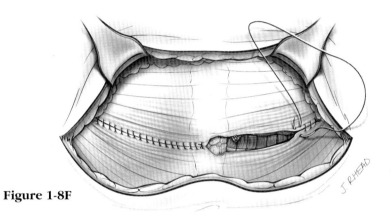

Figure 1-8F

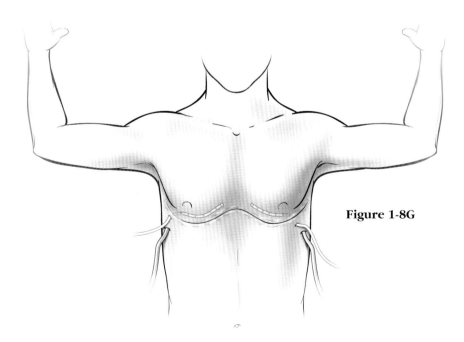

Figure 1-8G

Chapter 2

Minimally Invasive Approaches

2-1 Thoracoscopy

Thoracoscopic approaches to diseases of the chest were initially developed at the beginning of the 20th century. They are becoming popular due to increasing experience with the techniques and substantial technological improvements. Once used almost exclusively for diagnostic purposes, video-assisted thoracic surgical techniques now encompass almost all types of operations within the thorax with the current exception of lung transplantation. Benefits of thoracoscopy include less pain in the early postoperative period, improved shoulder girdle function, shortened hospital stay, an enhanced ability to view some operative regions, and better cosmesis. Potential benefits that have yet to be conclusively proven include reduced activation of mediators of inflammation, less interference with immune system function, and reduced overall costs of care. Some surgeons remain concerned about the use of minimally invasive techniques for cancer operations, arguing that regional nodal dissections are less complete. Initial reports suggest that thoracoscopic techniques have intermediate-term outcomes similar to those for standard open techniques for management of early stage lung cancer.

Because of the variety of problems for which thoracoscopy is suited, there is no standard for patient positioning or port site placement. For most procedures involving the lung, parietal pleura, esophagus, and middle or posterior mediastinum, the patient is placed in a lateral decubitus position (see Fig. 2-1A inset). In people (usually women) with wide hips it is often necessary to flex the distal half of the operating table downward, permitting the legs and ipsilateral hip to sink away from the plane of surgery. This is important in permitting adequate range of motion for instruments, especially telescopes used in the inferiorly located ports. Although not illustrated in this chapter, bilateral procedures for bleb resection, metastasectomy, or sympathectomy are often performed with the patient supine and the arms extended alongside the head. Similarly, procedures for problems of the anterior mediastinum, such as thymectomy, are performed with the patient supine. Most procedures are performed under a general anesthetic with single lung ventilation so that the ipsilateral lung can be collapsed, providing an adequate working space within the chest.

Port placement is crucial to the success of any thoracoscopic procedure. In general, port sites are placed close to the surgeon and relatively far from the area of interest so that thoracoscopic instruments have an adequate range of motion within the pleural space. The camera port is usually located between the working port sites so that the surgeon and the assistant are both aligned with the axis of the camera (Fig. 2-1A). The triangulation concept, with the camera and operating ports along the base of the triangle and the area of interest at the apex of the triangle, helps to avoid presenting either the surgeon or the assistant with an inverted view of the procedure, which invariably leads to difficulty in maneuvering instruments (Fig. 2-1B).

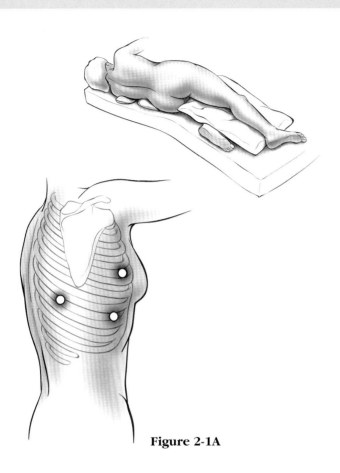

Figure 2-1A

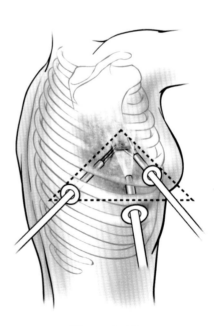

Figure 2-1B

The smallest ports that will permit safe performance of an operation are selected. The routine use of large rigid ports increases the likelihood of postoperative pain owing to impingement on the intercostal nerves. Infiltrating the skin, subcutaneous tissues, and pleura with a local anesthetic (preemptive analgesia) may help reduce postoperative pain. After incising the skin, a hemostat is passed into the pleural space, taking care to traverse the pleura slowly so as to avoid injury to the underlying lung. Once it is ascertained that there is a free pleural space, a camera port is placed and an initial exploration of the ipsilateral chest is accomplished (Fig. 2-1C). If there is no apparent free pleural space, the incision is enlarged enough to permit digital exploration of the pleural space. At times it is possible to sufficiently sweep away thin adhesions to permit telescope placement and further port placement. If dense adhesions are encountered, and there is no alternate region for initial telescope placement apparent on computed tomography, an open procedure may be required.

Some surgeons prefer to initially insufflate carbon dioxide to hasten the process of lung collapse. If insufflation is used, careful monitoring of cardiovascular status is important, as insufflation can cause hemodynamic instability and bradycardia if significant mediastinal shift occurs. Once the area of interest is defined, additional port sites are selected that are appropriate for the planned procedure. These additional ports are placed under direct observation through use of the telescope and camera (Fig. 2-1D). It is possible to perform most thoracic procedures using 5 mm instruments, permitting placement of 5 mm ports. This reduces the risk of acute and chronic postoperative pain resulting from injury to or impingement on the intercostal nerves. Use of a linear cutting stapler currently requires placement of a larger (12 mm or 15 mm) port. If possible, it is best to insert this port in the anterior chest wall, where the intercostal spaces are widest.

Telescope selection is based on the procedure being performed, the patient's anatomy, and the skill of the assistant who is handling the telescope. Sometimes adequate visualization is not possible with a 0-degree telescope because it is necessary to visualize the diaphragmatic surface of the lung, the posterior mediastinum, portions of the chest wall, or to look over the pulmonary hilum to visualize paratracheal lymph nodes. Use of a 30- or 45-degree telescope in such instances greatly facilitates performance of the operation. However, expertise is required for the use of angled telescopes because substantial distortion of the viewing perspective can occur. If the assistant who is handling the telescope is not skilled in the use of an angled telescope, the operation may be prolonged, obviating the potential benefit of that technology.

At the conclusion of the procedure one or more chest drains may be placed through the existing port sites. Ports are removed under direct visualization to ensure there is no bleeding, and port incisions for 5 mm or larger diameter ports are closed in layers including fascia and then skin. Smaller port sites may be closed only with surgical adhesive or tape.

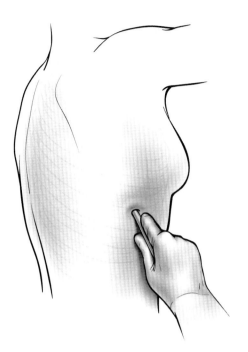

Figure 2-1C

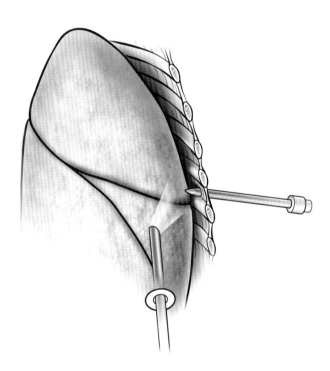

Figure 2-1D

2-2 Video-Assisted Thoracic Surgery

Video-assisted thoracic surgery (VATS) encompasses thoracoscopy and includes procedures that are performed, at least in part, with standard surgical instruments inserted through a small accessory incision. According to current convention, accessory incisions measure 5 to 8 cm in length and are used without benefit of rib spreading. The advantages of this hybrid approach include the ability to directly visualize, palpate, and manipulate regions of interest; the opportunity to use standard instruments for dissection and vessel closure; and the availability of an incision of sufficient size to permit removal of large resected specimens. The potential disadvantages are an increased severity of postoperative pain and loss of some of the cosmetic benefits of pure thoracoscopy. As the length of the accessory incision increases, the surgeon encroaches upon the zone of transition from VATS to a standard small thoracotomy, and this delineation is theoretically breached when a rib spreader is inserted.

The most challenging operation currently performed using a VATS technique is major lung resection. With the patient in a lateral position (Fig. 2-2A, inset) initial port locations are selected so that the accessory thoracotomy incision is located a sufficient distance from the port sites (Fig. 2-2A). In general, the camera port is placed in the eighth intercostal space; a location in the anterior axillary line is used for right lung resections, whereas the port is placed in the posterior axillary line for left lung resections because the heart prevents adequate visualization from the more anterior location. A second port is placed in the posterior axillary line or in the auscultatory triangle for retraction, and a third port is placed anterior to the camera port in the sixth or seventh interspace for use of a linear cutting stapler. The accessory incision is positioned just posterior to the pectoralis muscle so that the appropriate pulmonary vein is immediately deep to the incision (Fig. 2-2B). For upper and middle lobectomies the fourth interspace is effective, whereas the fifth interspace is best used for lower lobe resections. With appropriate retraction from the posterior port, standard surgical instruments are used to dissect the hilar structures and complete the fissures. This permits a standard anatomic lobectomy and mediastinal nodal dissection to be performed using a combination of minimally invasive techniques and traditional dissection through the small accessory incision (Fig. 2-2C).

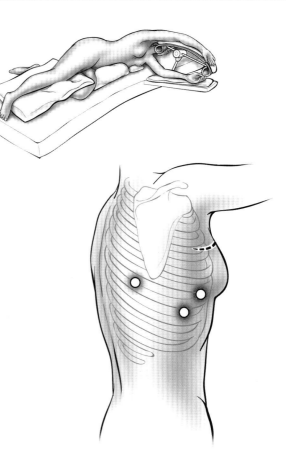

Figure 2-2A

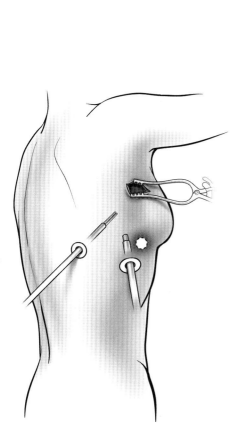

Figure 2-2B

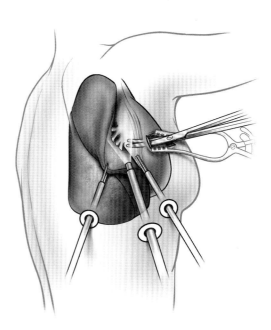

Figure 2-2C

2-3 Laparoscopy

General, thoracic, and transplant surgeons, and urologists (to name but a few specialists) now perform operations using laparoscopic techniques that formerly required open approaches. As a result, the field of laparoscopy is broad and continues to expand with each technological innovation. The operations of interest here focus primarily on foregut procedures of interest to general and thoracic surgeons, specifically those involving the esophagus and proximal stomach. Such operations include fundoplication for gastroesophageal reflux disease, myotomy for esophageal motility disorders, and resection for esophageal cancer.

As with thoracoscopy, port placement for laparoscopy is important in ensuring that the operation proceeds smoothly. Incorrect port placement may result in a prolonged procedure, injury to intraabdominal organs, the need to place additional ports, and possibly conversion of the procedure from a laparoscopic approach to an open one. Correct port placement requires a detailed knowledge of the anatomy of the abdominal wall and of the surface anatomy of the abdomen as it relates to intraabdominal anatomy.

The muscles of the abdominal wall include the rectus abdominis, which is in a paramedian location and is enveloped by anterior and posterior fascial sheaths (Fig. 2-3A). The rectus abdominis originates from the pubis and inserts on the xiphoid and on the costal cartilages of ribs 5 to 7. It is innervated by the lower branches of the thoracic nerves and the blood supply is from the superior and inferior epigastric vessels. Of note, these vessels course in the substance of the rectus muscle, making them vulnerable to injury from medially placed laparoscopy ports. Three layers of muscles overlap to form the lateral abdominal wall, each ending medially in its own aponeurosis that joins with the rectus sheath (Fig. 2-3B). These include, from superficial to deep, the external oblique, internal oblique, and transversus abdominis muscles, all of which are innervated by the lower branches of the thoracic nerves. The external oblique originates from the fifth to twelfth ribs and inserts on the iliac crest and inguinal ligament. The internal oblique muscle originates from the iliac fascia and crest and from the lumbar fascia, and inserts on ribs 10 to 12. The transversus abdominis originates from the lower ribs, the lumbar fascia, the iliac crest, and the inguinal ligament, and inserts primarily on the linea alba.

The optimal location for ports is dependent on the procedure being performed. For most operations involving the proximal stomach and lower esophagus, the port placements illustrated in Figure 2-3C provide good access to the upper abdomen and esophageal hiatus. The camera port is typically placed in the left upper quadrant about 5 cm from the umbilicus. In patients with very long torsos it may be appropriate to position this port even higher to permit adequate imaging of the hiatus. A liver retractor is usually required; the port for this is positioned either in the right flank or just inferior to the xiphoid, depending on the type of retractor used. Working ports are placed in the epigastrium, usually one near the midline and the other in the right subcostal region. Exact placement depends on a variety of factors, including whether the surgeon stands between the patient's legs or to the patient's right side, the size of the liver, and the procedure being performed. The right subcostal working port sometimes is passed through the falciform ligament to gain access to the upper abdomen. Finally, a retracting port is used by some surgeons and is best placed in the left flank.

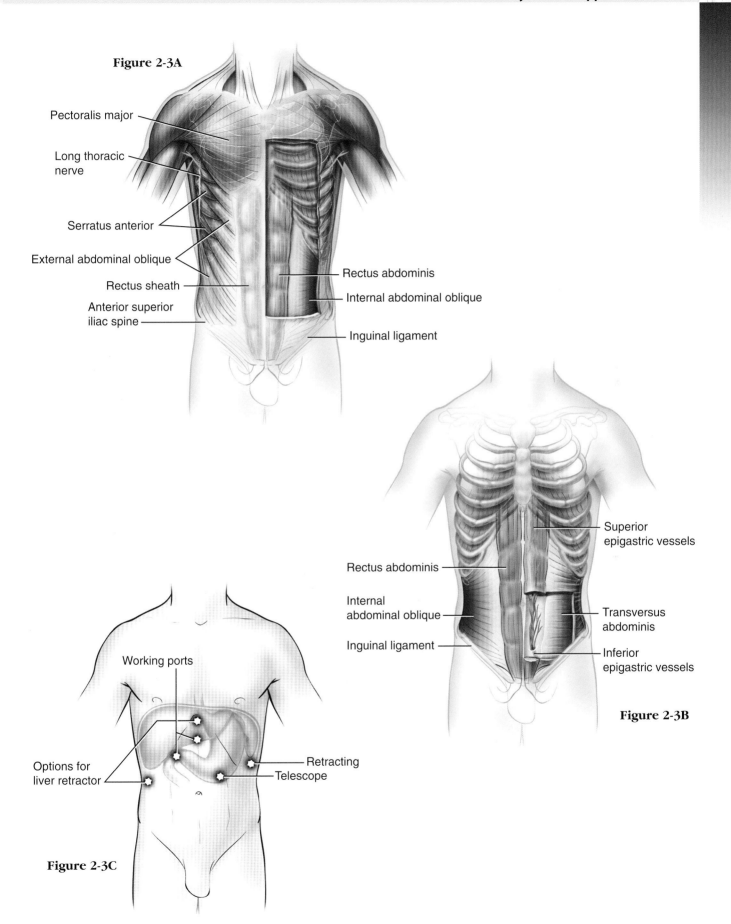

Figure 2-3A

Pectoralis major

Long thoracic nerve

Serratus anterior

External abdominal oblique

Rectus sheath

Anterior superior iliac spine

Rectus abdominis

Internal abdominal oblique

Inguinal ligament

Rectus abdominis

Internal abdominal oblique

Inguinal ligament

Superior epigastric vessels

Transversus abdominis

Inferior epigastric vessels

Figure 2-3B

Working ports

Options for liver retractor

Retracting

Telescope

Figure 2-3C

The technique for initial port placement is dependent on surgeon's preference, the type of procedure being performed, and whether it is anticipated that intraabdominal adhesions will be present. For patients who are undergoing routine procedures in which no adhesions are likely to be encountered, blind insertion of the camera trocar is the most common technique. The port site is identified and is infiltrated with a local anesthetic. After creating a skin incision appropriate to the size of the port, the abdominal wall is grasped and elevated, and a Veress needle is passed into the abdomen (Fig. 2-3D). It is typical to hear three separate clicks of the protective sheath of the needle as it passes through the anterior and posterior rectus sheaths and the transversus abdominis sheath/peritoneum. Carbon dioxide is insufflated to a maximum pressure of about 15 mm Hg. The flow rate on the insufflator should be observed to ensure that adequate gas flow is occurring. Flow rates much lower than the established maximum flow rate indicate that flow of carbon dioxide is encountering some obstruction. This may be because the needle tip is positioned against intraabdominal contents, in which case the needle needs to be repositioned, or because the needle has not completely traversed the abdominal wall, indicating the need to reinsert the needle.

Once a satisfactory pneumoperitoneum has been established, the camera port is inserted. The skin incision is opened to just accommodate the port. A disposable port with a trocar-type obturator covered with a spring-loaded retractable safety shield is then inserted gently with a twisting motion into the peritoneal cavity (Fig. 2-3E). The insufflation tubing is attached to a stopcock on the side of the port to maintain the pneumoperitoneum. The telescope and attached camera are inserted and a general inspection is performed to ensure that no injury has occurred and that the port position is satisfactory. An alternative to blind placement of the initial port after establishment of a pneumoperitoneum is passage of a small port under direct vision. Clear plastic-tipped obturators that accommodate a 0-degree telescope permit the surgeon to view the fascial and muscular layers as the port is inserted. This may help minimize the chance of injury to intraabdominal contents.

Once the camera port has been established, other port positions are identified relative to the intraabdominal anatomy. The objective is to place ports in such a way that there will be no interference between the working instruments or with the telescope. These additional ports are placed under direct imaging using the telescope and camera to avoid inadvertent injury to intraabdominal structures (Fig. 2-3F). The peritoneum is palpated to identify the location for insertion and the abdominal wall is anesthetized transmurally with local anesthetic. Once the optimal location is selected and the anesthetic has been administered, an appropriate sized skin incision is made. The trocar is inserted with a gentle twisting motion until the shaft of the port is within the peritoneum and the safety shield has deployed to cover the tip of the trocar. The obturator is removed, and an instrument is inserted. Care should be taken to ensure that the side port for insufflation is closed so that the pneumoperitoneum is maintained.

In some patients blind placement of the initial port is hazardous and use of an open insertion technique is safer. Such patients include those with previous abdominal surgery in the regions targeted for port placement and those likely to have diffuse abdominal adhesions. The most common open port placement technique is that of Hasson. A skin incision is made at the port site and dissection is carried down to the anterior fascial layer, usually the anterior rectus sheath. The fascia is grasped with two instruments, such as Kocher clamps, and is incised between the clamps (Fig. 2-3G).

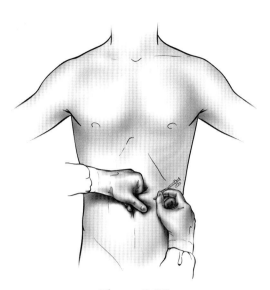

Figure 2-3D

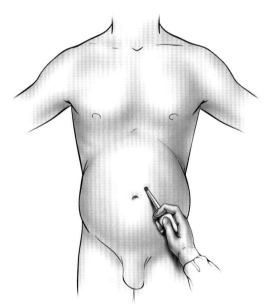

Figure 2-3E

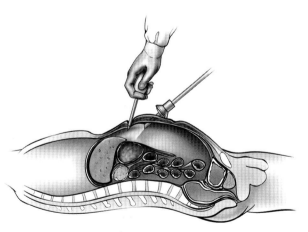

Figure 2-3F

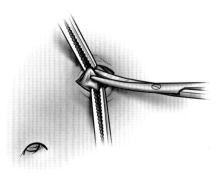

Figure 2-3G

A heavy suture is passed on each side of the incision, permitting the fascia (and abdominal wall) to be elevated (Fig. 2-3H). A hemostat or similar instrument is used to bluntly dissect through the remaining layers of the abdominal wall into the peritoneal cavity. The surgeon passes a finger through the resulting opening to ensure the existence of a free peritoneal space (Fig. 2-3I). A large port with a blunt-tipped trocar is inserted and is anchored in place using the heavy fascial stitches, which are snugly looped around side wings on the port (Fig. 2-3J). A pneumoperitoneum is established, and the telescope is inserted. Additional ports are placed under direct vision as described earlier, permitting division of abdominal wall adhesions as necessary to complete the placement of all ports.

As with thoracoscopic procedures, angled telescopes are often invaluable in performing many laparoscopic procedures in the epigastric region. Procedures such as fundoplication, for example, require lateral views for posterior elements of the dissection and performance of the wrap. Use of a 30-degree telescope is common, whereas the additional exposure obtained with a 45-degree telescope is not often required. As mentioned above, an assistant skilled in the positioning of an angled telescope is necessary if such a telescope is to be used. Attempting to perform complex procedures using an angled telescope managed by an assistant unfamiliar with the principles of such optics will invariably lead to frustration and will likely prolong the operative procedure.

Larger (10 mm, 12 mm, and greater) port sites pose a risk for hernia development of 1% to 5%, indicating the need for routine fascial closure. The use of small skin incisions makes standard suture techniques difficult and time consuming. A variety of innovative fascial closure techniques exists, most of which are based on the concept of passing a suture through the fascia into the abdomen, retrieving the suture laparoscopically, and passing it back through the surface at a point 180 degrees from the initial entry site. This effort is facilitated by special ports with guide holes that direct the suture 1 cm from the fascial defect, and by retrieval devices, including hooks and graspers. The process is begun by inserting the special guide port while maintaining the pneumoperitoneum. Alternatively, the skin can be retracted from the indwelling port, giving access to the surface of the fascia. Using the special small graspers or an angiocath or similar device, a tract is established through the fascia and a long heavy suture is guided into the abdomen under telescopic monitoring (Fig. 2-3K). The access process is repeated on the opposite side of the incision, and the suture is brought back through the abdominal wall (Fig. 2-3L). Additional sutures are placed for other port sites. Once closure materials for all port sites have been inserted, the ports are removed under telescopic monitoring to ensure that no bleeding occurs, and the pneumoperitoneum is evacuated. The sutures are then tied down, closing the fascial layers.

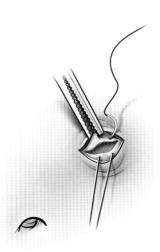

Figure 2-3H

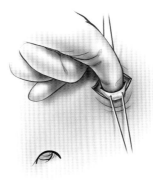

Figure 2-3I

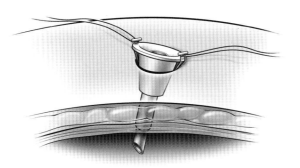

Figure 2-3J

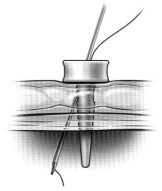

Figure 2-3K

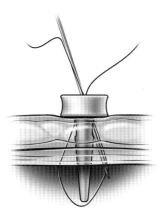

Figure 2-3L

Chapter 3

Pulmonary Procedures

▪ 3-1 Anatomy

A thorough knowledge of the complex and highly variable anatomy of the lungs is a prerequisite to performing safe and effective pulmonary surgery. There is some symmetry between the right and left lungs with regard to the segmental anatomy, which represents the gross functional subunits of the lung (Figs. 3-1A and 3-1B). The right lung comprises 10 segments: the right upper lobe has three (apical, anterior, and posterior), the right middle lobe has two (lateral and medial), and the right lower lobe has five (superior, and medial, lateral, anterior, and posterior basal segments). The left lung has nine segments: the left upper lobe has four (apicoposterior and anterior segments make up the left upper lobe proper, and the lingula has superior and inferior segments), and the left lower lobe has five segments, similar to those identified for the right lower lobe. The medial basal segment of the left lower lobe is smaller than the comparable segment in the right lower lobe, leading to the classification by some authors of the anterior and medial segments of the left lower lobe as a single segment. Each segment is numbered according to accepted standards, permitting unambiguous reference to specific bronchial or arterial anatomy.

Figure 3-1A

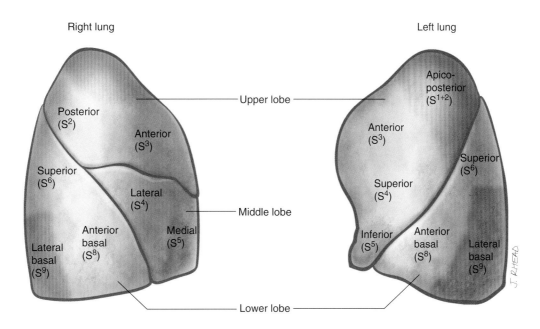

Figure 3-1B

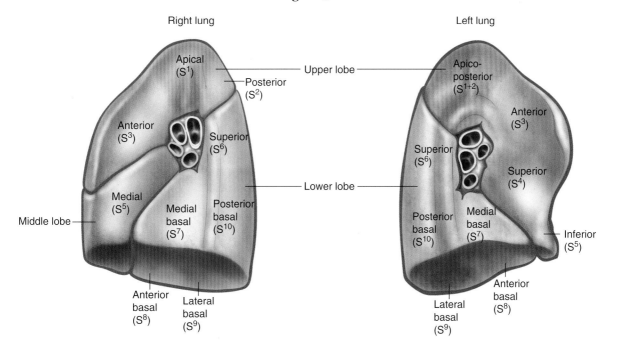

Each of the pulmonary segments has its own segmental bronchus (Fig. 3-1C). Some variability exists in the bronchial anatomy of the lungs. The right mainstem bronchus takes off from the trachea at a shallow angle (20 to 30 degrees) from the midline and measures about 1.5 to 2 cm in length and 15 mm in diameter. The right upper lobe bronchus arises from its lateral wall; some authors contend that the right upper lobe bronchus is the only lobar bronchus to originate outside of the pulmonary hilum, but careful dissection demonstrates that this usually is not the case. Although the right upper lobe contains three well-defined segments, more than half the time the right upper lobe bronchus initially bifurcates before subdividing into three segmental bronchi. The bronchus intermedius begins at the distal extent of the origin of the right upper lobe bronchus and measures 2 to 3 cm in length. The bronchus intermedius divides into the right middle lobe bronchus anteriorly and the right lower lobe bronchus posterolaterally. The right middle lobe bronchus extends for 15 to 20 mm before dividing into medial and lateral segmental bronchi in 80% of patients. The subdivision of the right lower lobe bronchus into the four basal segments is quite variable. There is a single bronchus to the right lower lobe superior segment in 95% of patients; it sometimes arises at the same level as the middle lobe bronchus.

The left mainstem bronchus arises at a sharper angle from the trachea than does the right mainstem bronchus, usually 40 to 50 degrees from the midline (see Fig. 3-1C). It is 4 to 5 cm in length, 11 mm in diameter, and reliably divides into two bronchi of equal diameter associated with the left upper and lower lobes. The left upper lobe bronchus subdivides into two branches in 75% of patients and trifurcates in 25% of patients. The superior branches—when a bifurcation is present—are associated with the left upper lobe proper, and further subdivide into apicoposterior and anterior segmental bronchi. In cases in which a trifurcation occurs, the superior and anterior branches are associated with the apicoposterior and anterior segments, respectively. The inferior branch subdivides into superior and inferior lingular segments. The left lower lobe bronchus is similar to the right lower lobe bronchus in that the basal segmental bronchi subdivide variably off of the inferior and anterior divisions; the bronchus to the medial basal segment sometimes arises from the anterior basal segment bronchus. The superior segment bronchus is a single branch in nearly 100% of patients. It arises somewhat more proximal to the basal segmental complex and extends posteriorly.

The vascular supply to the bronchial tree is quite variable. The most common pattern for the right bronchus is a single artery arising from the third right intercostal artery posteriorly, which branches directly from the aorta. At times the right bronchus is supplied by two arteries, and arteries may sometimes arise directly from the aorta or as branches from the left superior bronchial artery. The most common pattern for the left bronchus is one or two arteries arising directly from the anteromedial surface of the descending aorta. When two arteries are present, one is typically dominant. The takeoff of the superior branch is at the level of the carina, and the inferior branch arises at a point inferior to the left mainstem bronchus. The arteries form a peribronchial plexus and follow the bronchial tree deep into the lung parenchyma. They supply the visceral pleura and the walls of the pulmonary arteries and veins as vasa vasora. Venous drainage occurs partly through the azygos and hemiazygos veins. The bronchial arteries also form anastomoses to the pulmonary alveolar arterioles and thus drain through the pulmonary venous system.

Figure 3-1C

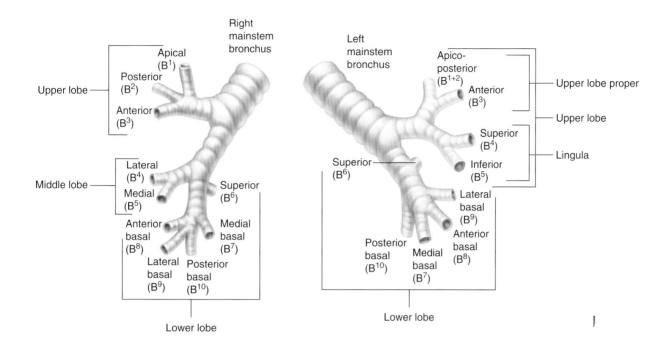

Table 3-1. Patterns of Arterial Supply to the Right Upper Lobe								
Anterior trunk to 1,3	*	*		*	*			
Anterior trunk to 1-3			*			*		
Anterior trunk to 1,2								*
Anterior trunk to 1							*	
Posterior ascending to 2	*	*				*	*	
Double posterior ascending to 2				*				
Posterior ascending from superior segmental					*			
Anterior ascending artery to 3		*					*	*
Incidence (%)	56	11	10	7	4	3	3	2

Data from:

Barrett RJ, O'Rourke PV, Tuttle WM: The arterial distribution to the right upper pulmonary lobe. J Thorac Surg 1958;36:117-119.

Boyden EA, Scannell JG: An analysis of variations in the bronchovascular pattern of the right upper lobe of fifty lungs. Am J Anat 1948;82:27-73.

Corey RAS, Valentine EJ: Varying patterns of the lobar branches of the pulmonary artery. Thorax 1959;14:267-280.

Milloy FJ, Wragg LE, Anson BJ: The pulmonary arterial supply to the right upper lobe of the lung based upon a study of 300 laboratory and surgical specimens. Surg Gynecol Obstet 1963;116:34-41.

The relationships of the pulmonary arteries to the bronchial tree are somewhat complex (Fig. 3-1D). The pulmonary trunk ascends from the pulmonary outflow tract and assumes a position posterior and to the left of the ascending aorta, from where the right and left pulmonary arteries arise. The right pulmonary artery passes posterior to the aorta and the superior vena cava, emerging lateral to the atria and anterior and slightly inferior to the right mainstem bronchus. After giving off right upper lobe branches, where it is anterior to the right upper lobe bronchus, the interlobar portion of the artery is lateral to the bronchial tree. In contrast, the origin of the left pulmonary artery is situated anterior to the left mainstem bronchus. It courses posteriorly, so that laterally it is superior to the bronchus and its branches. It is located lateral to the bronchus more distally, and is finally situated between the bifurcation of the bronchus into lingular and inferior lobe basal segmental branches.

The arborization of the right pulmonary artery is quite variable, particularly with respect to the right upper lobe (Table 3-1). The first branch of the right pulmonary artery is the truncus anterior, which supplies the apical, anterior, and sometimes the posterior segments of the right upper lobe (see Fig. 3-1D). The interlobar portion of the artery, which is anterior to the bronchus intermedius, gives rise to one or more posterior ascending branches to the posterior segment of the right upper lobe. At times there is a common trunk providing branches to the posterior segment of the right upper lobe and the superior segment of the right lower lobe. Sometimes there is an anterior ascending branch to the anterior segment of the right upper lobe. The interlobar portion of the right pulmonary artery then gives rise to one or two middle lobe arteries, and at this level or slightly more distal the superior segment of the right lower lobe is supplied by one (80% of patients) or two

branches. Finally, the interlobar portion of the artery terminates in the vessels to the basilar segments of the right lower lobe.

The left pulmonary artery is shorter than the right, but there is greater length available for dissection. The artery arises from beneath the aortic arch and courses posteriorly almost from its origin (see Fig. 3-1D). Just distal to its origin it is connected to the underside of the aortic arch by the ligamentum arteriosum. The arborization of the left pulmonary artery to the left upper lobe is more variable than that of the right pulmonary artery to the right upper lobe (Table 3-2). The anterior trunk arises from the superior and lateral surface of the vessel as one or sometimes two branches beginning 1.5 cm distal to the ligamentum arteriosum. This trunk usually supplies the apicoposterior and anterior segments of the left upper lobe. Typically, one or two posterior segmental arteries arise from the segment of the artery in the interlobar fissure. In two thirds of patients a single vessel arises from the posterior and lateral surface of the interlobar portion of the artery just distal to, or sometimes at the same level as, the posterior segmental arteries to the upper lobe, and supplies the superior segment of the lower lobe. Most of the remaining one third of patients have two vessels supplying the superior segment of the left lower lobe. One or possibly two arteries subsequently arise from the anterior surface of the interlobar portion of the artery to supply the lingula. Distal to this, the interlobar portion of the artery terminates in the branches to the basal segments of the left lower lobe.

The venous drainage from the lungs is also somewhat variable. The superior and inferior pulmonary veins on each side typically join at or near their junction with the left atrium, and usually this common area is intrapericardial. The right superior pulmonary vein drains the right upper and middle lobes, and the left superior pulmonary vein drains the left upper lobe including the

Figure 3-1D

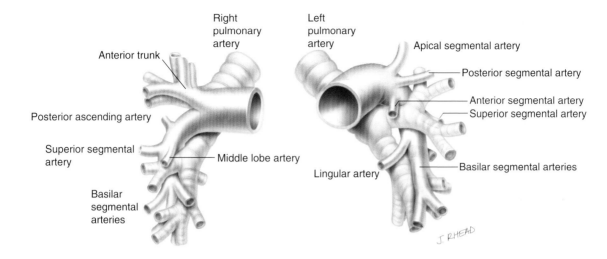

lingula. The inferior pulmonary vein on each side drains the associated lower lobe. At the segmental and subsegmental levels, the pulmonary veins lie in the intersegmental planes, and often cannot be specifically associated with a single segment.

The right upper lobe is drained by three primary veins: apical-anterior, inferior, and posterior (Fig. 3-1E). The apical-anterior vein is usually visible in its subpleural location on the mediastinal surface of the lung. The inferior vein is located inferior to the anterior segmental bronchus. The largest of the three veins, the posterior vein, is formed from a large central vein that drains the upper half of the right upper lobe and from a superficial vein that is located subpleurally on the interlobar aspect of the lobe. There is some variability in the regions drained by the apical-anterior and posterior vessels, leading to some overlap of drainage of these regions. The right middle lobe has a single draining vein in over half of patients and most of the remaining patients have two veins. The right lower lobe is drained by the inferior pulmonary vein, which has two principle tributaries: the superior vein drains the superior segment of the lobe, and the common basal vein that arises from the superior basal vein (draining segments 8,9) and the inferior basal vein (draining segments 9+10 or 7+10). Segment 7 is sometimes drained by its own vein leading to the common basal vein.

There are many similarities in the venous drainage patterns of the upper and middle lobes on the right and the left upper lobe. In three of four patients there are three veins draining the left upper lobe, including and apical-posterior vein, and anterior vein, and a lingular vein that comprises superior and inferior rami. The anterior vein variably joins the apical-posterior (35%) or the lingular (5%) veins, or enters the superior pulmonary vein individually (35%). In the remaining 25% of patients there are two anterior veins. On the left side the upper lobe draining veins are somewhat more complex than the right upper lobe veins because of their relationships to the bronchi. There is often a branch of the apical-posterior vein called the superior hilar vein, which wraps around the superior surface of the hilum. In addition, the posterior vein, a tributary of the apical-posterior vein, passes superior to the anterior segmental bronchus. The left inferior pulmonary vein is made up of two principal tributaries: the superior segmental vein, and the basal segmental vein, the latter being divided into superior and inferior branches. The patterns of venous drainage of the left lower lobe are similar to those of the right lower lobe.

The lungs are enveloped by the visceral pleura, which is contiguous with the parietal pleura as it reflects from the lateral surfaces of the mediastinum. Each lung is tethered within its hemithorax by the pulmonary hilum and by the pulmonary ligament, which is a double layer of pleura that extends caudad along the mediastinum from the inferior pulmonary vein to the diaphragm. The pleura somewhat obscures the anatomy detailed above, particularly when it has been affected by inflammation or fibrosis.

The lymphatic pathways of the lung are somewhat complex and have an important bearing on lung pathophysiology and on patterns of dissemination of pulmonary neoplasms. Traditionally the right lung lymphatics are thought to drain into intraparenchymal lymphatics and lymph nodes, then to peribronchial (hilar) lymph nodes, and subsequently to subcarinal and right tracheobronchial and paratracheal lymph nodes. The left upper lobe similarly initially drains to intraparenchymal and peribronchial (hilar) lymph nodes and subsequently to subcarinal, left tracheobronchial, left paratracheal, aortopulmonary, and prevascular (aortic arch) lymph nodes. The left lower lobe initially drains to intraparenchymal and peribronchial (hilar) lymph nodes and subsequently to subcarinal lymph nodes and primarily right tracheobronchial lymph nodes. The lymphatics eventually communicate with the venous system via the bronchomediastinal lymphatic trunk and thoracic duct or via the inferior deep cervical (scalene) lymph nodes. In 20% to 25% of people, some lymphatics from the pulmonary parenchyma, primarily from the upper lobes, bypass the hilar lymphatics and communicate directly with mediastinal lymphatics. The lymph node distribution has been classified for purposes of lung cancer staging (Fig. 3-1F). In general, lymph nodes with a single-digit classification are considered mediastinal nodes and those with a double-digit classification are within the visceral pleural envelope and are considered either hilar or intraparenchymal nodes (Table 3-3).

Figure 3-1E

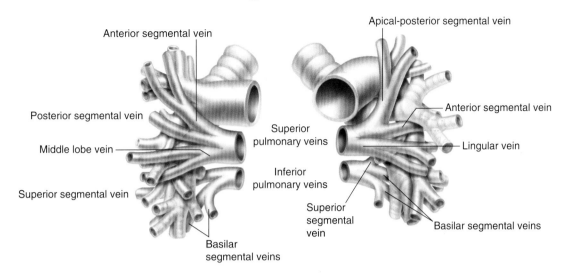

Anterior segmental vein

Apical-posterior segmental vein

Posterior segmental vein

Anterior segmental vein

Middle lobe vein

Superior pulmonary veins

Lingular vein

Superior segmental vein

Inferior pulmonary veins

Superior segmental vein

Basilar segmental veins

Basilar segmental veins

Figure 3-1F

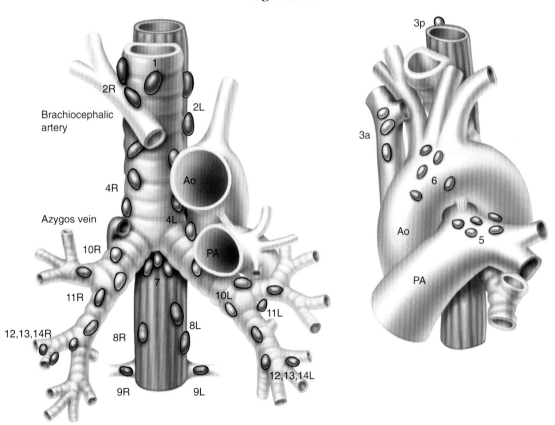

1

2R

2L

Brachiocephalic artery

Ao

4R

4L

Azygos vein

PA

10R

7

11R

10L

11L

12,13,14R

8R

8L

9R

9L

12,13,14L

3p

3a

6

Ao

5

PA

Table 3-2. Patterns of Arterial Supply to the Left Upper Lobe

Anterior trunk to 1–3		*	*	*				*
Anterior trunk to 1,2					*		*	
Anterior trunk to 1,3	*				*			
Anterior trunk to 1–5						*		
Anterior trunk to 2	*							
Interlobar to 1								
Interlobar ascending to 2				*		*		*
Interlobar ascending to 3		*	*	*		*		
Single branch to 4,5	*		*	*	*	*		*
Split branch to 3–5		*					*	
Incidence (%)	13	10	9	8	3	3	3	2

Data from:
Cory RAS, Valentine EJ: Varying patterns of the lobar branches of the pulmonary artery. Thorax 1959;14:267–280.
Milloy FJ, Wragg LE, Anson BJ: The pulmonary arterial supply to the upper lobe of the left lung. Surg Gynecol Obstet 1968;126:811–824.

Table 3-3. Lymph Node Classification for Lung Cancer Staging

Station	Description
1	Highest mediastinal lymph nodes
2	Upper paratracheal nodes, located above level of innominate artery (right) or aortic arch (left)
3	Prevascular and precarinal (3a) and retrotracheal (3p) nodes
4	Lower paratracheal nodes located between the lower border of level 2 and the superior margin of the azygos vein (right) or the carina (left)
5	Aorto-pulmonary nodes found lateral to the ligamentum arteriosum and proximal to the takeoff of the first branch of the left pulmonary artery
6	Pre-aortic nodes anterior to the ligamentum arteriosum
7	Subcarinal nodes
8	Paraesophageal nodes located inferior to the carina
9	Pulmonary ligament lymph nodes
10	Tracheobronchial lymph nodes located between the superior border of the azygos vein and the takeoff of the right mainstem bronchus (right) or between the carina and the takeoff of the left upper lobe bronchus, medial to the ligamentum arteriosum (left)
11	Interlobar nodes
12 (not shown)	Lobar bronchial nodes
13 (not shown)	Segmental nodes
14 (not shown)	Subsegmental nodes

Adapted from Mountain CF, Dressler CM: Regional lymph node classification for lung cancer staging. Chest 1977;111:1718–1723.

3-2 General Considerations

Preoperative Evaluation

Lung resection operations have the potential to create substantial cardiopulmonary dysfunction and are thus associated with a moderate risk of operative mortality. Selection of patients for lung resection is based on proper anatomic and physiologic evaluation. Although general guidelines exist for what types of tests should be performed and what test results are required to permit safe lung resection, there is no substitute for the judgment of the surgeon in patient selection.

In patients in whom non–small cell lung cancer is diagnosed or suspected preoperatively, staging studies are performed to eliminate the possibility of regionally advanced or distant metastatic disease. Such studies typically include computed tomography (CT) with intravenous contrast and possibly positron emission tomography (PET). Invasion of the spine, brachial plexus, or the great vessels and their branches can be assessed with magnetic resonance imaging (MRI) in selected patients. Some surgeons routinely perform mediastinoscopy to evaluate the status of mediastinal lymph nodes; others use the procedure selectively for patients with enlarged mediastinal or hilar lymph nodes or with advanced primary tumor stage (T3 or T4). Endoscopic esophageal ultrasonography (EUS), bronchoscopy with transbronchial needle aspiration, bronchoscopic ultrasonography, parasternal mediastinotomy, and thoracoscopy are other available techniques for establishing nodal status. If regionally advanced yet potentially resectable disease is identified, it is appropriate to consider other staging studies to eliminate the possibility of asymptomatic metastatic disease with a head CT or MRI and possibly bone scintigraphy.

Another indication for major lung resection is the presence of isolated pulmonary metastases, although lobectomy and pneumonectomy should be avoided unless one of these procedures is the only means for achieving a complete resection. Major lung resection is also appropriate for a variety of benign problems diagnosed in adults such as destroyed lung, persistent infection (mycobacterial, fungal, amebic, hydatid), pulmonary arteriovenous malformation, pulmonary sequestration, pulmonary artery aneurysms, and middle lobe syndrome. For isolated peripheral benign nodules and diffuse benign disease, simple wedge resection is usually sufficient for diagnosis.

Appropriate cardiovascular and pulmonary physiologic assessment is important in minimizing the risk of postoperative complications and mortality. In addition to being associated with immediate operative outcomes, cardiopulmonary status is also a determinant of quality of life after major lung resection. Patients are generally willing to accept immediate operative risks such as pneu-

monia, myocardial infarction, prolonged hospitalization, and even death. However, they are more averse to outcomes that affect their long-term quality of life, such as debilitating conditions including dyspnea, which limits ambulation or requires home oxygen use, chronic pain, and the need for assistance with activities of daily living. For these reasons, selection of patients using cardiopulmonary risk factors should be based on both expected perioperative risks and long-term outcomes.

Cardiovascular risk factors include coronary artery disease, diabetes, renal insufficiency, congestive heart failure, and poor performance status. The presence of coronary artery disease or the identification of two or more factors in the absence of known coronary artery disease should prompt noninvasive testing, such as an exercise or chemical stress test. Abnormal findings are further investigated with coronary angiogram, and, if indicated, appropriate percutaneous or surgical revascularization is performed prior to any planned lung resection.

Formal pulmonary function testing, rather than office-based spirometry, is necessary to critically evaluate lung volumes as well as airflow abnormalities. In addition, it is good practice to assess gas exchange and/or oxygen consumption as another measure of operative risk. This can be accomplished through assessment of diffusing capacity of the lung for carbon monoxide (DLCO), oxygen consumption during maximum exercise (VO_2max), or oxygen saturation during measured exercise, such as stair climbing. Some patients who have centrally located tumors or adenopathy that might impact on airflow or blood flow into the lung have marginal spirometry or gas exchange. In such patients additional assessment, including either quantitative ventilation-perfusion scanning or quantitative computed tomography to measure regional lung function, is appropriate to enable a more accurate estimation of risk. Generally accepted guidelines for normal risk for major lung resection are a) a postoperative predicted expiratory volume in the first second (ppoFEV1) of more than 800 mL or more than 40% of normal; b) a postoperative predicted DLCO (ppoDLCO) of 40% of normal; c) a VO_2max more than 15 mL/Kg/min; and d) a minute ventilatory volume of more than 50% of normal. Other factors that are often considered in assessing risk for major lung resection included arterial blood gas values indicating the presence of hypercarbia (>50 mm Hg) or hypoxia (<60 mm Hg).

Preoperative Preparation

Important goals in the preoperative preparation of patients for major lung surgery include optimizing performance status and cardiopulmonary conditioning. This is accomplished by ensuring smoking cessation for a period of several weeks preoperatively, and encouraging patients to perform walking exercise. Their goal in performing this exercise is to be able to walk 1 to 2 miles (1.5 to 3 km) nonstop. Patients who are at increased risk of complications owing to cardiopulmonary insufficiency may benefit from training in and use of incentive spirometry preoperatively. For those who are at substantially increased risk, a four-to-six-week period of cardiopulmonary rehabilitation may improve performance status and cardiovascular conditioning sufficiently to decrease their overall risks.

Pharmacologic management of patients is an important element of preoperative preparation. Most patients with two or more cardiovascular risk factors should be placed on beta-blocker therapy perioperatively to reduce the risk of perioperative myocardial infarction. Patients with obstructive airway disease who demonstrate a response to bronchodilators on pulmonary function testing are placed on such medications preoperatively. If possible, the dose of any systemic steroid should be reduced to the minimum possible that is still compatible with its desired therapeutic effect; high doses interfere with wound healing, which is a major concern when dealing with pulmonary parenchymal staple lines, bronchial stump closures, and bronchial anastomoses.

The use of perioperative antibiotics is controversial for routine major lung surgery. Most surgeons administer antibiotics preoperatively and postoperatively even though randomized studies have failed to demonstrate a clinical benefit. Antibiotics are probably indicated in patients undergoing pneumonectomy because of the challenging complication of postpneumonectomy empyema. Antibiotics should be routinely administered for operations for lung abscess, bronchopleural fistula, sleeve lobectomy, or other operations in which obvious pleural contamination exists or is likely to develop.

Patients are encouraged to maintain a healthy diet. Inadequate nutrition, including that present in the face of cancer cachexia, is associated with reduced immunologic function and can predispose patients to infection and wound healing complications. Unfortunately, it is very difficult to correct nutritional deficiencies during a short preoperative preparation period, even with the use of dietary supplements or intravenous hyperalimentation.

Anesthetic Considerations

Communication and collaboration with an anesthesiologist who is experienced with anesthetic techniques for lung resection is essential. Common issues include ipsilateral lung isolation, measurement of central venous and/or peripheral arterial pressure, intraoperative and postoperative analgesia, and administration of appropriate medications perioperatively. The surgeon's perspective on the technical requirements of the operation is important in enabling the anesthesiologist to select proper induction, monitoring, and ventilatory management techniques. The surgeon's input also provides

necessary background for the anesthesiologist to anticipate requirements for transfusion of blood and coagulation factors and to assess the timing of patient extubation after the procedure. It is the anesthesiologist's responsibility to ensure that the surgeon is aware of any issues that might affect the conduct of the operation, such as problems that arise during anesthetic induction, cardiopulmonary instability that develops intraoperatively, abnormal laboratory values obtained during the operation, and problems with maintaining adequate lung isolation.

The feature of anesthetic management that is most unique for major lung resection is the need for isolated lung ventilation and how best to achieve this. Major lung resection can be performed during ventilation of the ipsilateral lung, and use of this technique was routine during the early decades of major lung surgery. The current advantages of this technique include maintenance of optimal ventilation in patients with marginal lung function, less opportunity for airway trauma, quicker anesthetic induction, no need to change from a single lumen to a double lumen tube prior to repositioning the patient (if bronchoscopy is done under the surgical anesthetic but prior to thoracotomy), and a better ability to remove airway secretions.

The introduction of sophisticated lung isolation techniques, including the double lumen endotracheal tube and bronchial blockers, has substantially advanced the art of pulmonary surgery. Using this technology, major lung surgery can be performed through small open incisions or thoracoscopically. Performance of bronchial sleeve resections is greatly facilitated with isolated lung ventilation. The use of double lumen tubes helps prevent contamination of the dependent lung by infected secretions from a destroyed or abscessed lung or blood from bronchial hemorrhage during complex operations. Single lung ventilation is almost always necessary for management of patients with a large bronchopleural fistula to avoid loss of tidal volume. Overall, this technology saves time, enhances patient safety, and permits operations that could otherwise not easily be performed. It is used routinely for major lung resection and performing such operations without use of the technique should be reserved for isolated and special circumstances.

Most patients who undergo major lung surgery do not require monitoring of central venous pressures. Specific indications for central monitoring include anticipation of substantial blood loss, a history of congestive heart failure or other high-risk cardiac disease, pulmonary hypertension, renal insufficiency, the need for careful monitoring of fluid balances such as during pneumonectomy, and the need to surgically occlude the superior vena cava. In the latter instance, central venous pressure monitoring through a femoral vein is appropriate. In addition to the ability to measure central venous pressures, placement of a central venous line also enables rapid infusion of fluids if resuscitation is required during major lung resection. Central lines inserted in the subclavian vein or distal internal jugular vein are most appropriately placed on the same side as the thoracotomy to eliminate the risk of contralateral pneumothorax.

Continuous monitoring of arterial oxygen saturation with a pulse oximeter is standard in most operating rooms and provides a near–real time indication of the adequacy of ventilation, oxygenation, and perfusion. The accuracy of this technique may be reduced by poor perfusion and hypothermia. In addition, falsely elevated readings can occur in patients with elevated levels of methemoglobin or carboxyhemoglobin, and injection of intravascular dyes that absorb light in the red or infrared wavelengths may cause erroneous oxygen saturation readings.

Placement of a peripheral arterial catheter is common for major lung surgery and for lesser pulmonary operations in patients who are at increased risk for cardiopulmonary instability. It permits monitoring of blood pressure and sampling of arterial blood for assessment of blood gases. In high-risk patients it is often appropriate to confirm pulse oximetry and capnography readings with arterial blood gas assessment. Technological advances may soon permit routine real-time monitoring of pH, pO_2, and pCO_2.

Pain management for major lung resections begins prior to the operation and continues for several weeks into the postoperative period. The patient is informed that the operation often engenders considerable pain and that every effort will be made to minimize this. The patient is instructed to inform the caregivers when pain develops so that appropriate measures can be instituted. There is no benefit to the patient in trying to bear the pain and avoid appropriate analgesia. There may be some benefit in reducing activation of the cyclooxygenase (COX) pathway by preoperative administration of nonsteroidal anti-inflammatory drugs (NSAIDs), which provide nonspecific COX or more specific COX-2 inhibition. Adequate intraoperative analgesia is always necessary for lung resection operations. Multimodality analgesia is usually required in the early postoperative period using elements from at least two of three pain management categories: local anesthetics administered as intercostal block, continuous epidural infusion, etc.; oral or intravenous NSAIDs; and opiates administered orally, intravenously, and/or as part of an epidural infusion.

Postoperative Care

In addition to analgesic management that is described above, there are a number of important issues in the postoperative management of lung resection patients. Supplemental oxygen is administered using a face mask or nasal cannula. The adequacy of oxygenation is periodically monitored with a pulse oximeter both at rest and during exercise, and the supplemental oxygen is weaned (usually over a period of days) to ensure that arterial saturations above 92% are maintained. Clearance of secretions is encouraged by instructing patients to perform vigorous coughing maneuvers. The use of mucolytics is occasionally useful to facilitate this. All patients develop atelectasis intraoperatively, and performance of deep breathing and coughing exercises frequently helps to reverse this. Use of incentive spirometry may provide patients with feedback regarding the effectiveness of their efforts. Mobilization from bed to chair and early ambulation help prevent deep venous thrombosis. Intravenous fluids are generally restricted to avoid fluid overload and pulmonary edema. Oral alimentation is resumed as soon as possible after recovery from the anesthetic.

3-3 Right Upper Lobectomy

The patient is usually placed in a lateral decubitus position for lateral thoracotomy or in a semilateral position for anterolateral thoracotomy. Video-assisted lung resection is usually performed with the patient in a full lateral position. Under unusual circumstances, such as a concomitant cardiac procedure or for resection of a tumor invading the superior vena cava, a right upper lobectomy may be performed through a sternotomy incision with the patient positioned supine. The appropriate interspace for entry is identified after dividing the soft tissues overlying the chest wall. For access through a lateral thoracotomy, the fifth interspace is usually sufficient, and the fourth interspace is used if the patient is in a semilateral position. For patients who are obese with high diaphragms, an interspace higher than the one usually selected is appropriate to use. When extensive apical adhesions are anticipated, if the superior sulcus must be approached, or if there may be involvement of the superior vena cava, the fourth interspace is selected. If there is a possibility of chest wall involvement by a lung cancer the point of entry is selected to avoid this region so that it can be assessed prior to completing the thoracotomy.

A thorough exploration of the hemithorax is performed. In patients with a known or suspected lung cancer, appropriate lymph nodes are biopsied for intraoperative evaluation by frozen section to determine whether lung resection is appropriate. In general, confirmation of the diagnosis of lung cancer is advisable before performing a major lung resection. If not established preoperatively, this is accomplished with wedge resection or core needle biopsy of the lung abnormality. In some patients it is not possible to definitively exclude a diagnosis of lung cancer. If the patient has a normal risk level for lung resection and the clinical suspicion for

a lung cancer is high, it is appropriate to proceed with lung resection in such instances.

The visceral pleura surrounding the right upper lobe is divided from the inferior border of the superior pulmonary vein, extending superiorly around the hilum between the right mainstem bronchus and the azygos vein, and ending at the inferior border of the right upper lobe bronchus. The branches of the superior pulmonary vein to the right upper lobe are dissected circumferentially taking care to preserve the branch to the right middle lobe (Fig. 3-3A). The visceral pleura is divided in the fissure beginning at the confluence of the three lobes and the incision is extended posteriorly for a distance of 1 to 2 cm. Sharp dissection is carried deep to this to identify the interlobar portion of the pulmonary artery. The subadventitial plane is opened and the dissection is carried posteriorly in the plane lateral to the artery to permit identification of the branches to the basilar segment of the lower lobe, the superior segment of the lower lobe, and the posterior segment of the upper lobe (Fig. 3-3B). The dissection is extended anteriorly to identify the middle lobe vessel(s) and ensure their preservation.

The lung is retracted anteriorly exposing the takeoff of the right upper lobe bronchus and the bronchus intermedius. The pleura at the inferior margin of the right upper lobe bronchus origin is divided, exposing a level R11 lymph node that is fairly constant in this location. Completion of the major fissure is accomplished by continuing the dissection from the posterior margin of the arterial branches to this opening in the pleura posteriorly. This is sometimes accomplished by inserting the index finger from the posterior pleural opening into the plane of dissection; alternatively the scissors or a similar instrument is passed from anterior to posterior to complete the plane of dissection (Fig. 3-3C). The tissues that lie lateral to this plane of dissection comprise the major fissure and are divided with a linear cutting stapler (Fig. 3-3D).

Figure 3-3A

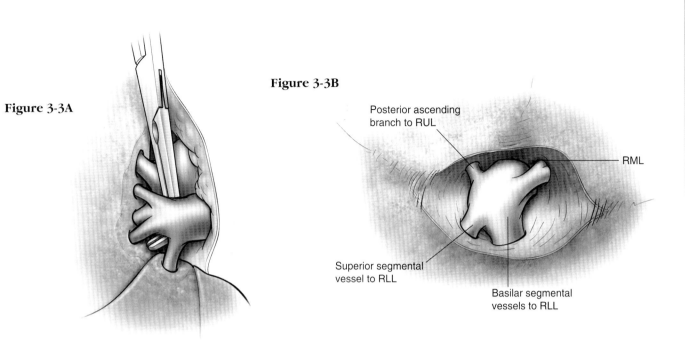

Figure 3-3B

Posterior ascending
branch to RUL

RML

Superior segmental
vessel to RLL

Basilar segmental
vessels to RLL

Figure 3-3C

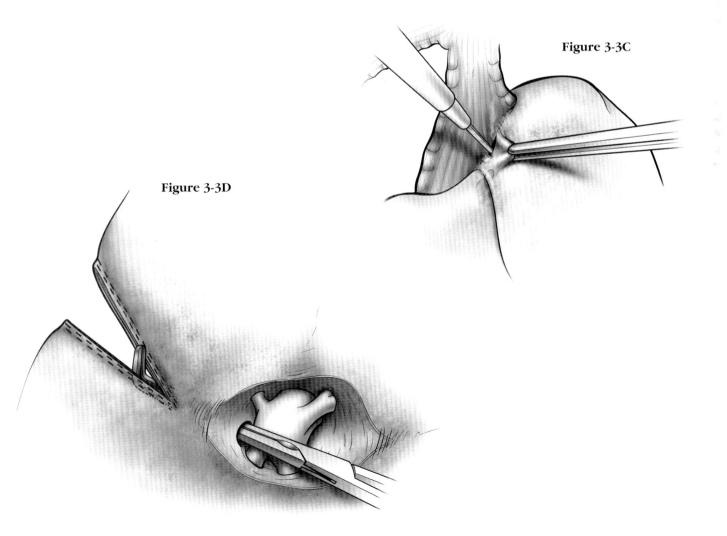

Figure 3-3D

Once it is ascertained that the lobectomy should proceed, the vein branches to the upper lobe are divided (Fig. 3-3E). Options for accomplishing this include division with a linear cutting stapler, sectioning of the vessel between two firings of a vascular stapler, or division after placement of two vascular clamps with oversewing or suture ligation of the vessel ends. Placement of a rubber catheter through the plane of dissection greatly facilitates positioning of the linear cutting stapler. The anvil of the stapler is placed within the wide end of the catheter, and the catheter is pulled through the opening with the attached stapler following behind, protecting the surrounding tissues from injury. Once the tip of the stapler has cleared the margins of the vessels the red rubber catheter is detached from the stapler and the stapler is fired. Simple ligation has been shown to result in an unacceptable rate of life-threatening hemorrhage owing to the ligature slipping off the vessel during surgery or in the early postoperative period.

The pulmonary end of the divided superior pulmonary vein is retracted laterally, exposing the right pulmonary artery and its first branch, the anterior trunk. This branch is dissected circumferentially (Fig. 3-3F). The anterior trunk sometimes has a large diameter and posterior branches can be missed during dissection, leading to injury when trying to pass an instrument around the vessel. One uncommon anatomic variation that can create technical difficulties is the origin of a branch of the anterior trunk that passes superiorly over the right mainstem bronchus to supply the posterior segment. Recognition of this anomaly prior to completing the dissection helps avoid its injury. The anterior trunk is closely approximated to the right upper lobe bronchus, which serves as a guide to the anatomic limits of the vessel but may also involve the vessel in a peribronchial inflammatory process that makes dissection difficult. Lymph nodes are frequently found in the bifurcation between the anterior trunk and the interlobar portion of the artery. Once completely dissected, the anterior trunk is divided using any of the techniques described above (Fig. 3-3G).

Figure 3-3E

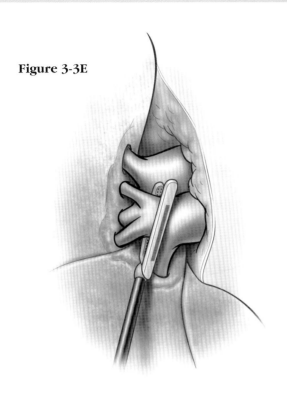

Figure 3-3F

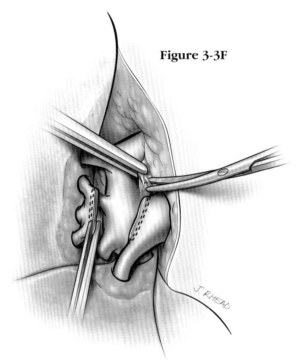

Figure 3-3G

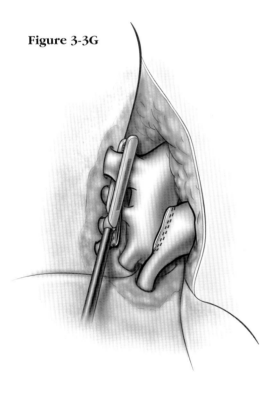

Dissection is continued along the interlobar portion of the pulmonary artery, taking care to preserve the artery to the middle lobe. Once this vessel is identified, the minor fissure can easily be completed. The plane along the interlobar artery is dissected laterally between the branches to the upper lobe and the middle lobe branch. A right-angled clamp is inserted superior to the venous branch from the right middle lobe to the superior pulmonary vein and is brought through the interlobar fissure superior to the middle lobe artery. All of the lung tissue anterior and lateral to this plane comprises the minor fissure and is divided with a linear cutting stapler (Fig. 3-3H).

The remaining one to three branches to the upper lobe are now easily seen and are divided between ligatures or with a linear cutting stapler (Fig. 3-3I). The bronchus is cleaned of surrounding soft tissues. This is accomplished by passing a right-angled clamp between the soft tissues and the bronchus and dividing the tissues with electrocautery. Bronchial arteries are controlled with electrocautery, small clips, or fine ligatures. Lymph nodes are dissected, taking care to dissect the nodes toward the upper lobe so that they are removed with the specimen (Fig. 3-3J). The bronchus is palpated to ensure that no foreign body, such as an endotracheal tube tip or temperature probe, lies within the lumen. The bronchus

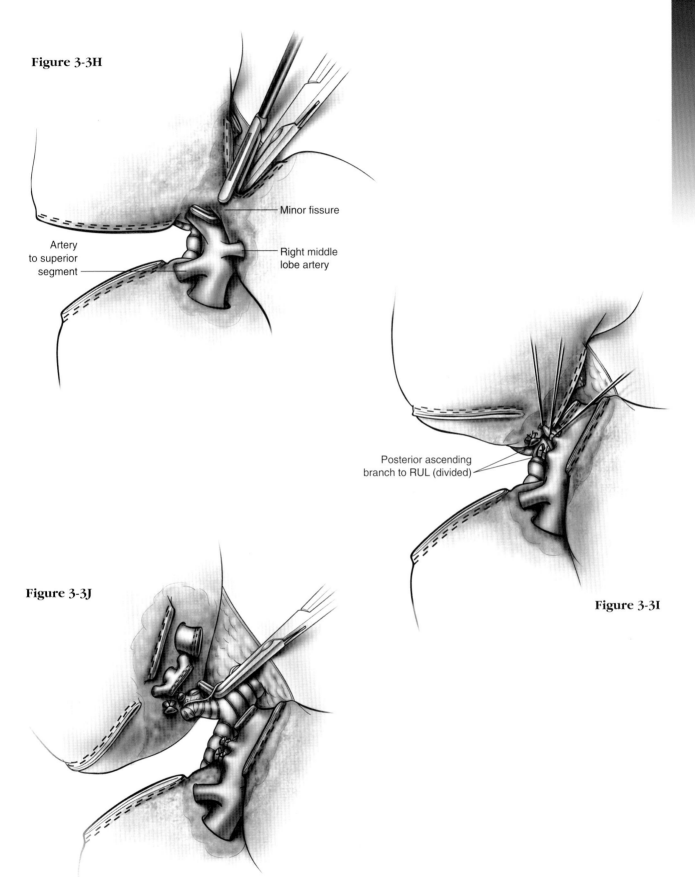

Figure 3-3H

Minor fissure

Right middle lobe artery

Artery to superior segment

Posterior ascending branch to RUL (divided)

Figure 3-3I

Figure 3-3J

is divided close to its origin from the mainstem bronchus to optimize the blood supply to the bronchial stump, maintain a maximum margin between any tumor and the cut end of the bronchus, and eliminate as much potential dead space as possible. This is accomplished with a linear cutting stapler, or the bronchus is stapled and transected (Fig. 3-3K). If the tumor is sufficiently proximal that placement of a stapler is not feasible, then the bronchus is divided and the stump is closed with interrupted sutures (Fig. 3-3L). The stump is covered with saline and tested under sustained intrabronchial pressure (40 cm H_2O) to ensure that the closure is airtight. If coverage of the stump is necessary this is accomplished after completion of the lymph node dissection.

In cases in which a primary lung tumor is resected for potential cure it is appropriate to perform a complete lymph node sampling at a minimum. There is some evidence to suggest that a complete lymph node dissection may provide more accurate surgical staging and improve long-term survival. For right upper lobe tumors the right lung hilum, subcarinal (level 7), low right paratracheal (level R4) and high right paratracheal (level R2) are dissected. Any additional suspicious nodes are also removed. The pulmonary ligament is divided, permitting the right lower and middle lobes freedom to ascend to the apex of the pleural space, helping to eliminate any space problem that might otherwise exist.

In patients in whom it is anticipated there will substantial technical difficulty with the hilar dissection due to the central location of a cancer, prior inflammation, or the effects of radiation therapy, it is often appropriate to get proximal vascular control prior to beginning the dissection. Obtaining proximal control of the right pulmonary artery is easily accomplished by mobilizing the superior vena cava medially and bluntly dissecting the artery in its subadventitial plane. There is no risk of injury to the main pulmonary artery when dissecting the right pulmonary artery in this location. It may also be appropriate to dissect the pulmonary veins to avoid problems with back bleeding should an injury to an arterial branch occur during dissection.

When there is difficulty in dissecting the branches of the pulmonary artery to the upper lobe, it is sometimes appropriate to divide the right upper lobe bronchus prior to attempting such dissection. This helps expose the branches to the posterior segment that normally require division of the greater fissure, and is a useful technique when the fissure is inflamed or very undeveloped. Finally, the "bronchus first" dissection is also useful when performing a right upper lobectomy thoracoscopically because of the added safety of dissection of the posterior segmental pulmonary artery branches and the lack of need to dissect the fissure prior to dividing the arterial supply to the upper lobe.

Figure 3-3K

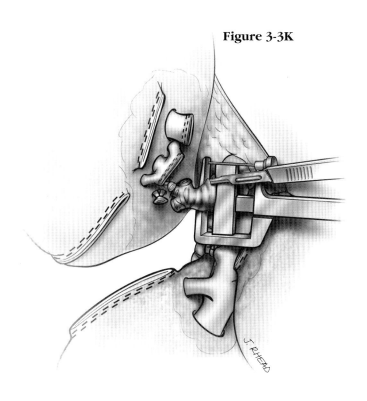

Figure 3-3L

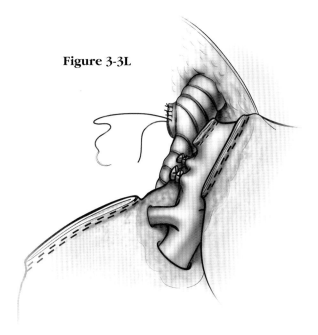

3-4 Right Middle Lobectomy

The patient is usually placed in a lateral decubitus position for lateral thoracotomy or in a semilateral position for anterolateral thoracotomy. Video-assisted lung resection is usually performed with the patient in a full lateral position. The appropriate interspace for entry is identified after dividing the soft tissues overlying the chest wall. For access through a lateral thoracotomy, the fifth interspace is usually sufficient, and the fourth or fifth interspace is used if the patient is in a semilateral position. For patients who are obese with high diaphragms, an interspace higher than the one usually selected is appropriate to use. A thorough exploration of the hemithorax is performed and appropriate biopsies are taken (see Section 3-3).

When it is determined that a middle lobectomy should be performed, the pleura is divided anterior to the superior pulmonary vein, just posterior to the phrenic nerve. The middle lobe vein branch is identified and dissected circumferentially. The space between the middle lobe branch and the branches to the upper lobe is developed, exposing the beginning of the interlobar portion of the right pulmonary artery. The right middle lobe vein is divided with a linear cutting stapler or between ligatures (Fig. 3-4A).

The pleura overlying the decussation of the interlobar portion of the artery in the fissure is divided and the subadventitial plane of the artery is dissected. The arterial branches to the middle lobe are identified. It is usually not necessary to do additional dissection of the branches to the upper and lower lobes. Using a right angle clamp, the plane superior to the middle lobe vein and artery and anterior to the artery is identified. Using

this as a target, the minor fissure is completed with a linear cutting stapler (Fig. 3-4B). Dissecting medial to the artery to the basilar segments of the lower lobe and the middle lobe bronchus, the plane is identified between the middle and lower lobes, sparing the underlying bronchus to the middle lobe. This portion of the major fissure is completed with a linear cutting stapler.

Having completed the fissures, the pulmonary artery branch or branches to the right middle lobe are divided with a linear cutting stapler or between ligatures (Fig. 3-4C). The right middle lobe bronchus is dissected circumferentially. This bronchus is of a much smaller caliber and thickness than other lobar bronchi, and is subject to injury if undo force is used to develop the peribronchial plane. Associated lymph nodes are dissected with the specimen. The bronchus is usually closed and divided with a linear cutting stapler or is closed with a linear stapler and then divided with a scalpel (Fig. 3-4D). Preservation of adequate ventilation to the lower lobe should be assessed after closing the middle lobe bronchus and before firing the stapler by asking the anesthesiologist to ventilate the right lung with two to three breaths. This helps to ensure that the bronchial division is being performed at the correct level.

If right middle lobe resection is done for lung cancer therapy, an appropriate nodal dissection is performed. A complete hilar nodal dissection is standard practice. Mediastinal stations 7 and 4R are most commonly involved by metastatic disease and should also be dissected completely. It is not usually necessary to divide the pulmonary ligament to mobilize the right lower lobe unless the right middle lobe is unusually large and there is concern about adequate capacity of the right lower lobe to fill the space without division of the ligament.

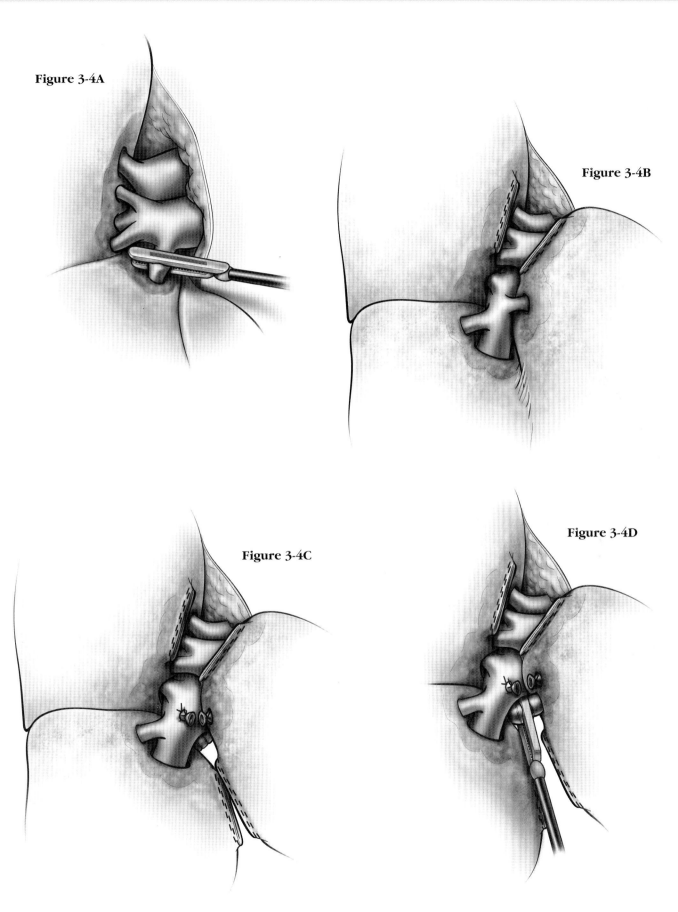

Figure 3-4A

Figure 3-4B

Figure 3-4C

Figure 3-4D

3-5 Right Lower Lobectomy

The patient is usually placed in a lateral decubitus position for lateral thoracotomy or in a semilateral position for anterolateral thoracotomy. Video-assisted lung resection is usually performed with the patient in a full lateral position. The appropriate interspace for entry is identified after dividing the soft tissues overlying the chest wall. For access through a lateral thoracotomy, the sixth interspace is usually sufficient, and the fifth interspace is used if the patient is in a semilateral position. For patients who are obese with high diaphragms, an interspace higher than the one usually selected is appropriate to use. If there is a possibility of chest wall involvement by a lung cancer, the point of entry is selected to avoid this region so that it can be assessed prior to completing the thoracotomy. A thorough exploration of the hemithorax is performed and appropriate biopsies are taken (see Section 3-3).

When it is decided to proceed with a right lower lobectomy, the pulmonary ligament is divided to the level of the inferior pulmonary vein (Fig. 3-5A). If there is direct tumor invasion into this region or if there is substantial inflammation and scarring of the ligament, the thoracic duct is identified and ligated to prevent the development of postoperative chylothorax. The pleura surrounding the right lower lobe is divided anteriorly to the level of the right middle lobe vein branch and the plane between the superior and inferior pulmonary veins is dissected. The visceral pleura is divided on the posterior aspect of the hilum to the level of the takeoff of the right upper lobe bronchus. The junction between the right upper lobe bronchus and the bronchus intermedius is identified and this plane is developed, keeping the lymph node that is constant in that location on the specimen side.

The inferior pulmonary vein is dissected circumferentially and is divided with a linear cutting stapler or between staple lines or suture lines (Fig. 3-5B). If there is tumor encroaching on the vein, it sometimes grows into the vein, giving rise to concerns about possible tumor embolus as the vein is manipulated. In such situations it is prudent to open the pericardium around the vein and dissect the vein on its left atrial end, controlling it with a vascular clamp as soon as it is feasible. The degree of risk for tumor embolization is determined by palpation. The vein is divided on the left atrial side of any palpable abnormality.

The pleura in the fissure overlying the decussation of the interlobar portion of the right pulmonary artery is opened and the subadventitial plane of the artery is identified. It is important that all major vessel branches be identified at this point, including the right middle lobe artery, the posterior recurring branch to the right upper lobe, and the superior and basilar segmental vessels to the right lower lobe. The major fissure is developed posteriorly (see Section 3-3) and anteriorly (see Section 3-4) and the fissure is completed either before or after the pulmonary artery branches to the right lower lobe are divided.

Staying in the subadventitial plane, the branches of the interlobar portion of the right pulmonary artery to the right lower lobe are dissected circumferentially. Care must be taken to ensure that the takeoff of the posterior recurring branch to the right upper lobe is not compromised, as it arises from the superior segmental artery in some patients. The superior segmental artery and combined takeoff of the basilar segmental arteries are usually divided as two separate vessels using a linear cutting stapler or by cutting the vessel after two sequential firings of a linear stapler or following placement of suture ligatures. Under some circumstances a single firing of a linear cutting stapler can encompass both branches at once (Fig. 3-5C).

The bronchus to the right lower lobe is circumferentially dissected. Hilar lymph nodes are completely dissected with the specimen. Care is taken not to injure the junction between the right middle and right lower lobe bronchi. As the specimen is retracted laterally from the hilum, the bronchus is clamped with a linear cutting stapler, a linear stapler, or a bronchial clamp. The right lung is insufflated with two or three breaths to ensure that there has been no compromise of the right middle lobe bronchus. The right lower lobe bronchus is then sealed and divided and the specimen is removed (Fig. 3-5D).

For patients undergoing right lower lobectomy for cancer, an appropriate nodal dissection is performed. A complete hilar nodal dissection is standard practice. Mediastinal stations 7, 8R, 9R, and possibly 4R are most commonly involved by metastatic disease and should also be dissected completely.

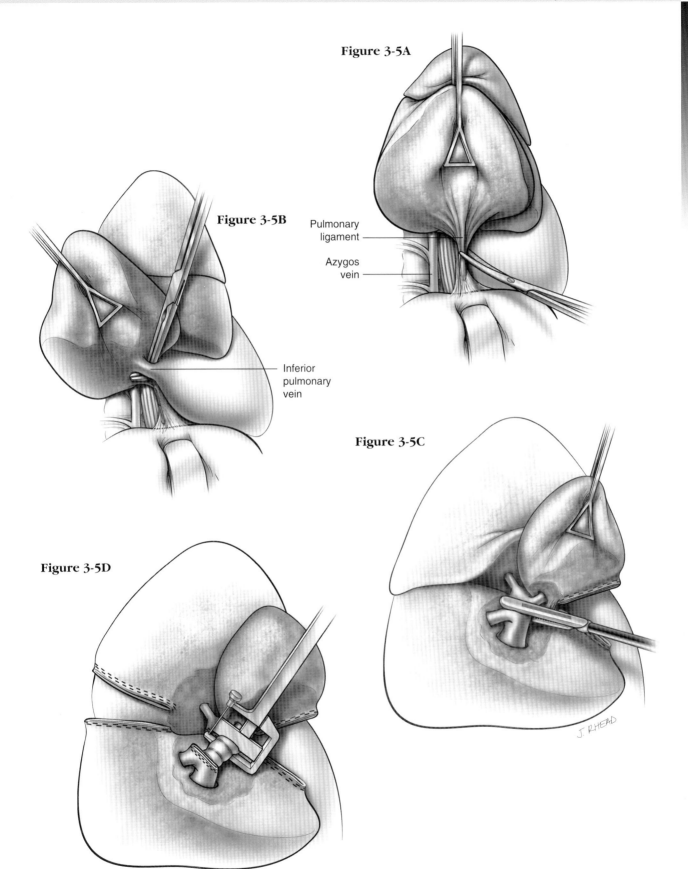

Figure 3-5A

Pulmonary ligament

Azygos vein

Figure 3-5B

Inferior pulmonary vein

Figure 3-5C

Figure 3-5D

J. R. HEAD

3-6 Left Upper Lobectomy

The patient is usually placed in a lateral decubitus position for lateral thoracotomy or in a semilateral position for anterolateral thoracotomy. Video-assisted lung resection is usually performed with the patient in a full lateral position. The appropriate interspace for entry is identified after dividing the soft tissues overlying the chest wall. For access through a lateral thoracotomy, the fifth interspace is usually sufficient, and the fourth interspace is used if the patient is in a semilateral position. For patients who are obese with high diaphragms, an interspace higher than the one usually selected is appropriate to use. If there is a possibility of chest wall involvement by a lung cancer, the point of entry is selected to avoid this region so that it can be assessed prior to completing the thoracotomy. A thorough exploration of the hemithorax is performed and appropriate biopsies are taken (see Section 3-3).

When the decision is made to proceed with left upper lobectomy, the pleura surrounding the left upper lobe is divided, taking care to preserve the phrenic nerve, vagus nerve, and left recurrent laryngeal nerve. The superior pulmonary vein is dissected circumferentially, opening the plane inferior to the left pulmonary artery and the plane anterior to the left mainstem bronchus (Fig. 3-6A). The pleura overlying the interlobar portion of the left pulmonary artery is divided and the dissection is carried into the subadventitial plane. This plane is dissected on the lateral surfaces of the artery and its branches superiorly to the edge of the lung tissue. The fissure is completed superiorly with a linear cutting stapler. The plane inferior to the lingular artery and medial to the basilar arteries is developed inferior to the left upper lobe bronchus. The space between the superior and inferior pulmonary veins marks the target for completing the inferior portion of the fissure (Fig. 3-6B), which is also performed using a linear cutting stapler.

Once it is ascertained that left upper lobectomy is technically feasible, the superior pulmonary vein is divided with a linear cutting stapler or between firings of a linear stapler. The pulmonary artery branches to the left upper lobe are dissected and divided individually. This may be performed in an antegrade or a retrograde direction, depending on the exposure and the tumor location. To perform an antegrade dissection, the subadventitial plane is developed at the level of the first branch of the left pulmonary artery. Care must be exercised so that undue traction is not applied to the lung tissue to gain adequate exposure of this vessel, which can result in its avulsion from the left pulmonary artery. Once the first branch is controlled and divided, the ensuing two or three remaining branches are similarly controlled (Fig. 3-6C). The retrograde approach is begun by circumferentially dissecting the lingular artery and dividing it between ligatures or with a linear cutting stapler. The next one or two branches proximal to this are similarly controlled. One advantage of this technique is that the left upper lobe bronchus can be divided at this point, prior to control of the most proximal one or two arterial branches to the left upper lobe. This is useful in patients who have tumor encroachment on these vessel segments. After dividing the bronchus, the arterial branches are well exposed, enabling placement of a linear cutting stapler tangentially across the takeoffs of the branches. Alternatively, it permits application of a side-biting vascular clamp, which enables resection of the lobe and oversewing of the vessel.

The left upper lobe bronchus is dissected circumferentially to the level of its origin, taking care to keep the regional lymph nodes with the specimen. The bronchus is then divided with a linear cutting stapler or is cut between two firings of a linear stapler (Fig. 3-6D). If the tumor is quite proximal in the left upper lobe bronchus, the bronchus is divided with a blade to ensure an adequate margin and is then closed with interrupted absorbable sutures.

In cases in which a primary lung tumor is resected for potential cure it is appropriate to perform a complete hilar lymph node dissection. For left upper lobe tumors, levels 7 and 5/6 nodes are also dissected. The pulmonary ligament is divided, permitting the left lower lobe freedom to ascend to the apex of the pleural space, helping to eliminate any space problem that might otherwise exist.

Figure 3-6A

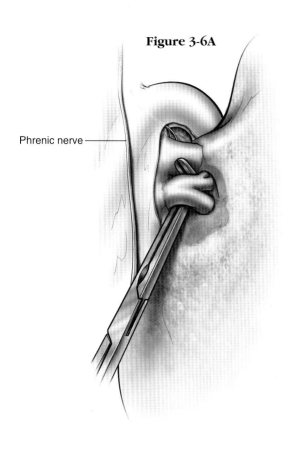

Phrenic nerve

Figure 3-6B

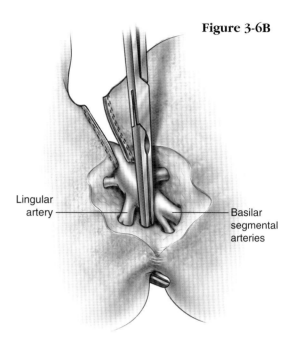

Lingular artery

Basilar segmental arteries

Figure 3-6C

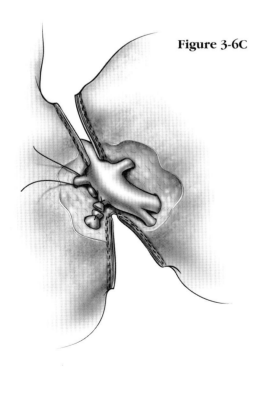

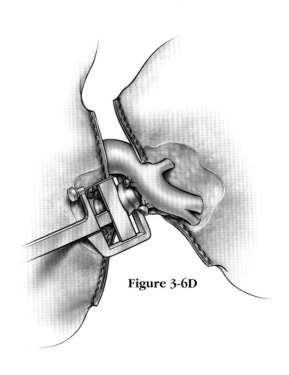

Figure 3-6D

3-7 Left Lower Lobectomy

The patient is usually placed in a lateral decubitus position for lateral or posterolateral thoracotomy or in a semilateral position for anterolateral thoracotomy. Video-assisted lung resection is usually performed with the patient in a full lateral position. The appropriate interspace for entry is identified after dividing the soft tissues overlying the chest wall. For access through a lateral thoracotomy, the sixth interspace is usually sufficient, and the fifth interspace is used if the patient is in a semilateral position. For patients who are obese with high diaphragms, an interspace higher than the one usually selected is appropriate to use. If there is a possibility of chest wall involvement by a lung cancer, the point of entry is selected to avoid this region so that it can be assessed prior to completing the thoracotomy. A thorough exploration of the hemithorax is performed and appropriate biopsies are taken (see Section 3-3).

When the decision to proceed with lobectomy is made, the pulmonary ligament is divided. The pleura surrounding the left lower lobe is divided to the level of the mainstem bronchus posteriorly and the superior pulmonary vein superiorly. The inferior pulmonary vein is dissected circumferentially (Fig. 3-7A). The pleura overlying the interlobar portion of the left pulmonary artery is divided and dissection is carried down to the subadventitial plane. The lateral surfaces of the pulmonary artery branches to the left lower lobe are dissected, helping to develop the fissure. Once it is confirmed that resection is technically feasible, the fissure is completed superiorly with a linear cutting stapler. The space

between the inferior and superior pulmonary veins is developed. The plane inferior to the takeoff of the lingular artery and medial to the basilar segmental vessels is developed, proceeding inferior and anterior to the lower lobe bronchus. The lung tissue anterolateral to this plane is divided with a linear cutting stapler, completing the inferior aspect of the fissure.

The inferior pulmonary vein is divided with a linear cutting stapler or between firings of a linear stapler. Issues pertaining to possible tumor invasion of the vein and tumor embolization described in Section 3-5 are pertinent here, as well. The superior segmental artery is dissected circumferentially and is divided with a linear cutting stapler or between ligatures (Fig. 3-7B). The trunk of vessels to the basilar segments is circumferentially dissected. It can usually be divided with a single firing of a linear cutting stapler, or can be divided between suture ligatures (Fig. 3-7C). The bronchus to the lower lobe is dissected circumferentially to the level of its takeoff, taking care to leave associated lymph nodes with the specimen. Bronchial artery branches are cauterized, clipped, or ligated. The bronchus is divided with a linear cutting stapler or is cut between firings of a linear stapler (Fig. 3-7D). When necessary, such as when a tumor encroaches on the takeoff of the left lower lobe bronchus, the bronchus is divided with a knife to ensure that an adequate margin exists. The stump is closed with interrupted 4-0 absorbable sutures.

For patients undergoing left lower lobectomy for cancer, an appropriate nodal dissection is performed. A complete hilar nodal dissection is standard practice. Mediastinal stations 7, 8L, 9L, and possibly 5 are most commonly involved by metastatic disease and should also be dissected completely.

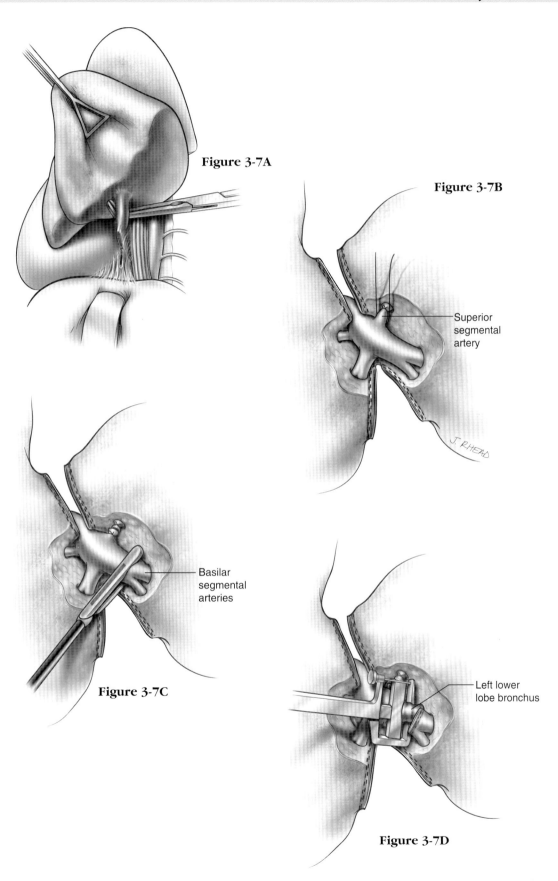

Figure 3-7A

Figure 3-7B

Superior
segmental
artery

J.R.HEAD

Basilar
segmental
arteries

Figure 3-7C

Left lower
lobe bronchus

Figure 3-7D

3-8   Right Pneumonectomy

The incision chosen for right pneumonectomy is similar to that selected for right upper lobectomy, although additional considerations are sometimes necessary. Airway complications such as bronchopleural fistula are more difficult to manage after pneumonectomy than following lesser lung resections. When they occur, it is advantageous to have methods for their control available, including muscle flaps such as those developed using serratus anterior or latissimus dorsi. As a result, it is often useful to employ a muscle sparing incision when possible for performing a pneumonectomy. Nevertheless, a wider field of exposure is sometimes necessary to accomplish a pneumonectomy because such procedures are necessitated by proximal tumors that require difficult airway or vascular dissections. The type and location of the access incision must be decided based on the characteristics of the patient and the preferences of the surgeon.

Lesser lung resection procedures sometimes must be performed in patients with centrally located abnormalities of uncertain etiology to establish a diagnosis. In contrast, pneumonectomy is a higher risk procedure that is usually much more debilitating than lesser lung resections, and should not be performed without first establishing a diagnosis. When the diagnosis has been established, a thorough exploration of the hemithorax is performed. In patients with a known or suspected lung cancer, the most common indication for pneumonectomy, appropriate lymph nodes are biopsied for intraoperative evaluation by frozen section to determine whether resection is appropriate. A full assessment of the hilar vessels is also appropriate to ensure that a complete resection is technically feasible.

Once the decision is made to proceed with right pneumonectomy, the pulmonary ligament is mobilized to the level of the inferior pulmonary vein and the pleura surrounding the hilum is divided. For an extrapericardial pneumonectomy, both pulmonary veins are dissected circumferentially. The right pulmonary artery is then dissected circumferentially to the level of the pericardial reflection (Fig. 3-8A). The veins are relatively resistant to injury during dissection, and if an injury occurs it is usually easy to repair. The pulmonary artery is a less forgiving vessel, and every effort is made to avoid injury. Such efforts include: avoiding grasping the vessel directly but instead handling the adventitia; grasping a large portion of the vessel circumference if use of tissue forceps is necessary; use of blunt, closed scissor tips or cotton-tipped dissectors (Kittner, push, peanut) for portions of the dissection; and not forcing a right angle clamp behind the vessel until it has been circumferentially dissected. Some surgeons emphasize that the safest instrument to use to encircle the pulmonary artery is their own index finger (see Fig. 3-8A inset).

If dissection of one of these three vessels is likely to be difficult, the other two vessels are dissected first and are then encircled with vessel loops and gently snared. If injury to the third vessel should occur, bleeding can be greatly reduced by closing the snares to occlude the other two vessels. Injuries to the proximal right pulmonary artery are challenging to control. There is very little room available to permit placement of an occluding vascular clamp, and positioning such a clamp too close to the point of injury may serve to extend the injury more proximally on the vessel. One technique for gaining control of the vessel is to dissect between the superior vena cava and the ascending aorta, entering the pericardium and cross clamping the right pulmonary artery at its takeoff from the pulmonary trunk. In other instances, particularly when there is no ready availability of cardiopulmonary bypass to support the patient, inflow occlusion obtained by snaring down both vena cavae may provide sufficient time and exposure to permit repair of the pulmonary artery injury.

In some situations it is appropriate to dissect intrapericardially to obtain control of the vessels. Typical indications include a tumor that encroaches on any of the three main vessels close to the pericardial reflection, pericardial involvement by a bulky proximal tumor (which often also engulfs the phrenic nerve), and extensive fibrosis and inflammation after radiation therapy. The pericardium is opened longitudinally from below the inferior pulmonary vein to above the pulmonary artery; under most circumstances the pericardiotomy is performed posterior to the phrenic nerve to spare it. With minimal dissection the veins and artery are usually easily encircled after proper exposure is obtained (Fig. 3-8B). After the vessels are dissected the anesthesiologist is alerted that the lung is going to be isolated from the circulation. It is wise to test clamp the pulmonary artery for a minute or two prior to permanently occluding it to ensure the patient can tolerate loss of the lung. The vessels are then occluded and divided using whatever means is most suitable. Under most circumstances the vessel is sectioned between two firings of a vascular stapler, or is divided using a linear cutting stapler (Fig. 3-8C). If cost is an important issue, or if there is not sufficient normal vessel dissected to permit placement of a vascular stapler, the medial portion of the vessel is clamped and is oversewn with a Blalock stitch using a permanent monofilament suture. The pulmonary end of the vessel is suture ligated (see Fig. 3-8C inset).

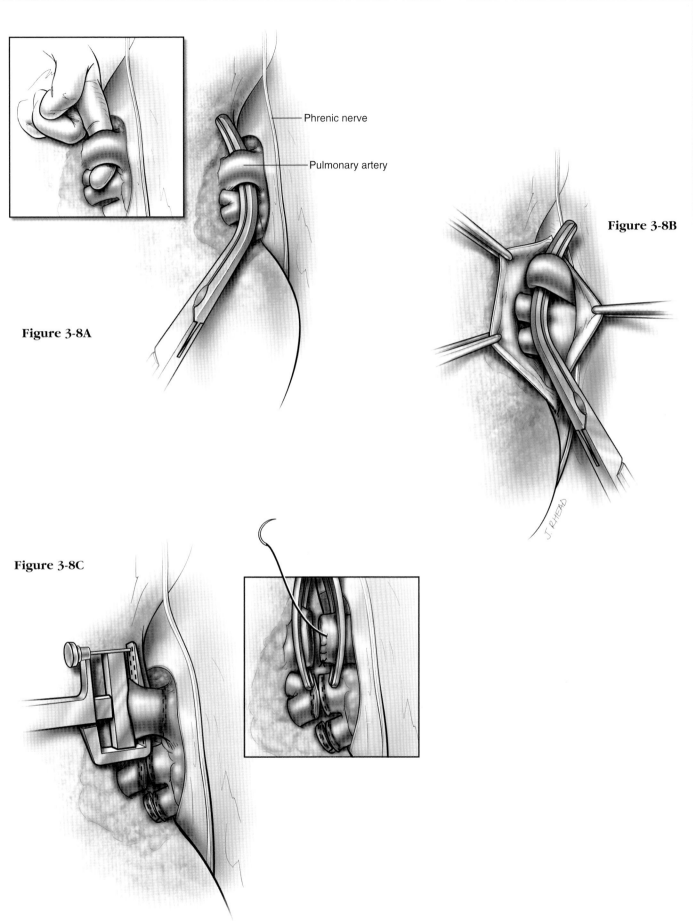

Phrenic nerve

Pulmonary artery

Figure 3-8A

Figure 3-8B

Figure 3-8C

The bronchus is dissected circumferentially at its origin, taking care not to devascularize the trachea or left mainstem bronchus. It is important to completely clear lymph nodes from the subcarinal (level 7) region to prepare the bronchus for division and closure, and this also serves to improve staging accuracy in patients with lung cancer (Fig. 3-8D). If the tumor is very proximal and encroaches on the azygos, the azygos arch is resected en bloc with the lung to provide better exposure of the origin of the right mainstem bronchus. Ensure that there is no foreign body in the right mainstem bronchus, such as an oropharyngeal temperature probe or bronchial suction catheter. If a right-sided double lumen tube has been used for lung isolation, which would be very uncommon in this setting, the tube must be withdrawn into the trachea at this time. The right mainstem bronchus is then closed with a stapler, occluded distally with a bronchial clamp, and divided (Fig. 3-8E). The surgeon must take care to select a cartridge containing staples of the proper length based on the thickness of the bronchial tissues to ensure that the bronchial closure is airtight.

An alternative to use of this stapled closure is application of a linear cutting stapler, which completely seals both ends of the cut bronchus and helps limit pleural space contamination as the bronchus is divided. The downside of this technique is that with currently available technology, the anvil and cartridge of the linear cutting stapler sometimes misalign when the stapler is fired. This leads to complete division of the bronchus but incomplete formation of the staples, leaving an incomplete bronchial closure. In patients in whom there is tumor close to the carina, the bronchus is divided with a knife at the carina without clamping across the tumor. The bronchus then is closed with interrupted absorbable sutures, taking care not to rupture the bronchial balloon of the left-sided double lumen endotracheal tube if such a tube has been used for isolating the right lung.

Figure 3-8D

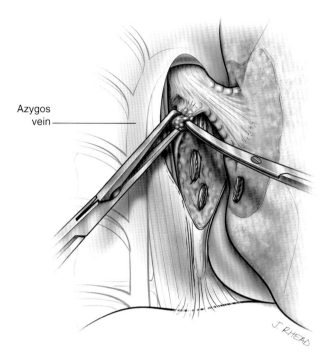

Azygos
vein

J. R. HEAD

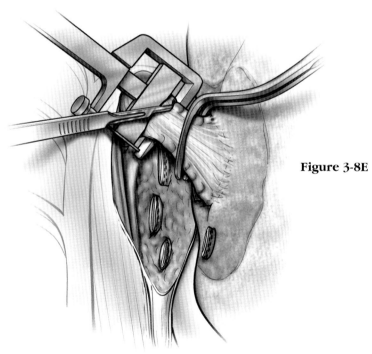

Figure 3-8E

The risk of stump leak can be reduced by covering the stump with a flap of vascularized tissue. Options for tissue flaps include pericardial fat, pleura, pericardium, azygos vein, and intercostal muscle; a variety of shoulder girdle muscle flaps are available for covering mainstem bronchus stumps that are at high risk for leakage (see Chapter 12). If there is insufficient soft tissue to permit its reapproximation to exclude the bronchial stump from the pleural space, one option is to raise a pleural flap lateral to the azygos based superiorly (Fig. 3-8F). It needs to be sufficiently wide to be sutured to viable soft tissue at the medial extent of the bronchial dissection, and sufficiently long to reach over the azygos vein to cover the stump without tension (Fig. 3-8G). Interrupted sutures are used to tailor the pleural flap coverage over the bronchial stump (see Fig. 3-8G inset).

It is important to remember that the pericardium must be closed after performing an intrapericardial pneumonectomy to avoid cardiac herniation. Primary closure is sometimes possible, but use of a patch to eliminate the pericardial defect has advantages. Pneumonectomy, particularly of the right lung, is associated with right heart dysfunction and right ventricular dilatation. Primary pericardial closure of necessity reduces the size of the pericardial space, restricting cardiac function. The effects of this are usually negligible in healthy people, but in the postpneumonectomy patient this can lead to restrictive effects that become evident 24 to 48 hours postoperatively and are poorly tolerated. Use of a small patch, such as expanded polytetrafluoroethylene (PTFE) that is sutured to the pericardial edges, prevents cardiac herniation and eliminates the risk of pericardial restrictive effects in the immediate postoperative period (Fig. 3-8H).

Meticulous hemostasis is vital because postoperatively there is no lung parenchyma to tamponade even the smallest bleeding vessels or oozing tissues. Whether or not to place a drain in the pneumonectomy space is controversial. One advantage of a drain is that it may be used after the thoracotomy incision is closed to balance the mediastinum in the center of the chest. This is done by first positioning the still-intubated and sedated patient supine on the operating table. The pleural drainage system is placed at the level of the right heart and on water seal only. The contralateral lung is inflated and maintained at a constant airway pressure of about 40 cm H_2O for 5 to 10 seconds. After excess air is evacuated from the pneumonectomy space during this breath, the drainage tube is clamped before the inspiratory cycle is terminated. The drainage tube is then left clamped unless a tension hemothorax develops on the side of the pneumonectomy, which can be relieved by temporarily unclamping the chest tube but nevertheless requires urgent return to the operating room. The problem with placing a chest tube is that there is increased risk of contaminating the pleural space, leading to postpneumonectomy empyema. An alternative method of balancing the mediastinum is to position a soft rubber catheter through the incision as it is being closed, weaving the catheter slightly through the layers as they are sutured so that the tube does not lie in a straight tract. Before the skin is closed but after an airtight seal is achieved, the tube is placed under water seal and the patient is given a sustained breath as previously described. Once excess air has been evacuated, the tube is quickly withdrawn and normal ventilation is resumed. The remainder of the incision is then closed.

If the mediastinum has not been adequately medialized with these techniques, based on the postoperative chest radiograph, and if there is hemodynamic compromise, the mediastinum is repositioned in the postanesthesia care area. A large bore angiocath attached to a stopcock is inserted in the fourth intercostal space in the midclavicular line under sterile conditions, and an appropriate volume of air (usually 500 to 1,000 mL) is added or removed as necessary to achieve the desired result.

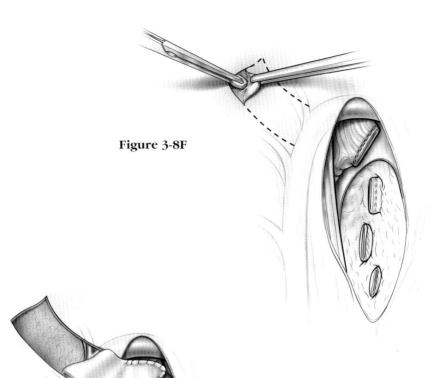

Figure 3-8F

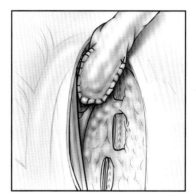

Figure 3-8G

Figure 3-8H

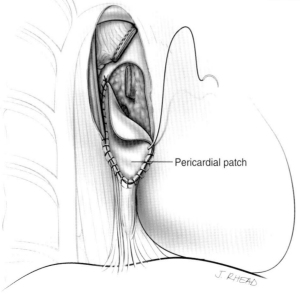

Pericardial patch

J. R. HEAD

3-9 Left Pneumonectomy

The incision chosen for left pneumonectomy is similar to that selected for left upper lobectomy, although additional considerations are sometimes necessary. As described earlier for right pneumonectomy, it is useful to employ a muscle sparing incision for performing a left pneumonectomy to provide options for managing postoperative surgical complications should they occur.

When the diagnosis has been established, a thorough exploration of the hemithorax is performed. Appropriate lymph nodes are biopsied in lung cancer patients for intraoperative evaluation by frozen section to determine whether resection is appropriate. A full assessment of the hilar vessels is also appropriate to ensure that a complete resection is technically feasible.

Once the decision is made to proceed with left pneumonectomy, the pulmonary ligament is mobilized to the level of the inferior pulmonary vein and the pleura surrounding the hilum is divided. Both pulmonary veins are dissected circumferentially. The left pulmonary artery is dissected circumferentially lateral to the ligamentum arteriosum (Fig. 3-9A). If the tumor involves the left main pulmonary artery it is sometimes necessary to divide the ligamentum arteriosum and complete the circumferential dissection of the left pulmonary artery close to its takeoff from the main pulmonary artery. If dissection of any of these three vessels is likely to be difficult, the other two vessels are dissected first and are then encircled with a vessel loop and gently snared. In some situations it is appropriate to dissect intrapericardially to obtain control of the vessels. Typical indications include a tumor that encroaches on any of the three main vessels close to the pericardial reflection, pericardial involvement by a bulky proximal tumor, and extensive fibrosis and inflammation after radiation therapy. The vessels are occluded and divided using stapler or oversewing techniques.

The bronchus is dissected circumferentially at its origin, taking care not to devascularize the trachea. Traction on the lung and left mainstem bronchus is sometimes required to enable the dissection to be developed medially enough to reach the carina (Fig. 3-9B). It is important to completely clear lymph nodes from the subcarinal (level 7) region to prepare the bronchus for division and closure; this also serves to improve staging accuracy in patients with lung cancer. Ensure that there is no foreign body in the left mainstem bronchus. The most common technique for left lung isolation is use of a left-sided double lumen endotracheal tube. Prior to applying a clamp or stapler to the bronchus, the surgeon must be sure that the endotracheal tube has been withdrawn into the trachea. Other foreign bodies that sometimes are positioned in the airway include oropharyngeal temperature probes or bronchial suction catheters. Palpation of the bronchus and verification with the anesthesiologist that the airway is clear is necessary prior to clamping the airway. The left mainstem bronchus is then closed with a stapler, occluded distally with a bronchial clamp, and divided (Fig. 3-9C). The surgeon must take care to select a cartridge containing staples of the proper length based on the thickness of the bronchial tissues to ensure that the bronchial closure is airtight.

When a right pneumonectomy is performed, during which a left-sided double lumen tube is used for lung isolation, division of the bronchus and oversewing the proximal stump is straightforward because of continued isolation of the right mainstem bronchus. If a left-sided double lumen tube is used for a left pneumonectomy, withdrawing the tube into the trachea prior to division of the left mainstem bronchus results in loss of isolation of the left lung, and the majority of the ventilatory volume will flow through the opened mainstem bronchus. This situation is obviously untenable because of inadequate ventilation of the patient and because of the contamination of the left pneumonectomy space by airway secretions. As a result, closed management of the left mainstem bronchus is most appropriate. When the margins are close for a lung cancer resection, initial consideration should be given to use of a right-sided double lumen tube for managing the airway.

In contrast to right pneumonectomy, development of specific tissue flaps for covering the bronchial stump is often not necessary. Assuming the mainstem bronchus is divided close to the carina, the stump will sink back into the mediastinum after the bronchus is divided. The soft tissues adjacent to the stump are easily closed over the stump with interrupted sutures (Fig. 3-9D). Under special circumstances, such as after induction chemotherapy and radiation therapy or in patients in whom the mediastinum is frozen and the stump fails to retract, a pleural or pericardial fat pad flap may be raised to reinforce the stump closure.

It is more important to close the pericardium after a left intrapericardial pneumonectomy to avoid cardiac herniation than after right intrapericardial pneumonectomy because the left ventricle is prone to herniate even through small pericardial defects. Use of a patch to close the pericardial defect eliminates the risk of creating an iatrogenic restrictive process, which is poorly tolerated in the postpneumonectomy patient. After obtaining adequate hemostasis, the incision is closed using one of the mediastinum centering techniques described earlier.

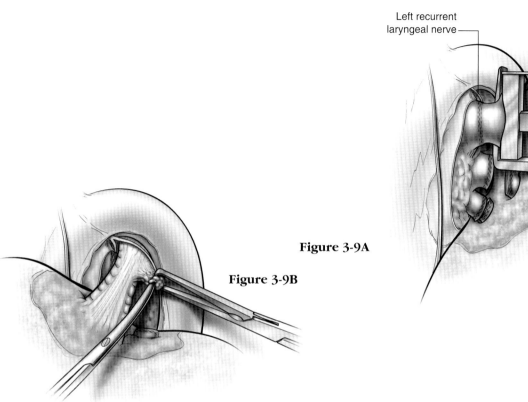

Left recurrent
laryngeal nerve

Figure 3-9A

Figure 3-9B

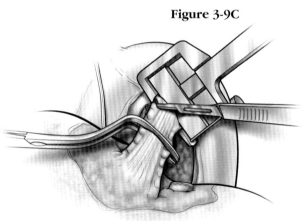

Figure 3-9C

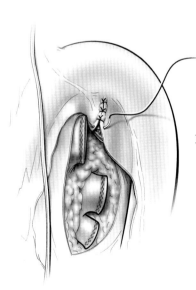

Figure 3-9D

3-10 Segmentectomy—Lingula

Resection of one or more anatomical and functional pulmonary subunits, or segments, with division of the corresponding individual bronchovascular structures, is referred to as segmentectomy. All other resections of less than a lung lobe that involve use of staplers, cautery, or laser for nonanatomic techniques are referred to as wedge resection or nodulectomy.

The lung is mobilized completely to enable assessment of hilar structures and to perform staging biopsies when appropriate. Once it is ascertained that segmental lingulectomy is appropriate, the lingular artery is identified in the fissure. The plane between the superior and inferior pulmonary veins is dissected. The plane inferior to the lingular artery and inferior to the upper lobe bronchus is developed to the plane between the pulmonary veins, and the fissure is completed with a linear cutting stapler. The lingular artery is dissected circumferentially in the fissure and is divided (Fig. 3-10A). This helps expose the left upper lobe bronchus and the segmental bronchi to the lingula.

The lingular bronchus is identified after development of the fissure deep to the stump of the lingular artery. One method of easily identifying the division between the lingular segments and the left upper lobe proper is by differential ventilation. After exposing the lingular bronchus, the lung is ventilated, inflating all segments. The lingular bronchus is then clamped and left lung isolation is resumed. As air in the left upper lobe

proper resorbs, the lingular segments remain inflated, creating a clear demarcation between these two regions. Alternatively, the bronchus is closed while the lung is deflated, and the remaining lung is then inflated, creating an inverse image of differential inflation. Maintaining inflation of the segments to be resected is an easier technique to use; working around the large amount of inflated lung when segments to remain in place are inflated can be problematic. In addition, the segment to be removed may become inflated using the technique of inflating the residual lung because of collateral airways crossing the intersegmental plane. The bronchus is divided and over-sewn, or is divided with a linear cutting stapler, taking care to avoid compromise of the bronchus to the left upper lobe (Fig. 3-10B).

The intersegmental vein drains adjacent segments and is preserved to maintain function of the parenchyma that remains after segmental resection. In the case of lingular resection, the intersegmental veins primarily drain the anterior segment of the left upper lobe proper, and must be preserved to retain adequate function of this segment. A clamp is applied to the bronchial stump of the lingular segments and traction is applied in an inferior direction (Fig. 3-10C). Initially using scissors or cautery, the plane between the segments is developed along the line demarcated by differential inflation. Small strands that interfere with development of the plane, which likely represent small arteries or bronchi, are divided with cautery or are clipped and divided. Once the plane is established, it is further developed using finger dissection along the path of least resistance.

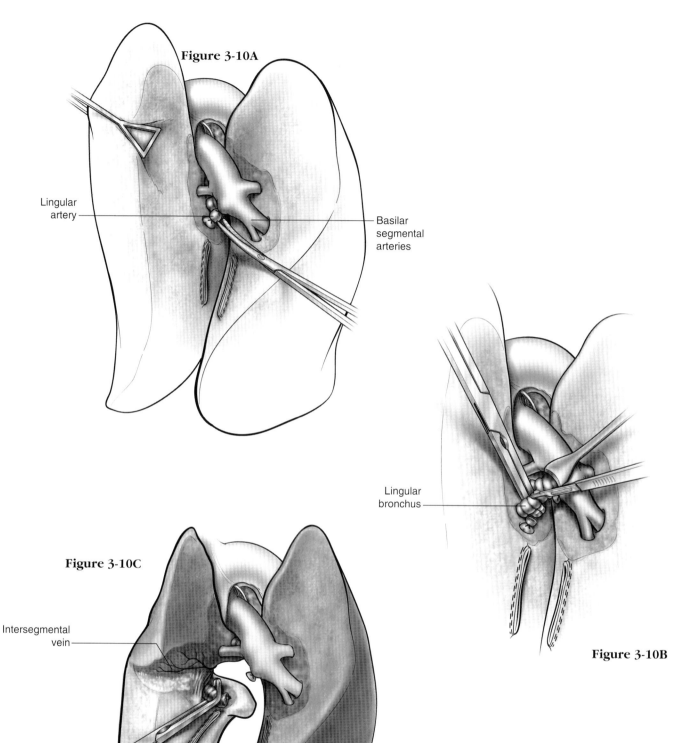

Figure 3-10A

Lingular artery

Basilar segmental arteries

Lingular bronchus

Figure 3-10B

Figure 3-10C

Intersegmental vein

J. RHEAD

The vein branch to the lingula is usually easily identified by carefully dissecting the most inferior branch of the superior pulmonary vein. In this situation, it may be divided prior to beginning development of the intersegmental fissure. If there is any question about which vein branch should be divided, it is best to wait until the fissure has been completely developed (Fig. 3-10D). This technique is most likely to preserve the intersegmental vein outflow path. Care should be taken not to compromise the veins draining the segments of the left upper lobe proper.

Once the plane is developed to the level of the visceral pleura, the pleura is divided and the specimen is removed. The raw surface of the remaining lung is compressed with a sponge for several minutes to help achieve hemostasis. As the lung is ventilated, any small bronchial branches that have been cut are cauterized or suture ligated. Bleeding vessels are cauterized, ligated, or clipped. Air leakage may be further reduced by reapproximation of the pleural edges with a running suture, but this may compromise full expansion of the lobe (see below). Alternative techniques for managing the raw surface include use of biological glues, suturing the raw surface to the pleura of the adjacent lung, or by suturing a broad flap of visceral pleura over the raw surface. Prolonged chest tube drainage is often necessary after segmental resection.

The objective of segmental resection is to preserve the maximum amount of functioning lung tissue while executing an anatomic resection. Generally speaking, even if the demarcation between segments is carefully identified and the bronchovascular structures are individually divided, separation of the lung parenchyma using a linear cutting stapler is not advisable. It unnecessarily compresses normal lung tissue and thus compromises postoperative lung function in patients in whom preservation of lung function is critical.

Perhaps the single exception to this guideline is lingulectomy in carefully selected patients. The lingula is particularly suitable for a stapled approach for two reasons. First, its bronchovascular structures are usually easily identified and individually controlled without extensive dissection of the lung parenchyma. Second, in some individuals the lingula is a long, thin appendage of the left upper lobe proper, making them ideal candidates for this technique. The principles of individual dissection and ligation of bronchovascular structures outlined earlier in this section apply. Once those steps have been accomplished, a long linear cutting stapler is applied at the demarcation between the lingula and the left upper lobe proper, completing the lingulectomy (Fig. 3-10E). The advantage of this technique is a resultant airtight margin of the parenchymal resection, which likely shortens the patient's hospital stay compared to leaving the usual raw parenchymal margin after standard segmental resection.

Figure 3-10D

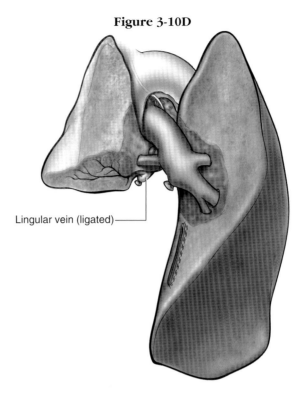

Lingular vein (ligated)

Figure 3-10E

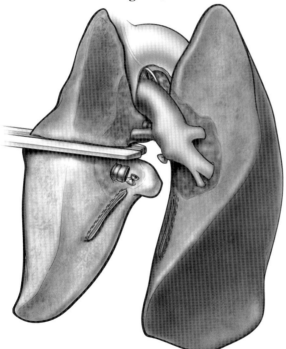

3-11 Segmentectomy—Basilar

The basilar segments of the lower lobes are usually resected as a group rather than individually, especially in the case of benign disease, which tends to collectively affect the basilar segments rather than involving a single basilar segment. For purposes of illustration, right basilar segmentectomy is described here, but the operative steps are similar for left basilar segmentectomy.

The lung is mobilized completely to enable assessment of hilar structures and perform staging biopsies when appropriate. Once it is ascertained that basilar segmentectomy is appropriate, the basilar segmental artery trunk is dissected circumferentially in the fissure and is divided (Fig. 3-11A). Care is taken to ensure that the superior segmental artery is preserved; this artery arises very close to the basilar arterial trunk in the right lung and is often distant from the trunk in the left lung. Division of the basilar artery trunk helps expose the lower lobe bronchus. After developing the fissure deep to the stump of the basilar artery, the basilar segmental bronchi are dissected, preserving the bronchus to the superior segment. Care must be taken to avoid injury to the vein to the superior segment, which often crosses the basilar segmental bronchus from the inferior segment to the bronchus. Differential inflation is accomplished and the bronchus is divided, taking care to avoid compromise of the bronchus to the lower lobe superior segment (Fig. 3-11B).

A clamp is applied to the bronchial stump of the basilar segments and downward traction is applied. The plane between the basilar and superior segments is developed along the line demarcated by differential inflation. Small arteries or bronchi are divided with cautery or are clipped and divided. Once the plane is established, it is further developed using finger dissection along the path of least resistance (Fig. 3-11C). After the plane is developed to the level of the visceral pleura, the pleura is divided sharply. The vein branches to the basilar segments are identified and individually ligated or stapled and divided, ensuring that the vein branches draining the superior segment are not compromised (Fig. 3-11D). The specimen is removed.

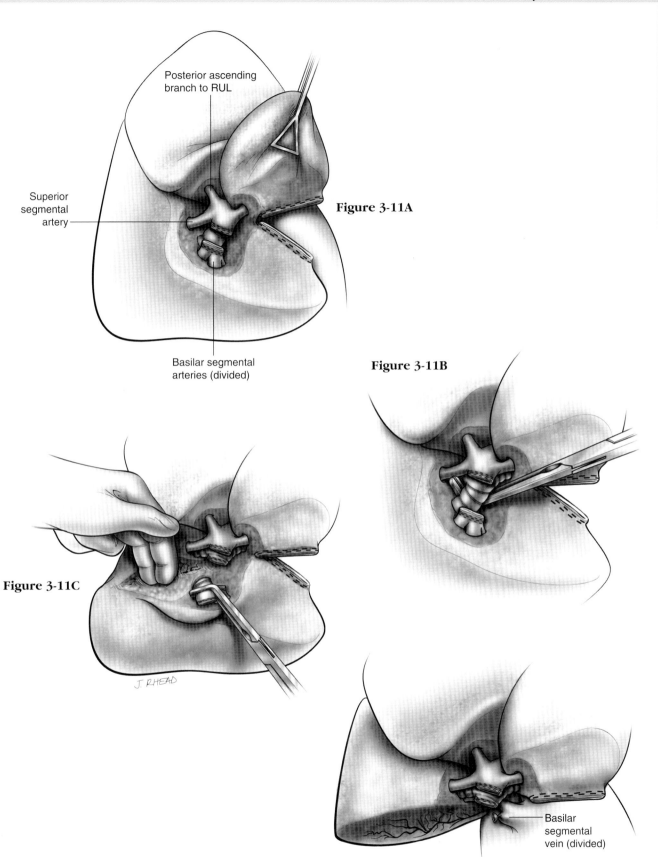

Posterior ascending
branch to RUL

Superior
segmental
artery

Figure 3-11A

Basilar segmental
arteries (divided)

Figure 3-11B

Figure 3-11C

J. RHEAD

Basilar
segmental
vein (divided)

Figure 3-11D

3-12 Segmentectomy—Superior

Superior segmentectomy is one of the more commonly performed anatomic segmental resections. This is partly because of the ease with which the operation is performed, and is due also to the distribution pattern of benign and malignant diseases that affect the lung. Although the anatomy varies slightly between the right lower lobe and left lower lobe superior segments, the techniques of superior segmentectomy are very similar. Right superior segmentectomy is illustrated.

The pleura surrounding the lower lobe is divided, as is the pulmonary ligament. The oblique fissure is opened in the right lung posteriorly beginning from the confluence of the lobes, whereas in the left lung the dissection extends inferiorly from the apex of the fissure. The superior segmental artery is dissected and divided (Fig. 3-12A). On the right, care must be exercised to avoid injury to the recurring artery to the posterior segment of the upper lobe, which sometimes arises from the superior segmental artery. On the left, there are sometimes two superior segmental arteries, both of which must be dissected.

The most superior branch of the inferior pulmonary vein drains the superior segment and is isolated. Preferably it is divided before beginning the bronchial and parenchymal dissection (Fig. 3-12B), or it can be divided at the conclusion of the parenchymal dissection. The bronchus to the superior segment is easily identified and is divided, taking care to avoid injury to the basilar segmental bronchi (Fig. 3-12C). A clamp is applied to the superior segmental bronchus and gentle upward traction is applied as the plane between the superior and basilar segments is developed along the line demarcated by differential inflation. Small arteries or bronchi are divided with cautery or are clipped and divided. Once the plane is established, it is further developed using finger dissection along the path of least resistance. After the plane is developed to the level of the visceral pleura, the pleura is divided sharply. If the superior segmental vein has not already been taken care of, the segment is rotated anteriorly and this vein is divided. Small bronchi and vessels that have been divided are oversewn or cauterized (Fig. 3-12D).

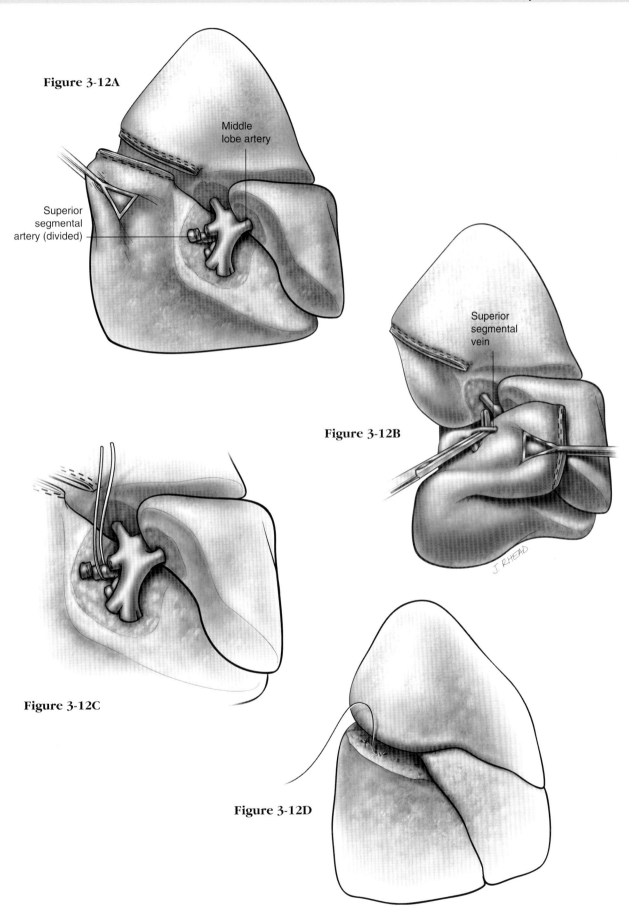

Figure 3-12A

Middle lobe artery

Superior segmental artery (divided)

Figure 3-12B

Superior segmental vein

Figure 3-12C

Figure 3-12D

J. RHEAD

3-13   Segmentectomy—Apical, Posterior, Anterior

Apical segmentectomy is the most commonly performed segmental resection owing to the predilection of this region of the lung for bullous disease, extensive damage from inflammatory and infectious processes, and lung cancer. Right apical segmentectomy is illustrated. A similar approach is used for left apical-posterior segmentectomy, and variances in the two techniques are described. Anterior and posterior segmentectomy are described but are not illustrated.

The pleura surrounding the right upper lobe is divided. The truncus anterior is dissected. The most superior branch of the truncus anterior supplies the apical segment, and this is divided (Fig. 3-13A). The most superior branch of the superior pulmonary vein crosses the inferior branch of the truncus anterior (which supplies the anterior segment of the right upper lobe) and this vein branch is divided.

The lobe is reflected anteriorly. The posterior aspect of the upper lobe bronchus is dissected sharply, eventually enabling exposure of the most superior branch of the bronchus, which represents the bronchus to the apical segment. Clamping this bronchus and using differential inflation confirms that the bronchus supplies the apical segment. This is divided and oversewn or is stapled if this can be accomplished without compromise to the rest of the bronchial tree (Fig. 3-13B). The parenchymal division is commenced sharply as traction is applied on the divided bronchus in an upward direction (Fig. 3-13C). Separation of the superior segment is continued bluntly with finger dissection along the plane identified by differential inflation (Fig. 3-13D). The pleura is divided sharply once the parenchymal dissection is completed.

Right upper lobe anterior and posterior segmental resections are accomplished using techniques similar to those for apical segmentectomy. For anterior segmentectomy, the inferior branch of the truncus anterior is identified, but is usually more easily dissected and divided after the vein to the segment is divided. The apical vein crossing this arterial branch is preserved. The anterior segmental vein joins it to form the upper trunk of the pulmonary vein draining the upper lobe, and this anterior segmental vein is divided. The anterior segmental artery is then divided. The lesser fissure is divided after identification of the interlobar artery. Occasionally an additional arterial branch to the anterior segment is identified and requires division. The base of the upper lobe is dissected posterior to the interlobar artery toward the bronchus to the right upper lobe, permitting identification of the anterior segmental bronchus. Identification of this is confirmed by differential inflation, after which the bronchus is divided. The plane between the segments is then dissected as described previously.

Right upper lobe posterior segmentectomy begins with identifying the interlobar portion of the artery and then completing the major fissure posteriorly. The artery to the posterior segment usually arises from the interlobar artery but may arise from the superior segmental artery to the lower lobe. The artery is divided. The right upper lobe bronchus is dissected, identifying the branch to the posterior segment. After confirmation of appropriate identification through differential inflation, the bronchus to the posterior segment is divided. The plane between the segments is dissected as described previously. The vein draining the posterior segment is divided last to avoid injury to the veins draining the anterior and superior segments.

Apicoposterior and anterior segmental resection of the left upper lobe are begun by subadventitial dissection of the left main pulmonary artery proximal to the first branch of that artery. Gaining control of this vessel permits control of bleeding, should such ensue during dissection of the branches, which are typically shorter and broader than those supplying other lung segments. The superior pulmonary vein is dissected; the uppermost branch drains the apicoposterior segment, the middle branch drains the anterior segment, and the inferior branch drains the lingula. The superior portion of the fissure is completed, exposing the arterial branches to the posterior segment and the lingula. Because there are often anatomic variations in the arterial supply to the left upper lobe, no arterial branches should be divided until all branches have been dissected. Traction on the appropriate segment will help identify which segmental arteries require division. Once this is accomplished, the appropriate vein branch is divided. Division of the segmental arteries exposes the underlying segmental bronchi, and the appropriate bronchus is clamped and its identification is verified by differential inflation of the lung segments. The bronchus is then divided, and the parenchymal plane is developed as described above.

Figure 3-13A

Ligated superior branch of
truncus anterior artery

Ligated superior branch of
anterior segmental vein

Figure 3-13B

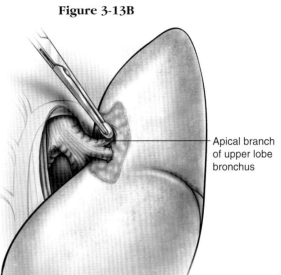

Apical branch
of upper lobe
bronchus

Figure 3-13C

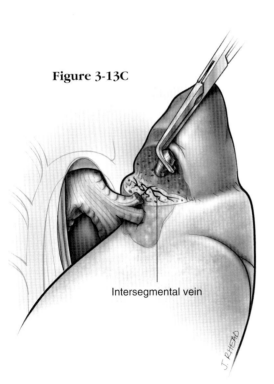

Intersegmental vein

Figure 3-13D

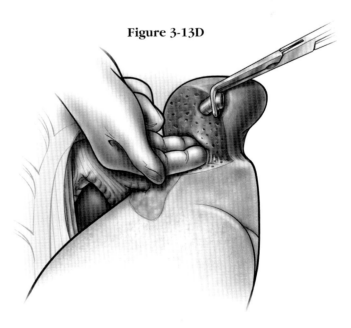

3-14 Bronchial Sleeve Resection

Bronchial sleeve resection for malignant disease should be considered as an alterative to pneumonectomy whenever an adequate lobar bronchial margin cannot be obtained. Historically the technique was reserved for patients with compromised lung function who were unable to tolerate pneumonectomy. Currently bronchial sleeve resection is appropriate to use whenever clear bronchial margins can be obtained and in the absence of extensive hilar or mediastinal adenopathy.

Suitability for sleeve lobectomy is initially determined by preoperative staging studies including computed tomography (CT) and possibly positron emission tomography (PET). The presence of abnormal mediastinal lymph nodes is an indication for cervical mediastinoscopy for pathologic evaluation of such nodes. The presence of macroscopic disease, multiple-involved lymph node stations, and contralateral nodal involvement are all contraindications to sleeve lobectomy. Bronchoscopy is an essential part of the initial evaluation that provides important information regarding the proximal extent of tumor and the technical feasibility of sleeve lobectomy. It should be performed by or witnessed by the operating surgeon.

The final decision regarding the appropriateness of sleeve lobectomy is not made until intraoperative exploration of the hilum and mediastinum, with appropriate pathologic staging, is completed. This is performed through a lateral or posterolateral thoracotomy, and isolation of the ipsilateral lung by anesthesia is essential. The presence of matted hilar lymph nodes or involved mediastinal lymph nodes precludes successful sleeve lobectomy. Once it has been determined that a patient is suitable for sleeve lobectomy, dissection of the hilar structures begins. A right upper lobe sleeve lobectomy, being the most commonly performed sleeve resection, is illustrated. Techniques used for other sleeve resections are similar.

The pleura surrounding the hilum of the right upper lobe is divided. The next step is careful dissection of the arterial branches, which often are in close proximity to or are involved by the tumor. It is wise to first dissect the right main pulmonary artery and encompass it with a vascular tourniquet prior to proceeding with dissection of the arterial branches if tumor involvement is suspected. Dissection of the arterial branches may reveal the need for pneumonectomy, sleeve arterial resection, or patch arterioplasty. When it has been determined that division of the arterial branches to the right upper lobe is possible, the branches are individually controlled and divided. The portion of the right superior pulmonary vein draining the right upper lobe is isolated and divided. The pulmonary ligament is divided to permit the lower and middle lobes to ascend during creation of the bronchial anastomosis, limiting tension on the suture line.

The bronchus is dissected proximal to the site of tumor. Careful attention is paid to preserving the bronchial arterial supply to the airways. There is usually one larger bronchial artery medial and anterior to the right mainstem bronchus that may be injured during tracheobronchial nodal dissection, whereas the bronchial artery at the level of the mid mediastinum that arises posteriorly and supplies the bronchus intermedius is usually easy to preserve. Typically the bronchial artery that courses through the region of the subcarinal lymph nodes must be sacrificed (Fig. 3-14A). The right mainstem bronchus is transected distally with a knife at a right angle to its main axis to provide a clean, straight margin (Fig. 3-14B). A similar cut is made across the proximal bronchus intermedius. No special effort is made to cut between or through bronchial cartilaginous rings. The points of division are selected to provide adequate tumor-free margins without placing excessive tension on the subsequent anastomosis. The margins are marked separately prior to passing off the specimen to enable the pathologist to confirm the absence of malignancy for each on frozen section.

The anastomosis is performed with absorbable monofilament or braided 4-0 sutures. All sutures are tied so that the knots are outside of the bronchial lumen. The initial stitches align the ends of the cartilaginous rings of the proximal stump to the ends of the cartilaginous rings of the distal stump (Fig. 3-14C). Careful alignment of the airways at this point helps prevent any torsion on the

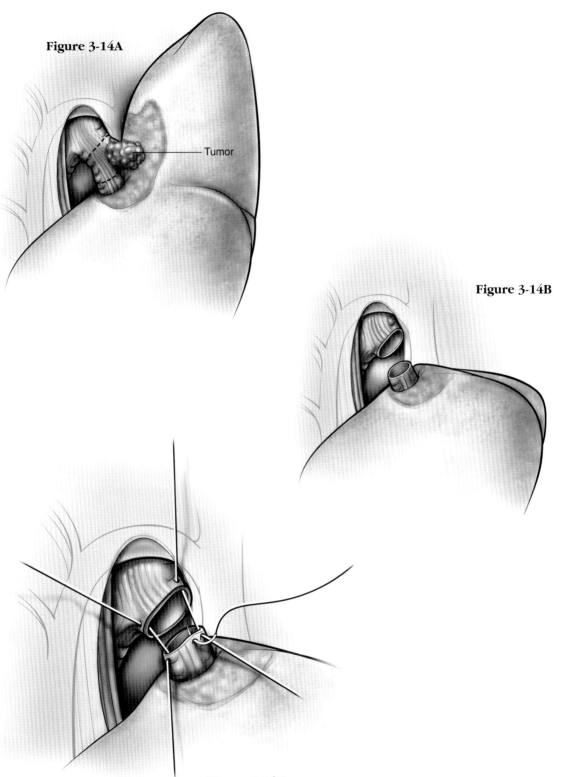

Figure 3-14A

Tumor

Figure 3-14B

Figure 3-14C

anastomosis as the lung is re-expanded. Tying these sutures takes tension off of the next set of stitches, which are placed to approximate the edges of the membranous portions of the airways. Once the back of the anastomosis has been completed, simple interrupted sutures are placed across the front of the anastomosis, leaving all of them untied until the final stitches have been placed (Fig. 3-14D). While tying the anterior row of sutures it is possible that a portion of the bronchus intermedius, having a smaller lumen, will partially telescope into the larger diameter mainstem bronchus. Once the anastomosis is completed it is observed for air leak by testing under saline while the lung is reinflated. Occasionally an additional suture is required to seal an evident leak. The anastomosis is wrapped with a generous flap of pleura or pericardial fat to isolate it from the pulmonary artery (Fig. 3-14E). This helps protect the vessel if the anastomosis breaks down, and may seal any small air leak that develops between sutures. Intraoperative flexible bronchoscopy is performed to evaluate the anastomosis.

Sleeve resections of the middle lobe and right lower lobe are not commonly performed. Middle lobe sleeve lobectomy is typically feasible only for patients with appropriately situated carcinoid tumors. Right lower lobe sleeve lobectomy, intended to preserve the middle lobe, is technically difficult. Because it preserves only a small amount of functioning lung tissue, it is more appropriate to perform a right lower and middle lobe bilobectomy in situations in which right lower lobe sleeve lobectomy is contemplated.

Left upper and left lower lobe sleeve lobectomies (Fig. 3-14F) are commonly performed using techniques similar to those described earlier in this section. For left upper lobe sleeve resection, the tendency to dissect the entire length of the left mainstem bronchus should be avoided, and the bronchial arteries to that bronchus need to be preserved during dissection of level 5 and level 7 lymph nodes. The mainstem bronchus is transected just proximal to the most proximal extent of tumor, close to the takeoff of the left upper lobe bronchus. The division between the left upper and left lower lobe bronchi must be performed carefully to preserve the superior segmental bronchus. If an adequate cuff of tissue is not left in place, the anastomosis may cause partial obstruction of the superior segment, resulting in atelectasis. Similarly, lack of careful alignment of the membranous portions of the bronchi during performance of the anastomosis may result in torsion on the left lower lobe bronchus and result in kinking of the superior segmental bronchus.

Left lower lobe sleeve resection is technically difficult primarily because of the size mismatch between the left upper lobe bronchus and the left mainstem bronchus. In addition, the lack of a clearly defined membranous portion of the left upper lobe bronchus makes alignment of the anastomosis challenging. Finally, the anastomosis must be performed adjacent to the left pulmonary artery, making placement of the posterior sutures difficult. If necessary, the few most posterior sutures may be tied with the knots inside the bronchial lumen to ensure their correct placement.

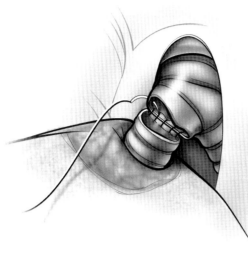

Figure 3-14D

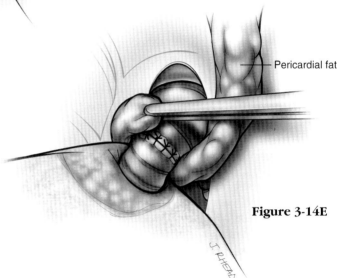

Pericardial fat

Figure 3-14E

Figure 3-14F

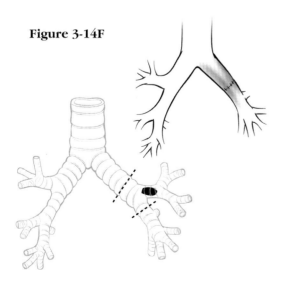

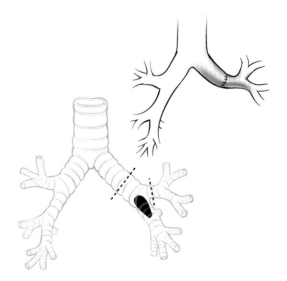

3-15 Pulmonary Arterioplasty, Bronchovascular Sleeve Resection

Proximal invasion of the pulmonary artery by a lung malignancy often indicates that the tumor is inoperable. However, in selected instances of more distal invasion, pulmonary artery sleeve resection or pulmonary arterioplasty can be performed, sometimes in conjunction with bronchial sleeve resection, as a potentially curative procedure. Although the left main pulmonary artery is shorter than the right main pulmonary artery, more of the length of the left pulmonary artery is exposed prior to its entering the fissure, and the interlobar portion of the artery is typically easily dissected along its full length. This makes the left pulmonary artery more amenable to arterioplastic procedures than the right pulmonary artery.

When pulmonary artery resection is contemplated, proximal and distal control of the vessel is obtained. Whenever complete cessation of blood flow is anticipated for more than a few minutes, temporary heparinization is advisable. Placing a tourniquet or vascular clamp around the origin of the left pulmonary artery is straightforward, and intrapericardial dissection of the vessel is not usually necessary except in cases of a very centrally located tumor. When such a situation is encountered, division of the ligamentum arteriosum and entry into the pericardium to gain proximal control are appropriate. Care must be taken under those circumstances to ensure that the left pulmonary artery, and not the main pulmonary artery, is dissected. In contrast, obtaining control of the right pulmonary artery in the presence of a centrally located tumor is more challenging, given its relatively short extrapericardial length. It is often necessary to dissect the vessel intrapericardially, and occasionally proximal control has to be obtained by dissecting the vessel intrapericardially between the superior vena cava (SVC) and the aorta (Fig. 3-15A).

Distal control can be obtained more caudad on the pulmonary arteries, but it is usually easier to simply place tourniquets on both pulmonary veins. This technique permits some flow from the bronchial artery circulation to contaminate the field during repair or reconstruction of the pulmonary artery, but the amount of flow is usually negligible.

In some instances the lung tumor invades only a portion of the pulmonary arterial wall, often close to or surrounding a pulmonary artery branch to the affected segment. In this situation partial resection of the pulmonary artery enables complete extirpation of the tumor (Fig. 3-15B). The appropriate pulmonary vein is divided, and any other pulmonary arterial branches to the affected lobe are divided. If possible, the bronchus to that lobe is divided as well, leaving the specimen tethered to a small segment of the pulmonary artery. This permits resection of only that portion of the pulmonary artery that is necessary to achieve an adequate margin. The resultant defect, if small, is closed with 4-0 or 5-0 running nonabsorbable monofilament sutures (Fig. 3-15C). If any compromise of the vascular cross-sectional area is anticipated, a patch angioplasty is performed using a piece of autologous pericardium or polytretrafluoroethylene (PTFE) (Fig. 3-15D). As with all vascular procedures in which the lumen is widely opened, exposing patients to the risk of embolism when flow is restored in the repaired vessel, air is evacuated from the lumen by permitting back bleeding prior to finalizing the closure.

Figure 3-15A

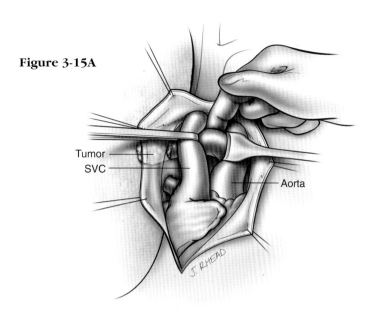

Tumor

SVC

Aorta

J. RHEAD

Figure 3-15B

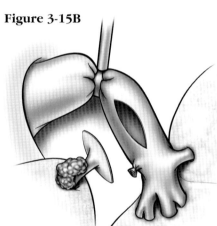

Figure 3-15C

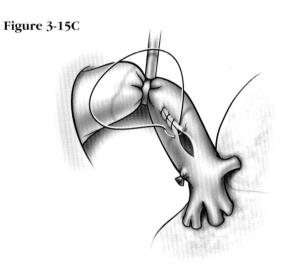

Figure 3-15D

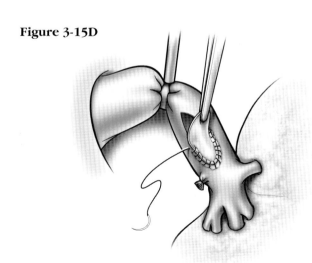

For patients whose tumors involve a greater length of the pulmonary artery, or in whom there is confluent involvement of the artery and bronchus precluding individual dissection of the structures, sleeve resection of the artery and bronchus is sometimes appropriate. This is particularly true for patients who will not tolerate pneumonectomy. Division of the artery proximally provides access to the bronchus for its division and reconstruction. Performing the bronchial anastomosis first limits the amount of subsequent manipulation necessary on the pulmonary artery during its repair, and reduces tension placed on the vascular anastomosis. Proximal control may be obtained with use of a tourniquet as described above, but if the resection margin is relatively close to the origin of the pulmonary artery, use of an atraumatic vascular clamp causes less distortion of the geometry of the vessel, enabling a more accurate anastomosis. For resections that involve a short segment of the artery, a simple end-to-end anastomosis is performed with running 4-0 or 5-0 monofilament sutures (Fig. 3-15E). If a segment greater than 1 to 2 cm is excised, an interposition graft of autologous vein, Dacron, or PTFE is used for reconstruction (Fig. 3-15F). It is easiest to perform the proximal anastomosis first using 4-0 or 5-0 running monofilament sutures. This enables the surgeon to cut the graft to an ideal length and provides optimal exposure for performing the distal anastomosis. Both a primary end-to-end anastomosis and an interposition graft, if performed in conjunction with a bronchial sleeve resection, need to be separated from the airway repair by a soft tissue flap of pericardial fat or pleura.

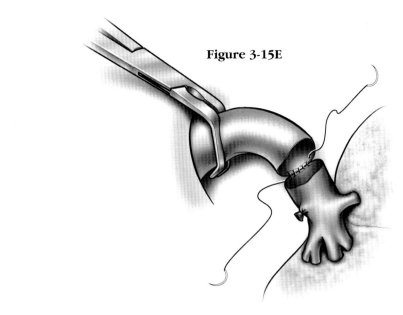

Figure 3-15E

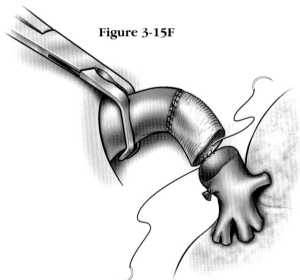

Figure 3-15F

3-16 Lung Volume Reduction Surgery

Lung volume reduction surgery, or LVRS, was originally introduced in the late 1950s as a treatment for end-stage emphysema. After being reintroduced in the mid 1990s, it has become an accepted therapy for patients with end-stage emphysema and also serves as a bridge to lung transplantation. The pathophysiology of end-stage emphysema is characterized in part by destruction of alveolar septum causing loss of elastic recoil in the lungs, resulting in air trapping. This causes hyperexpansion of the thoracic cage with flattening of the diaphragms, resulting in inefficient diaphragmatic breathing and forcing patients to use accessory muscles of respiration. Lung volume reduction surgery removes the most damaged areas of the lung, permitting improvement in elastic recoil and a reduction in residual volume. The diaphragms return to a more normal domed configuration, allowing them to function within the optimal part of the length-tension curve, relieving the accessory muscles of respiration of some of their burden.

Careful selection of patients is vital for a successful outcome. Patients must have severe emphysema characterized by substantially increased total lung capacity and residual volume (indicating air trapping), severely reduced expiratory airflow as measured by spirometry, and decreased diffusing capacity. Radiographic evaluation must show a heterogeneous pattern of disease distribution, with the worst disease typically confined to the upper lobes and perhaps the superior segments of the lower lobes. There should be some preservation of pulmonary vascularity in the lower pulmonary regions evident on computed tomography. Preoperative preparation of candidate patients for lung volume reduction surgery includes an extended period of monitored cardiopulmonary rehabilitation. Most patients exhibit a substantial improvement in forced expiratory measurements resulting from strengthening of their respiratory muscles. Timed walking distance is also typically increased.

Patients with severely compromised diffusing capacity (less than 20% of predicted) or with homogeneous distribution of their emphysema are generally excluded from consideration of lung volume reduction surgery because of the high early mortality postoperatively. Patients who otherwise qualify for lung volume reduction surgery on average experience a better quality of life and have a longer life expectancy than similar patients who are treated medically.

Lung volume reduction is typically performed bilaterally during a single anesthetic. The most common approaches include bilateral thoracoscopy (alternating lateral decubitus positions) and median sternotomy.

There are no important differences in the incidence of operative complications between these two approaches, but patients who undergo thoracoscopic lung volume reduction tend to experience a somewhat faster recovery compared to those having median sternotomy. Based on computed tomography and possibly lung scintigraphy, target areas for resection are established preoperatively. Target areas are regions of the lungs most severely affected by emphysema. These are typically identified in the upper lobes, and sometimes may affect the superior segment of the lower lobes (Fig. 3-16A). The objective of the operation is to remove approximately 30% of the lung volume by excising the target areas, preserving more normally functioning lung regions.

Excision is begun from inferior and extends in a curvilinear fashion over the apex of the upper lobe. Linear cutting staplers are required for a thoracoscopic approach, and are also typically used during open procedures performed through a sternotomy. It is important to map the planned staple line prior to beginning the resection. It is tempting to try to remove all the abnormal appearing tissues, which can result in a nearly complete nonanatomic lobectomy. Alternatively, following a curvilinear staple line sometimes results in an extremely long resection margin that does not end until the margin of the lung is reached at the fissure posteriorly. Mapping thus helps to avoid removing either too little or, more commonly, too much tissue.

Severely emphysematous tissues tend to tear through staple lines when reinflated, causing substantial and prolonged air leaks. To help minimize this risk, surgeons often reinforce the staple lines with biological glue, autologous tissues, or commercially available preserved bovine pericardium, expanded polytetrafluoroethylene, preserved porcine intestinal submucosa, and polyglycolic acid felt. The commercially available substances are manufactured to permit mounting on the stapler cartridge, and are incorporated into the staple line as the device is fired. At the conclusion of the procedure the lung assumes a more normal size, with a curvilinear reinforced staple line extending over the dome of the reconfigured lung (Fig. 3-16B).

Postoperative care of patients after lung volume reduction surgery is more challenging than after anatomic major lung resections. Patients tend to enter the operations in much poorer overall physical condition, and often experience problems with healing because of nutritional depletion, steroid administration, and poor tissue quality. Immediate resumption of cardiopulmonary rehabilitation postoperatively is useful in preventing cardiopulmonary complications. Prolonged air leaks are common, and discharge with pleural drainage tubes in place is not uncommon. Patients are often discharged to rehabilitation facilities rather than to home.

Figure 3-16A

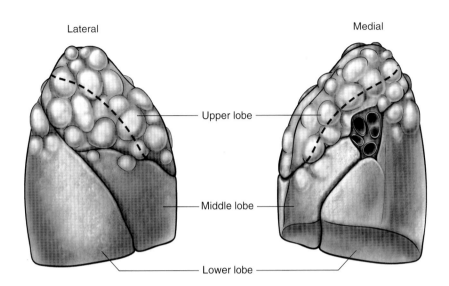

Lateral

Medial

Upper lobe

Middle lobe

Lower lobe

Figure 3-16B

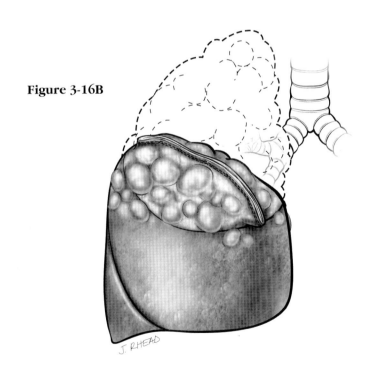

J. R. HEAD

3-17 Management of Giant Bullae

Giant bullae constitute an uncommon confined form of severe emphysema. Patients often have relatively normal lung tissue apart from their obvious bullous disease. Giant bullae that are preferentially ventilated and result in hypoventilation of the remaining lung are the best surgical targets. Careful selection of patients for resection is important so that outcomes are optimized. Patients typically must have at least 30% to 50% of the pleural space occupied by the bullous disease and should have moderate to severe dyspnea. Hypoventilation of the remaining lung is usually evidenced by the presence of vascular crowding visible on computed tomography. Patients who are deconditioned require preoperative cardiopulmonary rehabilitation similar to that recommended for patients with end-stage emphysema. If there is evidence of reactive airways disease or bronchitis, appropriate medical management is appropriate prior to bullectomy.

Options for surgical approaches are similar to those for lung volume reduction surgery. Patients with unilateral disease are better treated by thoracoscopic resection or open thoracotomy, whereas patients with bilateral giant bullae may undergo either bilateral thoracoscopy under a single anesthetic or median sternotomy. Intraoperatively the lung is examined during partial ventilation and while completely unventilated to enable clear demarcation of the limits of the giant bullous disease. It is often useful to deflate the giant bullae, especially when using minimally invasive techniques, to provide space within the pleural cavity to operate.

Sometimes it is useful to twist the bulla to help identify its stalk, which can be quite narrow. If a bulla has a narrow neck, it is ligated and the bulla is then excised. Special reinforcement techniques for the line of excision are rarely necessary. More often, bullae coalesce into a clump of abnormal tissue at the apex of the upper lobe. Manipulation of the abnormal tissues, including twisting,

helps to identify what is commonly a somewhat diffuse junction with more normal lung tissue. Once the limits of resection are identified, linear cutting staplers are used to excise the abnormal lung tissue. Figure 3-17A shows a linear cutting stapler defining the inferior limits of giant bullous disease after the bullae have been collapsed to permit their thoracoscopic treatment. Note that the majority of the upper lobe is relatively normal, underscoring the need to carefully define the limits between the bullae and the normal lung tissue prior to beginning resection. In contrast to lung volume reduction surgery, a defined percentage of lung tissue is not removed when treating isolated giant bullae. Rather, the principle is to preserve all relatively normal lung tissue while removing as much abnormal tissue as possible. When in doubt resect less, rather than more, tissue. As with stapling techniques for diffuse emphysema, use of reinforcement techniques for the staple lines may help reduce the incidence and duration of postoperative air leaks (Fig. 3-17B).

In addition to giant bullae, patients with limited bullous emphysema often have many smaller blebs or bullae in addition to their giant bullae. It is not necessary to completely excise these lung regions. The smaller blebs are typically confined to the surface of the lung. Although they may pose a small future risk of spontaneous rupture and pneumothorax, is it unlikely that these small blebs will progress to giant bullous disease resulting in pulmonary compromise. For these reasons, relatively conservative management of the more minor areas of disease is appropriate. One conservative technique is to use electrocautery applied very gently to the surface of the bleb or arcing the energy to the surface of the bleb without creating actual physical contact. Alternatively an argon beam coagulator may be used. The heat generated in the wall of the bleb causes contraction of the tissues, flattening the bleb to the level of the normal lung surface (Fig. 3-17C). No further management of these areas is required.

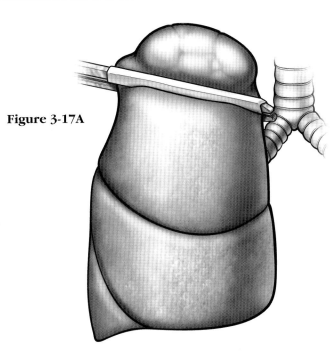

Figure 3-17A

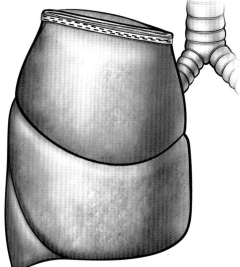

Figure 3-17B

Figure 3-17C

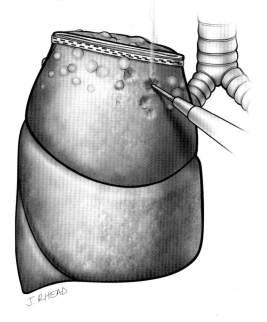

J. RHEAD

3-18 Wedge Resection and Nodulectomy

There are a wide variety of reasons to perform limited nonanatomic wedge resection of the lung, including diagnosis of nodules that represent benign processes, diagnosis, and sometimes therapy for early-stage lung cancer, treatment of metastasis from a known extrapulmonary malignancy, and diagnosis of diffuse parenchymal disease. The principles of wedge resection vary depending on the indication for surgery. For isolated nodules for which only a diagnosis is required, simple wedge resection with clear surgical margins is appropriate, minimizing the amount of normal lung tissue removed. Perhaps slightly wider normal margins should be achieved when excising metastases as a potentially curative procedure. And even wider margins are appropriate when limited resection is performed as a curative procedure for early-stage lung cancer in patients with impaired pulmonary function or other contraindication to anatomic resection.

In contrast, sampling of tissues for parenchymal disease requires a somewhat different approach. Target areas are identified based on the extent of disease evident on computed tomography. In some patients the disease is quite focal, dictating biopsy of a carefully identified and isolated portion of lung tissue. More commonly the disease is diffuse, often involving all five lobes of the lung, although there may be a predominance of abnormalities peripherally, at the lung bases, or at the lung apex. When diffuse parenchymal disease is present, it is best to obtain biopsies from multiple lung regions to obtain the best possible representation of the underlying process. In patients who are clinically stable and an elective lung biopsy is planned, a thoracoscopic approach is most appropriate. Operating on the patient's right lung provides more room for a minimally invasive approach and offers edges for biopsy from three lung lobes rather than the two that are present on the left side. In patients who are unstable and in whom thoracoscopy is not advisable because of inability to tolerate intubation with a double lumen tube or isolated lung ventilation, a limited open approach, usually through an inframammary incision, is best. In this instance a left-sided approach is sometimes preferred because of the ease with which the lingula can be accessed.

In patients in whom a small nodule is located very close to the pleural surface, a single firing of a linear cutting stapler is usually sufficient to excise the nodule. The nodule is gently grasped with a Lockwood lung clamp, Allis clamp, or Babcock clamp, minimizing the amount of normal lung tissue included in the clamp. The tissue is elevated above the level of the remaining lobe. A linear cutting stapler is positioned just under the clamp, encompassing the entire nodule in the tissue to be excised (Fig. 3-18A). It is sometimes useful to retract the lung tissues toward the nodule with a cotton peanut so that the edge of the lung tissue is included in the staple line, avoiding the need to fire another cartridge to complete the staple line. The resultant staple line lies flush with the lung surface (see Fig. 3-18A inset).

In most patients it is necessary to take a wedge-shaped segment of lung tissue to obtain an adequate specimen or to adequately encompass the region of abnormality. The area of interest is grasped and an initial staple line is established at an angle, aiming for the apex of the intended pattern of resection (Fig. 3-18B). The second staple line is created from the other side of the specimen (Fig. 3-18C). The result is a wedge-shaped defect in the lung (Fig. 3-18D). The staple lines are usually free of bleeding and air leak owing to the high efficiency of the staplers. In instances in which the parenchymal process is very advanced, the staple lines may pull through the tissue because it cannot be sufficiently compressed, resulting in air leakage but rarely in bleeding. Use of longer staples for such tissues may help prevent this complication.

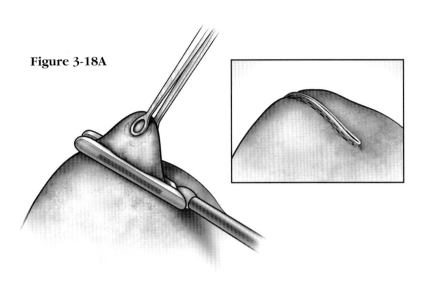

Figure 3-18A

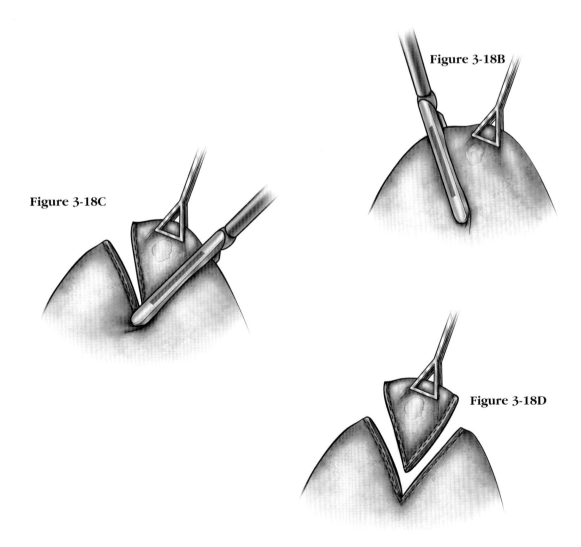

Figure 3-18B

Figure 3-18C

Figure 3-18D

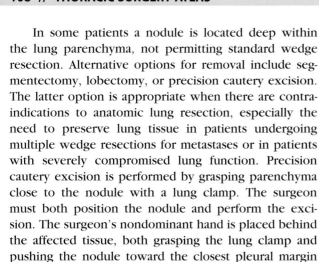

In some patients a nodule is located deep within the lung parenchyma, not permitting standard wedge resection. Alternative options for removal include segmentectomy, lobectomy, or precision cautery excision. The latter option is appropriate when there are contraindications to anatomic lung resection, especially the need to preserve lung tissue in patients undergoing multiple wedge resections for metastases or in patients with severely compromised lung function. Precision cautery excision is performed by grasping parenchyma close to the nodule with a lung clamp. The surgeon must both position the nodule and perform the excision. The surgeon's nondominant hand is placed behind the affected tissue, both grasping the lung clamp and pushing the nodule toward the closest pleural margin (Fig. 3-18E). The pleura is scored directly over the nodule (see Fig. 3-18E inset). Using electrocautery and occasional blunt dissection, the surface of the nodule is exposed. Larger bronchioles and arterioles that are encountered are cauterized or clipped. Smaller nodules can be grasped; alternatively, retraction is achieved by putting a heavy suture through the nodule. It is sometimes useful to dissect around the margin of the nodule with a right angle to expose any vascular supply. Most vascular and bronchial structures can simply be dissected bluntly to the side, permitting complete removal of the nodule, leaving a cavity in the lung parenchyma (Fig. 3-18F).

If the cavity is deep, it can be closed after all bronchial and vascular structures have been controlled. A funnel-type stitch is used to close the cavity from its base. The stitch is placed in a circular fashion, concentrically extending upward until the pleural surface is reached. Once the parenchymal defect is obliterated, the pleural defect is closed with a separate continuous suture (Fig. 3-18G).

Figure 3-18E

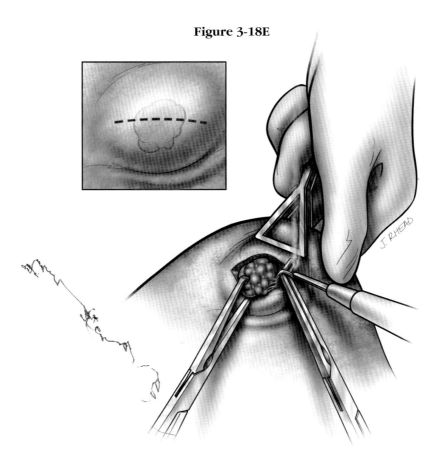

Figure 3-18F

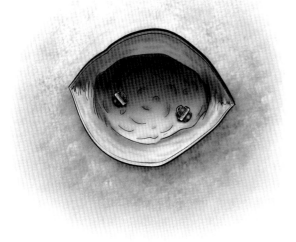

Figure 3-18G

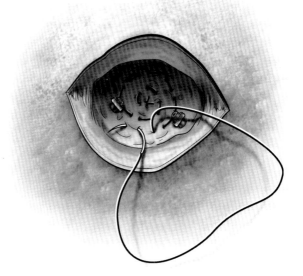

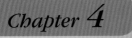

Chest Wall

Operations on the chest wall are performed for a wide variety of indications. Many such procedures, such as rib resections, are done simply to provide adequate exposure for more complex intrathoracic procedures. Chest wall resections are sometimes required for oncologic purposes, such as for lung cancers invading the superior sulcus or vertebral bodies, and primary tumors of the bony and cartilaginous chest wall. Resections are also sometimes performed for benign problems such as osteomyelitis and thoracic outlet compression syndromes. Occasionally rib resections are performed for thoracoplasty as part of the solution to intrathoracic space problems. Finally, chest wall procedures are often required for congenital deformities of the chest wall including a variety of pectus-type conditions. The relevant anatomy of the bony chest wall is outlined in Chapter 1, Figures 1-1D through 1-1F.

4-1 Rib Resection

Rib resection is most commonly performed by some surgeons as part of a standard thoracotomy. Removal of a rib segment improves exposure of intrathoracic contents and reduces the amount of rib distraction by rib spreaders necessary to accomplish an intrathoracic procedure. Limiting the amount of rib distraction lessens the pressure on intercostal nerves and may reduce acute and long-term post-thoracotomy pain. Rib resection is also useful when reoperative thoracotomy is necessary. Frequently the initial post-thoracotomy healing process causes fibrosis of the intercostal spaces, making them narrow and fixed, limiting the ability to distract ribs and provide operative exposure. This situation is often compounded by the presence of dense adhesions between the lung and pleura. The typical small pleural space entry common to initial intrathoracic procedures that permits a preliminary assessment of the condition of the lung and

pleural space is no longer sufficient for this purpose when reoperative surgery is performed. Rib resection with entry into and dissection of the pleural space through the bed of the resected rib provides the working space needed to perform adhesiolysis and proceed with the planned operation.

Simple individual rib resection is begun by scoring the periosteum of the selected rib with electrocautery. The periosteal opening is "tee'd" off at the limits chosen for rib resection. For most thoracotomy access procedures the limits of rib resection should extend to the limits of the thoracotomy, providing maximal exposure. For more limited procedures, such as axillary thoracotomy for bleb resection, removal of a 5-cm segment is sufficient to provide exposure. A periosteal elevator is used to strip the periosteum from the underlying bone on the lateral surface of the rib (Fig. 4-1A). The corner of the elevator is used to begin to separate the periosteum from the superior and inferior edges of the rib, taking care to preserve the neurovascular bundle when angling around the inferior rib edge. Because the external intercostal muscle fibers are oriented from posterosuperior to anteroinferior, it is easiest to strip the superior rib edge from posterior to anterior and the inferior rib edge from anterior to posterior. Once the subperiosteal plane is developed on the deep surface, a curved periosteal elevator (raspatory), such as a Doyen, is used to develop this plane completely around the rib. The Doyen is drawn anterior and posterior to complete this plane to the desired limits of the periosteal dissection (Fig. 4-1B). A rib cutter is used to transect the rib at the limits of the periosteal dissection. Depending on the rib angle and available exposure, an angled rib cutter (Fig. 4-1C) or a guillotine-type rib cutter is used. If the correct plane of periosteal dissection is developed and if the neurovascular bundle is preserved, there is typically little need for hemostasis after simple rib resection. Occasionally there is some bleeding from the transected ends of the ribs that requires electrocautery.

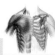

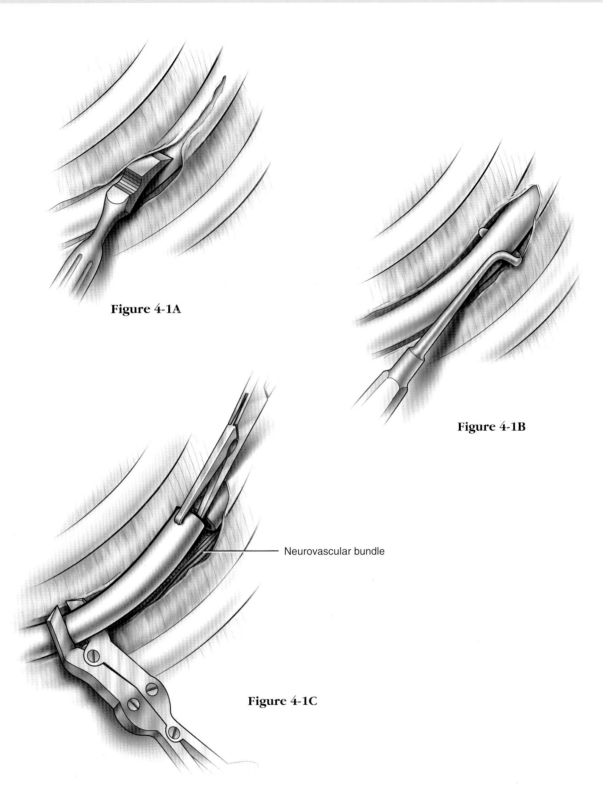

Figure 4-1A

Figure 4-1B

Neurovascular bundle

Figure 4-1C

4-2 Sternal Resection

Resection of the sternum is performed most often for treatment of osteomyelitis. This is usually owing to postoperative complications after sternotomy for cardiac procedures, but may arise spontaneously as a result of tuberculosis or due to joint seeding from blood-borne infections. The most likely scenario for the latter condition is intravenous illicit drug use. The other common indications for resection are primary tumors of the sternum and radiation-induced necrosis of tissues after intensive treatment for breast cancer.

The amount of tissue resected is determined by the disease process and its extent. Although one's index of suspicion must be high, simple sternal dehiscence may sometimes be a result of mechanical factors alone and will heal with appropriate sternal rewiring. Similarly, it is possible to have a superficial sternal wound infection without sternal osteomyelitis that responds appropriately to systemic therapy and open drainage. When positive blood cultures develop, or when there is a deep sternal wound infection or mediastinitis, the likelihood is strong that sternal osteomyelitis is present and that aggressive therapy is necessary.

Sternal osteomyelitis that occurs after sternotomy typically involves most of the sternum and the adjacent costal cartilages, necessitating their complete removal. Occasionally the manubrium and first costal cartilages can be preserved, thus providing shoulder girdle stabilization. The previous incision is opened completely, and all purulence is evacuated. After appropriate drainage

has been accomplished, the sternum is assessed for viability and the degree of involvement. In acute situations the extent of bone infection is not always evident. However, use of sternal conserving measures in the presence of a deep sternal wound infection, obvious mediastinitis, or positive blood cultures is not recommended.

Sternectomy for poststernotomy infection is performed through the existing standard sternotomy incision; occasionally "T" or "H" extensions are necessary to provide adequate exposure to permit both resection and reconstruction (see Fig. 4-2A inset). The pectoralis muscles are elevated off the sternum and costal cartilages (Fig. 4-2A). After adequate mediastinal debridement is performed, the perichondrium is elevated from the costal cartilages, and the cartilages are disarticulated from their costal and sternal attachments and are removed. The sternal halves are resected, including the manubrium if necessary (Fig. 4-2B). It is not usually necessary to resect the first costal cartilages. If drainage of the mediastinum is sufficient to permit primary closure of the wound, the pectoralis muscles are mobilized bilaterally based on the thoracoacromial arteries (Fig. 4-2C). It is often necessary to divide their humeral attachments to permit advancement of the muscles into the wound. The muscle with the most mobility is folded into the mediastinal defect, and the other muscle is layered over it (Fig. 4-2D). Alternatively, if the mediastinal space is relatively small and the internal mammary vessels are intact, the pectoralis muscles can be mobilized based on perforators from these vessels, detached from their lateral insertions, and flipped over into the mediastinal space. The skin edges are approximated over drains.

Figure 4-2A

Figure 4-2B

Figure 4-2C

Thoracoacromial artery

Figure 4-2D

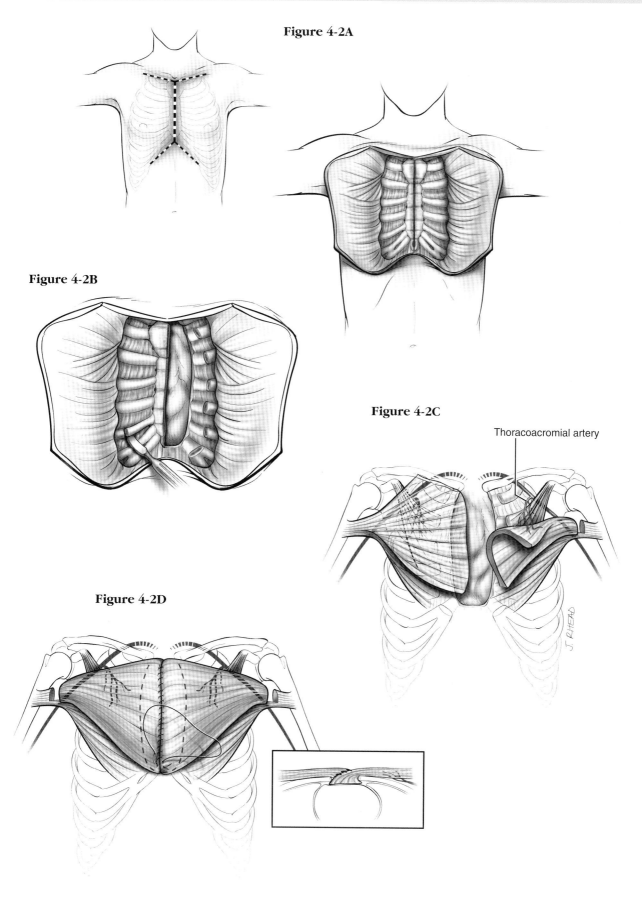

More limited infections of the sternum can occur, most commonly sternoclavicular osteomyelitis. Although decades ago this often arose spontaneously owing to tuberculosis, the usual scenario in the present era is intravenous drug abuse or the presence of an infected subclavian catheter. The infection arises in the joint space and then spreads to contiguous bones, including the first rib, clavicle, and manubrium. Treatment usually requires a combination of intravenous antibiotics and wide resection of the affected tissues, including the manubrium, clavicle, and portions of two or three ribs (Fig. 4-2E). A trapdoor incision is made extending along the clavicle, down the sternum, and out the third interspace (see Fig. 4-2E inset). The sternum is divided with a saw to the level of the third interspace, and the pectoralis major is mobilized off of the chest wall. The third intercostal space is opened with electrocautery for a distance of 5 to 10 cm, taking care to ligate the internal mammary vessels. The third and second ribs are divided. The clavicular muscle attachments (platysma, sternocleidomastoid) and deeper muscles (middle scalene) are divided. The clavicle is divided lateral to the extent of infection. The first rib is then cleared superiorly of remaining muscle attachments (subclavius, anterior scalene) and is divided lateral to the extent of the infection (Fig. 4-2F). Drains are placed, the pectoralis flap is rotated into the defect, and the incision is closed.

Primary tumors of the sternum are among the most common cancers of bone and cartilage. Potentially curative therapy requires en bloc resection with adequate tumor-free margins. The principles of resection are similar to those noted above with two exceptions. It is usually necessary to obtain a wider bony/cartilaginous margin for primary tumors of the sternum and adjacent chest wall than it is for benign disease. In addition, resection of overlying soft tissues, including pectoralis muscle and sometimes skin, is occasionally necessary depending on the degree of penetration of the tumor. When soft tissue resection is required, it is useful to have options for soft tissue reconstruction available (see Chapter 12). The extent of bone/cartilage resection is dependent upon the location of the tumor. Preservation of as much normal bone as possible is appropriate, within the constrictions of a curative resection, to maintain stability of the anterior chest wall. Options for resection are seen in Figure 4-2G.

Figure 4-2E

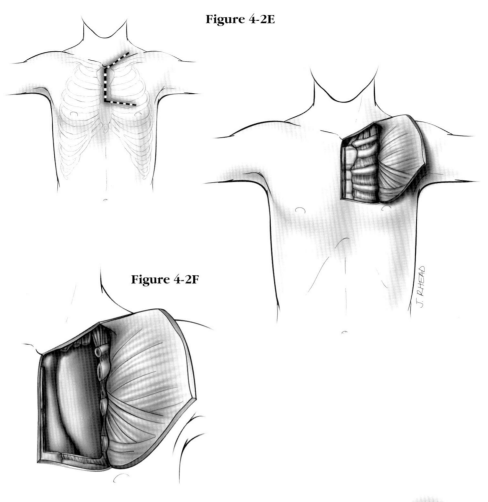

Figure 4-2F

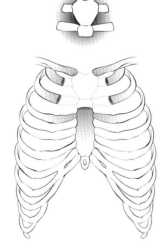

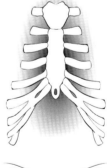

Figure 4-2G

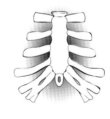

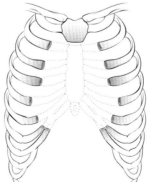

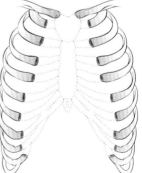

Manubrial resection   Resection of sternum proper   Complete sternectomy

4-3 Anterior Approach to Superior Sulcus Tumors

Tumors of the superior sulcus arise at the apex costovertebral gutter and usually originate in the lung. They involve structures of the apex of the chest wall above the level of the second rib and are technically challenging cancers to treat surgically. There are substantial differences of opinion about how aggressive surgical therapy should be. However, there is general agreement that patients with superior sulcus tumors should undergo preoperative therapy, including radiation therapy and chemotherapy, as part of multimodality treatment. This increases complete resection rates and possibly improves long-term survival.

Both posterior (historically the most common) and anterior approaches to surgical resection have been described. Tumors that extend cephalad to the apex of the lung and invade the thoracic inlet anteriorly or laterally are best approached through an anterior incision. Tumors that are located more posteriorly, including those that cause symptoms compatible with Pancoast's syndrome, are resected through a posterior approach. In some patients a combined approach is necessary. Relative contraindications to resection include extensive vertebral body involvement and involvement of the subclavian vessels or carotid artery. Absolute contraindications to resection include involvement of mediastinal or supraclavicular lymph nodes, total venous obstruction, invasion of the spinal canal, invasion of the brachial plexus above the lower trunk, the presence of distant metastatic disease, and involvement of more than two or three vertebral bodies.

For anterior approaches to resection of superior sulcus tumors, the patient is positioned supine with a roll under the upper chest and with the head turned to the opposite side. Arterial pressure is monitored in the contralateral upper limb, and venous access is provided both in the contralateral limb and in the lower extremities if necessary. Several types of incisions may be used, but the transclavicular approach provides the best exposure for most tumors. The incision is L-shaped, extend-ing from near the mastoid process along the anterior margin of the sternocleidomastoid muscle, inferior to the level of the second intercostal space, and laterally to the deltopectoral groove (Fig. 4-3A). The sternal attachments of the sternocleidomastoid are divided, the medial half of the clavicle is cleared of its muscular attachments, and a musculocutaneous flap is developed and folded laterally, exposing the neck and upper chest. The scalene fat pad is dissected, preserving the phrenic nerve, and the superior mediastinum is digitally explored to assess tumor resectability after division of the sternal strap muscles.

If the tumor appears resectable, the medial half of the clavicle is resected. The internal jugular vein, subclavian vein, and innominate vein are dissected. It is often useful to ligate and divide the internal jugular vein to provide exposure to the underlying structures. If there is involvement of the subclavian or innominate vein, proximal and distal control are obtained and the vein is divided. For left-sided tumors the thoracic duct usually must be divided as well. The anterior scalene muscle is divided from the first rib. The subclavian artery is dissected and small branches are isolated and divided to provide additional mobilization. If the artery is involved by tumor, it is controlled proximally and distally and the involved portion is divided (Fig. 4-3B). After removal of the surgical specimen, the artery is primarily anastomosed or an interposition graft of reinforced polyfluorotetraethylene (PFTE) is performed. The endothoracic fascia is opened into the pleural space. The middle scalene muscle is divided and the T1 and C8 nerve roots are dissected from lateral to medial to the confluence of the lower trunk of the brachial plexus. The T1 nerve root is ligated medial to the tumor, whereas the C8 nerve root is preserved if possible (Fig. 4-3C). The first and second ribs are divided laterally and at the costosternal junction. A segment of the third rib is similarly divided if necessary, and the appropriate interspace inferior to the portion of chest wall being excised is opened (Fig. 4-3D). A formal lung resection is performed. With some care this can be accomplished through the transclavicular opening rather than repositioning the patient for a standard lateral or posterolateral thoracotomy.

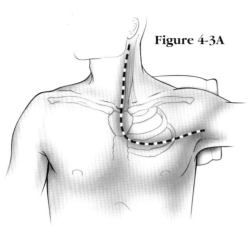

Figure 4-3A

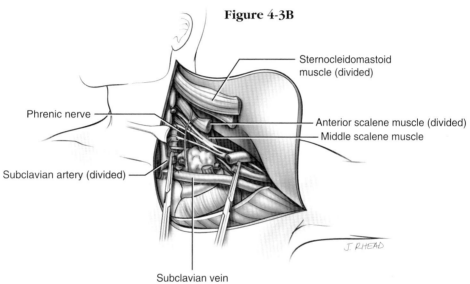

Figure 4-3B

Sternocleidomastoid
muscle (divided)

Phrenic nerve

Anterior scalene muscle (divided)

Middle scalene muscle

Subclavian artery (divided)

J. RHEAD

Subclavian vein

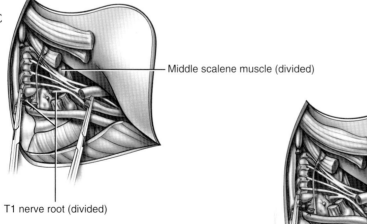

Figure 4-3C

Middle scalene muscle (divided)

T1 nerve root (divided)

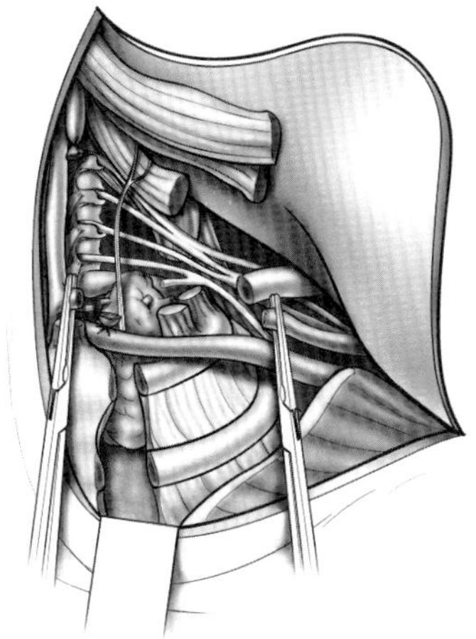

Figure 4-3D

4-4 Posterior Approach to Superior Sulcus Tumors

Superior sulcus tumors that involve the uppermost ribs near their junction with the spine are typically resected through a posterior approach. Although it is feasible to resect posteriorly situated tumors that extend to or involve the subclavian vessels and reconstruct those vessels through this incision, tumors with subclavian vessel involvement are more easily approached through an anterior incision (see Section 4-3). In contrast, tumors with posterior involvement, including those with involvement of the lower branch of the brachial plexus, are best managed through a posterior incision because of the ability to control nerve roots and, if necessary, perform partial vertebrectomy. As for anterior approaches to superior sulcus tumors, the possibility of mediastinal nodal involvement should be eliminated before embarking on an aggressive surgical approach such as this.

The patient is placed in the lateral decubitus position (see Fig. 4-4A inset) and a standard posterolateral thoracotomy is performed. The serratus anterior muscle may be preserved and retracted anteriorly, but the latissimus dorsi muscle must be divided. An interspace is opened that is two intercostal spaces below the caudad extent of tumor, and the chest cavity is explored to determine the resectability of the tumor. If there are no contraindications to resection, the incision is extended midway between the inner margin of the scapula and the spinous processes to the level of the C8 or C7 vertebral body. The trapezius, rhomboid major and minor, and occasionally the levator scapulae are divided. A large rib retractor is positioned with its inferior blade in the opened interspace, and the upper blade is placed under the scapula, elevating it off of the chest wall (Fig. 4-4A).

The scapula is dissected off of the chest wall and the thoracic inlet is exposed by division of the anterior and middle scalene muscles off of the first rib. The extent of tumor involvement is assessed. If no vascular involvement is identified and there are no other contraindications to resection, the chest wall resection is begun. The ribs involved by the tumor and one rib below the most caudal extent of tumor are divided 4 to 5 cm lateral to the extent of tumor involvement. It is sometimes useful to excise a 1-cm length of rib at each level of division to permit the cut rib ends to move freely. The dorsal scapular nerve and artery, which run deep to the rhomboids, are preserved. The interspace incision is developed medially to the rib head after the paraspinal muscles are elevated off of the ribs to be resected.

Two techniques are available for the medial portion of the chest wall resection. Under most circumstances the rib heads are disarticulated from the transverse processes. A periosteal elevator is insinuated between the rib head and spinous process, and gentle pressure using the transverse process as a fulcrum permits the rib head to be gradually disarticulated from the spine. This exposes the intercostal nerve and accompanying vessels emerging from the spine, which must be ligated with a vascular clip and divided (Fig. 4-4B). This obviates the possibility that a cerebrospinal fluid leak will develop postoperatively. If there appears to be more medial involvement by the tumor, the rib and transverse process may be transected en bloc with an osteotome. It is still imperative that the intercostal nerve be controlled and ligated during this maneuver (see Fig. 4-4B inset).

Disarticulation of the ribs continues cephalad until the first rib is reached. The T1 nerve root is divided if it is involved by tumor, and the cut end typically requires ligation rather than clipping owing to its larger diameter (Fig. 4-4C). Loss of the T1 nerve root sometimes causes temporary intrinsic hand muscle weakness with preserved hand function. The C8 nerve root may be divided if necessary, but this is avoided if at all possible because of the permanent, disabling, intrinsic hand muscle weakness that results. This is particularly bothersome if the patient's dominant hand is affected. Any existing attachments of the tumor to the subclavian artery are dissected, freeing the chest wall segment en bloc with the lung (Fig. 4-4D). A standard lung resection is performed and is usually accompanied by a complete mediastinal nodal dissection.

If segments of no more than three ribs are resected posteriorly, chest wall reconstruction is not required because the defect is adequately covered by the scapula. If more than the first three ribs are resected, it is usually necessary to reconstruct the bony chest wall using artificial material. Failure to do so may result in bothersome paradoxical motion of the chest wall. More importantly, the level of the defect permits the tip of the scapula to herniate into the pleural space, trapping it and restricting range of motion of the affected extremity. Reconstruction is accomplished using a 2-mm sheet of expanded polytetrafluoroethylene, which is sutured to the surrounding bony margins. Careful closure of the individual muscle layers is accomplished after appropriate chest drains are inserted.

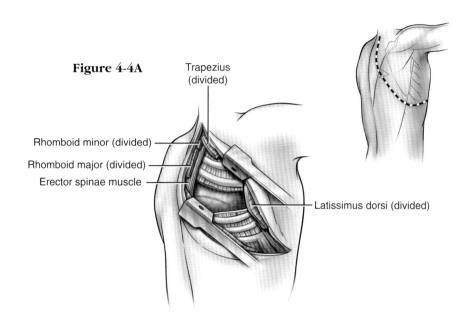

Figure 4-4A

Trapezius (divided)

Rhomboid minor (divided)

Rhomboid major (divided)

Erector spinae muscle

Latissimus dorsi (divided)

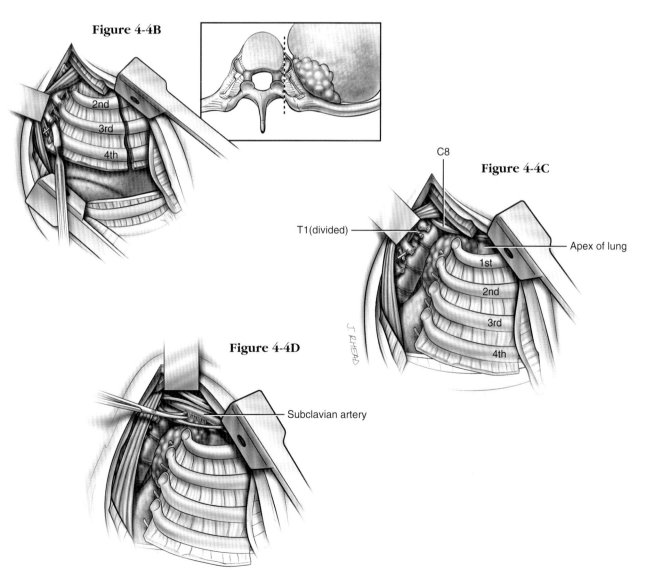

Figure 4-4B

2nd
3rd
4th

C8

Figure 4-4C

T1(divided)

Apex of lung

1st
2nd
3rd
4th

J. RHEAD

Figure 4-4D

Subclavian artery

4-5 Resection of Cancer Invading Vertebral Bodies

Tumors that invade the vertebral bodies and that sometimes are amenable to resection are almost exclusively non–small cell lung cancers. Until the late 1980s the presence of vertebral body involvement by a lung cancer was usually an absolute contraindication to resection. Since then, increasing experience with more aggressive surgical approaches to locally advanced lung cancers has helped to define a select population of patients who might benefit from such intervention. Patients who are currently thought to be candidates for resection of lung cancer invading the vertebral bodies must have: disease that is felt to be completely resectable; the ability to tolerate a major lung resection; no evidence for distant metastatic disease; no evidence for involvement of the brachial plexus higher than C7; involvement of no more than two or three vertebral bodies; no involvement of the anterior spinal artery; and documentation of absence of mediastinal nodal involvement by either mediastinoscopy or some other reliable means of pathologically staging the mediastinum. The benefits of induction therapy including chemotherapy, radiation therapy, or a combination of these modalities in patients with lung cancer invading the vertebral bodies are unproven. Similarly, the benefits of such modalities in a postoperative adjuvant setting are unproven. There is general agreement that management of patients with lung cancer and vertebral body involvement should include multimodality therapy, but the optimal timing and dosing of those modalities remains to be determined.

The procedure may be performed in several ways. Regardless of the approach, it is appropriate to operate in conjunction with an experienced orthopedic or neurosurgical spine surgeon. One initial description recommends partial vertebrectomy with tangential excision of the vertebral body using an osteotome in conjunction with en bloc standard lobectomy through a posterolateral thoracotomy. Unfortunately, the local recurrence rate after partial vertebrectomy in the presence of vertebral body involvement is relatively high using this technique. This finding leads to the general recommendation for hemicorporectomy, or even total vertebrectomy, if surgery is performed with curative intent. Some authors recommend beginning with an anterior approach similar to the anterior approach used for superior sulcus tumors to separate cervical structures from the tumor and assess resectability. The actual resection is then performed, first consisting of a standard lobectomy through a posterolateral thoracotomy, and then removing the lobe, tumor, and vertebral bodies en bloc through a posterior midline incision. Refinements of this approach include the use of a transmanubrial incision for access to the anterior spine and hilum, and a posterior midline incision for resection of the involved bone elements.

Another approach for resecting a lung cancer invading the vertebral bodies is through a single incision combining a posterolateral thoracotomy and a posterior midline incision (see Fig. 4-5A inset). The patient is placed in a true lateral position with the head immobilized in tongs and a bean bag is used to ensure that there is no rotational deformity of the spine that would interfere with placement of spinal instrumentation. For posterior tumors the intersection of the incisions is at the level of the T1 spinous process. Laminectomies of the involved vertebrae are performed and nerve roots that are affected are controlled. If the tumor extends from the vertebral bodies to or lateral to the costovertebral junction, the affected ribs are divided lateral to the tumor to achieve a 5-cm margin (Fig. 4-5A).

If the tumor is peripheral, the lung parenchyma is divided between the tumor and the hilum with a linear cutting stapler. This permits visualization of the mediastinal structures, including the azygos vein, esophagus, and aorta, which are dissected from the anterior surface of the vertebral bodies. For tumors that extend more proximally towards the hilum, this maneuver is not possible. In such situations blind dissection of the esophagus is sometimes facilitated by placement of a large bougie. If rib segments are to be removed with the tumor, the rib heads and transverse processes are divided en bloc with an osteotome. In the absence of rib involvement, the costovertebral and costotransverse ligaments are divided and the ribs are disarticulated from the transverse processes with an osteotome. The anterior longitudinal ligament and pleura are reflected off the vertebral bodies, and the bulk of the tumor is separated from the spine, providing a clear picture of the degree of vertebral body involvement (Fig. 4-5B). Although en bloc resection of the vertebral bodies is not possible with this technique, the risk of local recurrence is quite low. The advantages are that optimal exposure of the spine enables proper assessment of the extent of bone involvement and of the dural sac, and there is no need to rotate the specimen on the axis of the spinal cord to complete an en bloc resection.

If inspection reveals that only the foramen or pedicles are involved by tumor, the abnormal tissue is removed with a high-speed drill. This maintains the structural integrity of the vertebral column and avoids the necessity for instrumentation. When there is involvement of the cancellous bone, local recurrence is minimized by performing vertebrectomy or complete spondylectomy using high-speed drills, rongeurs, and curettes (Fig. 4-5C). Either approach requires anterior instrumentation with spacer grafting and posterior instrumentation for stabilization (Fig. 4-5D). A standard lobectomy is performed after resection of the tumor if the patient's pulmonary function permits.

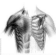

Figure 4-5A

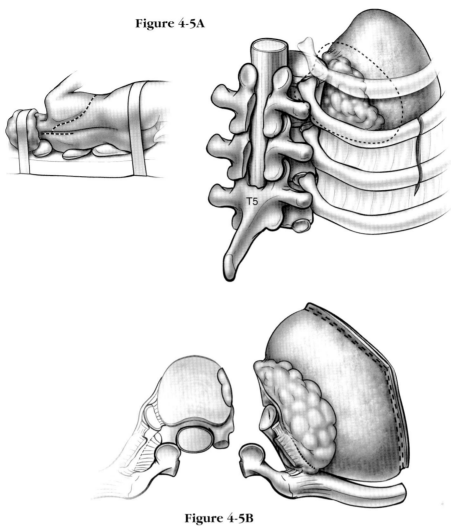

T5

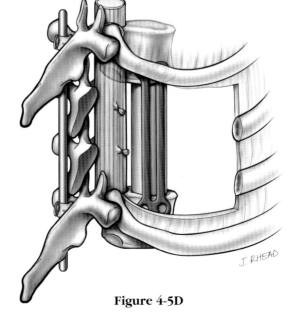

Figure 4-5B

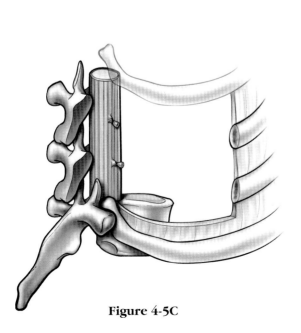

Figure 4-5C

Figure 4-5D

J. R. HEAD

4-6   Reconstruction of the Bony Chest Wall

There are numerous reasons to reconstruct bony defects of the chest wall. Defects of the upper anterior chest wall that may be exposed by certain types of clothing may be made more cosmetically acceptable when reconstructed. Underlying structures, especially the heart and great vessels, may benefit from rigid reconstruction for protection from blunt trauma, particularly in younger and more active individuals. In some patients the instability of formerly rigid chest wall structures may lead to pain that can be minimized with reconstruction. Large chest wall defects can result in paradoxical motion of soft tissues of the chest wall, resulting in respiratory embarrassment. Defects of the upper chest wall located posteriorly may permit the tip of the scapula to slip inside the rib cage, sometimes leading to entrapment and often causing pain.

The need for reconstruction of bony chest wall defects and the methods chosen for reconstruction thus depend on the size and location of the defect, the age and functional status of the patient, whether there is underlying respiratory compromise, the patient's physical lifestyle, and the desire of the patient for an optimal cosmetic result. Many bony defects of the chest wall do not require reconstruction, including small defects (segment of a single rib) and defects that underlie the scapula. Generally speaking, defects of three or fewer contiguous rib segments that lie posteriorly and are covered by the scapula do not require reconstruction unless there is risk of scapular entrapment. In contrast, defects that are anterior typically require reconstruction when three or more contiguous rib segments are involved.

The need for bony reconstruction of the sternum depends on a number of factors, including the need for protection of the underlying organs in patients who are physically active, and the degree of stability of mediastinal structures. Patients with large sternal defects who wish to participate in active sports should undergo rigid reconstruction for protection against direct trauma to mediastinal structures. It may be argued that every patient with a sizeable defect should be reconstructed if only to reduce the risks entailed as the driver of a motor vehicle involved in a head-on collision. In contrast, patients who suffer poststernotomy mediastinitis requiring near-total or complete sternectomy often have very good stability of their underlying mediastinal structures because of the degree of inflammation and subsequent fibrosis that result from this process. In such patients adequate functional and cosmetic results may be obtained from pectoralis flap rotation to fill the bony defect.

Most chest wall bony defects are satisfactorily repaired with flexible nonabsorbable synthetic materials such as a 2-mm patch of expanded polytetrafluoroethylene (PTFE) or a mesh of polypropylene. The former material has the advantage of permitting less fluid to pass from the pleural space to the soft tissues of the chest wall and can immediately seal the pleural space from air entry if carefully sutured around its periphery. A synthetic mesh has the advantage of permitting adequate drainage when used in the setting of previous contamination or even active infection. Both materials can be sutured under substantial tension, a requirement for adequate bony chest wall reconstruction.

After chest wall resection is complete and adequate hemostasis is obtained, the rib margins on all sides are identified. Any necessary pleural drains are placed before the chest wall reconstruction is begun. It is usually best to drill holes in the ribs for suture placement in a mattress fashion rather than merely suturing the synthetic patch to the surrounding soft tissues. Suturing the patch to the ribs permits placement of more tension on the patch, thus providing better chest wall stability, and helps to ensure that the sutures will not tear out during movement of the muscular tissues of the chest wall. The suture ends are brought to the outside so that the patch is fastened to the outer surface of the ribs (Fig. 4-6A). If the chest wall defect includes the first rib or the costal margin, leaving no rib to suture to along one margin of the defect, suitable fascia is used for suture placement instead.

The patch is deliberately oversized and is trimmed only after suturing is complete. The most difficult edge to access is sutured first, beginning in the center and working to the corners. Before suturing the adjoining sides, the opposite edge is sutured at one or two locations under tension to stabilize the ribs and to help assess appropriate suture placement for the rest of the patch. Tension is maintained as the sides adjoining the initial suture line are sewn, and the final side is completed (Fig. 4-6B). The patch is then trimmed, leaving a 5-to-10-mm margin beyond the tied sutures. The free edge of the patch may be sewn with a running suture to the underlying soft tissues to help create a seal between the pleura space and the soft tissues of the chest wall.

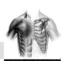

Figure 4-6A

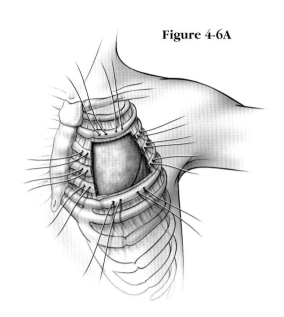

Figure 4-6B

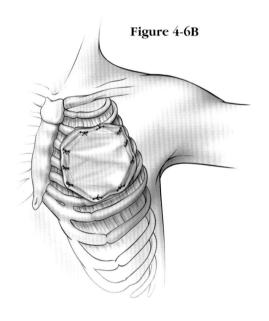

If a large span of chest wall requires reconstruction, use of a pliable patch may be disadvantageous. Rather than conforming to the convex shape of the chest wall, the relatively flat surface of the patch may displace some intrapleural volume, creating a cosmetic defect and a potential physiologic disadvantage. Instead, autologous rib segments can be used to span the gap. A long length of a single rib is harvested from the contralateral chest wall. The rib is split longitudinally, and each end of each rib segment is wired or sutured to the free ends of cut ribs on either side of the defect (Fig. 4-6C). Further stabilization is then gained by use of a synthetic patch overlying the rib struts.

Rigid stabilization of chest wall defects may also be accomplished with use of a combination of polypropylene mesh forming two outer layers with a layer of methylmethacrylate cement in the center. The mesh provides a sewing rim for suturing the structure to the chest wall, while the cement provides the desired rigidity. Sutures are placed through the soft tissues and boney structures as illustrated in Figure 4-6A. The size and shape of the defect are transferred to a paper template; a surgical glove wrapper works well for this purpose. Two pieces of mesh are cut to size, extending 1 cm or more beyond the defect to be filled. The methylmethacrylate is mixed and is applied to one surface of the mesh, matching the size of the defect rather than the size of the mesh. The other piece of mesh is applied over the cement. The construct is placed over the defect in the chest wall and is formed to the appropriate contours of the chest wall as the cement cures. Once the patch has hardened, the mesh edge extending beyond the cement is sutured to the bone and soft tissues as described above (Fig. 4-6D).

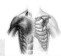

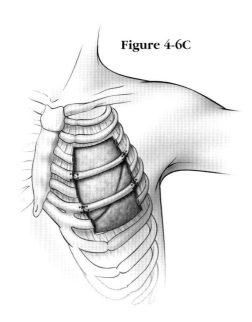

Figure 4-6C

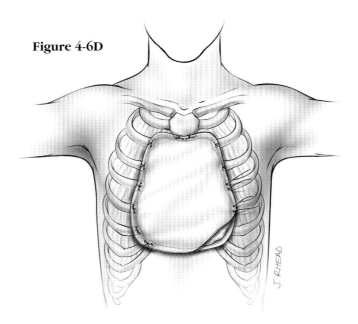

Figure 4-6D

4-7 Correction of Pectus Deformities

Pectus deformities are most commonly corrected in early childhood but may be corrected into the late teens or early adulthood. Surgery for pectus abnormalities generally has good cosmetic results regardless of the timing of the procedure. Correction of pectus deformities for treatment of physiologic limitations has variable success, but is more likely to be beneficial if performed in early childhood, particularly for pectus carinatum deformities. Two techniques are available for repair of pectus excavatum deformities. In the open method, originally described in the 1950s and 1960s, abnormal costal cartilages are excised and a sternal osteotomy is performed to permit correct repositioning of the sternum. This technique may also be used for correction of pectus carinatum deformities (not illustrated). The other common technique, described in the 1980s, involves a minimally invasive technique for insertion of a metal bar beneath the sternum and abnormal costal cartilages to permit their elevation. This technique is not applicable to pectus carinatum deformities.

The open technique is performed though a bilateral submammary incision that extends superiorly in the midline (see Fig. 4-7A inset). Careful placement of this incision is important in young female patients to avoid injury to breast tissue and provide an optimal cosmetic result later in life. Skin flaps are developed to the level of the manubrial-sternal junction superiorly, inferiorly to the xiphoid, and laterally almost to the midclavicular line. The pectoralis muscles are elevated from the chest wall beginning in the midline and extending laterally to the costochondral junctions. The intercostal neurovascular bundles are preserved to avoid excessive bleeding and to provide adequate blood supply to the perichondrium for future cartilaginous regrowth. The perichondrium over the affected depressed costal cartilages is scored from the sternum to the costochondral junctions of ribs 3 through 5. It is almost always necessary to perform this maneuver bilaterally. Rarely the second costal cartilages are involved and also must be treated.

The costal cartilages are elevated with a periostial elevator and are excised taking care to preserve the posterior perichondrium (Fig. 4-7A). Wider resections of cartilages six and seven are performed to a point where the depressions level off. There are often cartilaginous bridges between the fifth and sixth rib and lower that also require resection.

The sternum remains depressed because of the abnormal angle of the sternum inferior to the manubrial-sternal junction (see Fig. 4-7B inset). Correction of this depression is accomplished by performing an osteotomy of the anterior table using an oscillating saw (Fig. 4-7B). Sufficient material is excised to permit the affected portion of the sternum to be brought forward. The rectus muscles are dissected from the inferior sternum to permit blunt dissection of the substernal plane. The xiphoid process is often abnormally angled anteriorly, and this is excised with electrocautery. The sternum is elevated to a normal level as the posterior table is fractured. In some instances a strut is placed posterior to the sternum to hold it in place. This is most often necessary when there is significant sternal depression or angulation and when there are connective tissue abnormalities. Occasionally the most inferior one or two intercostal bundles are divided to permit the sternum to float freely and without tension. However, this may leave a depression lateral to the inferior sternum, which can adversely affect the ultimate cosmetic result. The osteotomy is fixed with heavy sutures as the sternum is held in an overcorrected position (Fig. 4-7C).

The area of dissection is flooded with saline as the lungs are ventilated to check for any possible entry into the pleural cavity. Any pleural entry can be managed with insertion of a pleural drainage catheter, which is removed after closure of the incision. One or two flat suction drains are placed over the beds of the resected costal cartilages. The pectoralis muscles are reapproximated in the midline and may be sutured to the underlying sternum as well (Fig. 4-7D). The rectus muscles are sutured to the pectoralis muscles and may also be tacked to the inferior sternum.

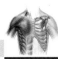

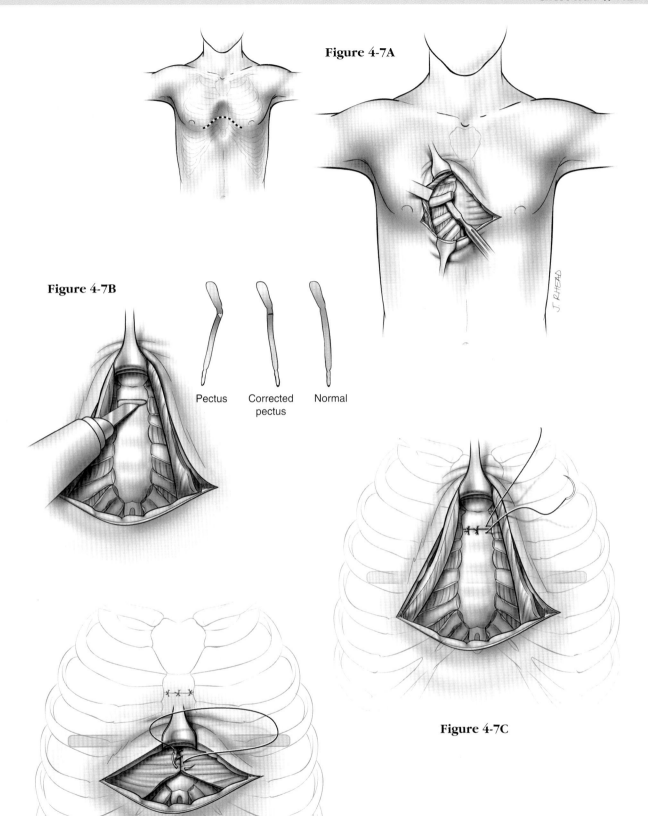

Figure 4-7A

Figure 4-7B

Pectus

Corrected
pectus

Normal

Figure 4-7C

Figure 4-7D

The minimally invasive approach to correction of pectus excavatum deformities is applicable to most patients, including young adults. With the patient in a supine position, the point of maximum depression of the sternum is identified and the depth of the depression is measured (Fig. 4-7E). This is usually located near the junction of the sternum and the xiphoid process. The distance between the midclavicular lines is also measured to enable selection of the appropriate sized bar to use for correcting the deformity. These data are used to shape a malleable template to conform to a slightly over-corrected shape of the corrected deformity, and the template is then used to shape a stainless steel bar of appropriate size.

Small incisions are made bilaterally in the midaxillary lines at the level of maximum sternal deformity, taking care to ensure that a line between the incisions is at the level of bony sternum rather than the xiphoid process. The incisions are taken down to the level of the chest wall, and pockets are developed bluntly posterior to them. These pockets will accommodate the tips of the bar after its insertion, which will lie deep to the chest wall muscles and superficial to the ribs and the intercostal muscles.

The bilateral incisions are opened through the intercostal space at the level of maximum sternal deformity but are limited to the extrapleural space if possible. Tunnels are created medially that join in the substernal space, taking care not to injure the internal mammary vessels. Although the original description of this procedure entailed blind creation of these tunnels, it is proba-bly safer to observe their creation through use of a thoracoscope that is inserted through a separate, inferior intercostal incision (Fig. 4-7F). This technique requires use of a double lumen endotracheal tube or a bronchial blocker to permit lung isolation. Alternatively, endo-scopic vein harvesting technology may be used to create the tunnels bilaterally (see Fig. 4-7F inset). After the tunnel is completed a large curved clamp is passed through it, grasping an umbilical tape, which is drawn through the tract. Successively larger thoracostomy tubes are passed through the tunnel, using the tape as a guide, to gradually dilate the tract.

A large thoracostomy tube or flat silastic mediastinal drain tube is brought through the tunnel and the tip of the prepared stainless steel bar is inserted partially into the tube. The tube and bar are slowly passed through the tunnel until the bar is positioned from through one incision and out the other, with the ends facing anteri-orly and the convexity of the bar facing posteriorly (see Fig. 4-7G inset). The ends of the bar are flared inward bilaterally with a heavy tool. The bar is then rotated so that the convexity faces posteriorly (Fig. 4-7G) and the ends of the bars are tucked into the pockets created previously. This forces the sternum anteriorly and straightens the abnormal shape of the associated costal cartilages. The bar is fixed to the adjacent ribs to prevent derotation and the incisions are closed (Fig. 4-7H, Fig. 4-7H inset). The bar is left in place for one to two years, depending on the age of the patient and the degree of deformity that was originally present. It can be subse-quently removed under sedation.

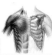

Figure 4-7E

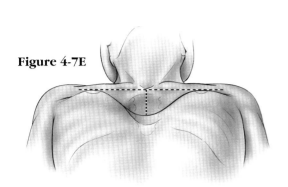

Figure 4-7F

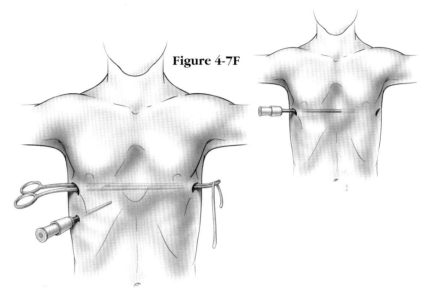

Figure 4-7G

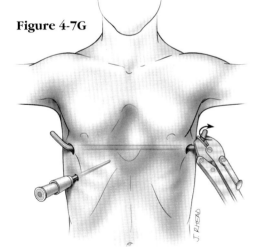

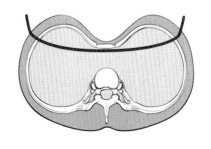

Figure 4-7H

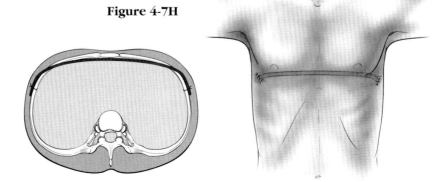

4-8 Surgery for Thoracic Outlet Syndrome

Surgery is indicated for patients with thoracic outlet syndrome who suffer from nerve compression or vascular complications. Nerve compression syndromes that are mild to moderate usually respond to conservative therapy and do not require surgical intervention. More severe sensory or motor deficits often require surgical decompression. Vascular compromise is less likely to respond to conservative management and surgical therapy should be considered early in the course of the process. Such compromise may include arterial narrowing or occlusion, possibly with peripheral emboli, or thrombosis of the subclavian vein (Paget-Schroetter syndrome).

The common operations for correction of thoracic outlet syndrome include the transaxillary and the supraclavicular approaches. Results of both procedures for first-time operations are similar in the hands of experts. Advocates of the transaxillary approach cite the improved ability to resect the first rib and the lack of need for retraction of the nerve roots during the dissection. Proponents of the supraclavicular approach suggest that exposure for neurolysis is improved and that there is better access for resection of a cervical rib should such exist.

The transaxillary approach is performed with the patient in a semilateral or lateral position with the ipsilateral arm elevated over the head. An incision is performed just inferior to the level of the axillary hair line, transversely between the pectoralis muscle anteriorly and the latissimus dorsi muscle posteriorly (see Fig. 4-8A inset). The dissection is carried directly down to the chest wall initially and then is directed superiorly until the first rib is encountered. During dissection the intercostal brachial nerve is identified between the first and second ribs and is retracted to avoid injury. The first rib is dissected in a subperiosteal plane. As the anterior scalene muscle is encountered, it is divided at its insertion on the first rib; this helps to avoid injury to the phrenic nerve, which lies more superiorly on its anterior surface (Fig. 4-8A). This is most easily accomplished by first passing a right angle behind the muscle, taking care not to injure the subclavian artery, which lies just deep to the muscle.

A wedge of first rib is excised permitting the free anterior end to be retracted slightly anteriorly. Dissection is carried along this segment of the rib, dividing the costoclavicular ligament, to the level of the costochondral junction, and this segment of the rib is excised (Fig. 4-8B). The middle scalene muscle is divided taking care not to injure the C8 and T1 nerve roots. The posterior segment of rib is dissected subperiosteally to the level of the transverse process and is divided (Fig. 4-8C). A large articulated rongeur is used to resect the head and neck of the rib, which helps to prevent its regeneration (Fig. 4-8D). The scalene muscles are resected superiorly. Neurolysis of the C7, C8, and T1 nerve roots is performed. Adhesions to the subclavian vessels are divided. This portion of the procedure may be facilitated with use of a thoracoscope, which provides better illumination and improves visualization.

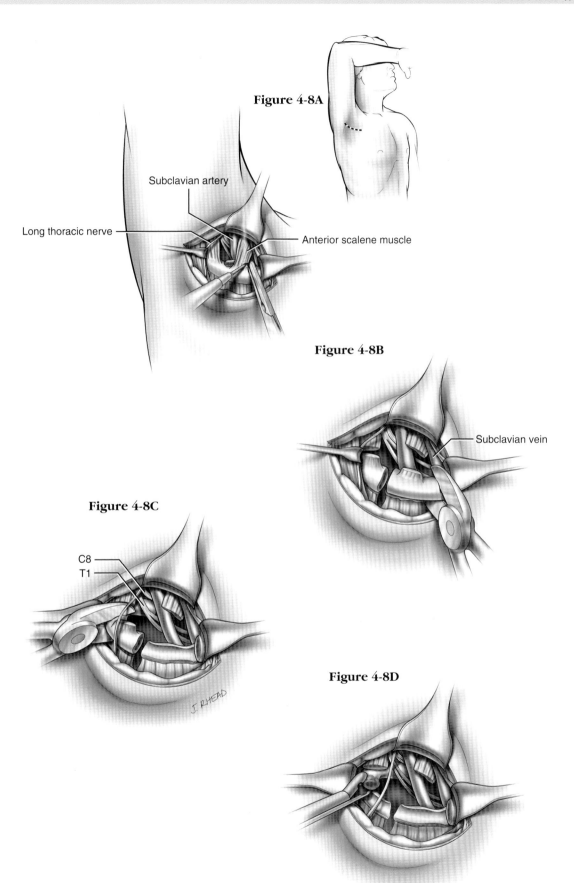

Figure 4-8A

Subclavian artery

Long thoracic nerve

Anterior scalene muscle

Figure 4-8B

Subclavian vein

Figure 4-8C

C8

T1

J. RHEAD

Figure 4-8D

The supraclavicular approach is performed with the patient supine through an incision performed parallel to the clavicle (see Fig. 4-8E inset). The sternocleidomastoid muscle is retracted medially, which sometimes entails partial division of the lateral head. The scalene fat pad is dissected. The anterior and middle scalene muscles are identified, with the brachial plexus evident between their bellies. Care is taken to avoid injury to the phrenic nerve that passes from lateral to medial across the anterior scalene muscle and to the long thoracic nerve that is identified emerging just lateral to the middle scalene muscle (Fig. 4-8E). The anterior scalene muscle is divided at its insertion to the first rib and the bulk of the inferior portion of the muscle is resected. Care is taken to avoid injury to the subclavian artery, which lies immediately deep to the muscle. The nerve roots are gently retracted anteriorly, exposing the first rib. The middle scalene muscle is divided at its insertion on the first rib and the body of the muscle is resected (Fig. 4-8F). The first rib is dissected subperiosteally and a short segment of the rib is excised (Fig. 4-8G).

The anterior segment of rib is dissected subperiosteally and is disarticulated at its costochondral junction. An extrapleural plane is maintained throughout the dissection. The posterior portion of the rib is excised in its entirety using rongeurs, including the neck and head, to prevent new bone formation (Fig. 4-8H). Neurolysis of the C7, C8, and T1 nerve roots is performed. The subclavian vessels are mobilized free of any adhesions. The incision is closed in a standard fashion; drainage is not usually required.

Figure 4-8E

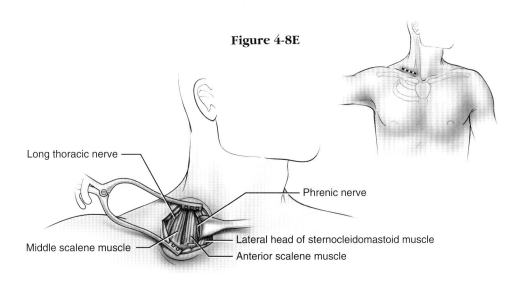

Long thoracic nerve

Phrenic nerve

Middle scalene muscle

Lateral head of sternocleidomastoid muscle

Anterior scalene muscle

Figure 4-8F

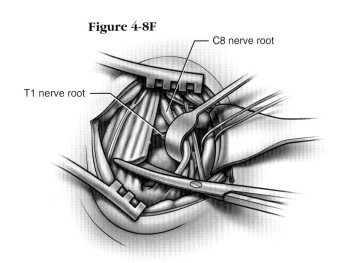

C8 nerve root

T1 nerve root

Figure 4-8G

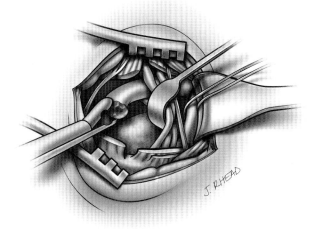

Figure 4-8H

J. RHEAD

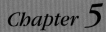

Chapter 5

Mediastinum

5-1 Anatomy

The mediastinum is among the most complex anatomical regions of the human body. A thorough understanding of its components and their three-dimensional relationships is a necessary precursor to safe and effective surgery of the mediastinum. It is useful to consider the mediastinum as a collection of compartments, each containing a collection of related structures. A variety of definitions of these compartments has been offered over the past several decades. From a purely surgical perspective it is appropriate to consider three compartments: anterior, visceral (middle), and paravertebral (posterior) (see Fig. 5-1A inset). The anterior compartment extends from the diaphragm to the thoracic inlet and is bounded by the posterior plate of the sternum anteriorly, the pericardium and anterior surfaces of the great vessels posteriorly, and by the pleura laterally. It contains pericardial fat, thymus gland, possibly parathyroid glands, lymphatic tissues, and sometimes portions of the thyroid gland. The middle, or visceral, compartment is bounded by the pleura laterally, the diaphragm and thoracic inlet proximally and distally, and by the anterior surface of the vertebral bodies posteriorly. This compartment contains most of the important structures in the mediastinum, including the heart and great vessels, lymphatics, the esophagus, the airways, and many of the important neural structures of the mediastinum. The paravertebral compartment extends from the anterior surface of the vertebral bodies to the paravertebral sulci, and primarily contains neural structures including the sympathetic chain.

From the perspective of a right thoracotomy a number of important anatomic structures are evident (Fig. 5-1A). From posterior to anterior, they begin with the sympathetic chain, which lies subpleurally over the heads of the ribs. A ganglion is evident at each rib level, the highest being the confluence of the C8 and T1 ganglia, which is termed the stellate ganglion. The intercostal vascular structures normally are deep to the sympathetic chain, but, particularly on the right side, there is often a superior intercostal vein that is superficial in the region of the T2 ganglion. The size and shape of the ganglia inferior to this level are quite variable. Each ganglion gives off gray and white rami communicans that connect it with the corresponding spinal nerve. The upper five or six ganglia give off small medial branches that supply the aorta and its branches, the pulmonary plexus, and the cardiac plexus. The latter two plexi give off branches to the esophagus and trachea. The medial branches from the lower seven ganglia are large, coalescing to form the greater (fifth to ninth or tenth ganglia) and lesser (ninth and tenth ganglia) splanchnic nerves. The splanchnic nerves course diagonally down the vertebra bodies and penetrate the ipsilateral diaphragm or pass posterior to the arcuate ligament to enter the retroperitoneal space. The sympathetic chain on the left side is quite similar to that described on the right side.

The azygos vein has a variable origin below the diaphragm, often arising from the lumbar azygos, which is joined by right ascending lumbar and inferior diaphragmatic veins as it passes through the diaphragm. Within the chest the azygos vein lies medial and anterior to the sympathetic chain on the right lateral surface of the vertebral bodies. Throughout its intrathoracic course the azygos accepts intercostal veins at each vertebral level. The arch of the azygos vein is usually located at the level of the fourth vertebra, having received the highest intercostal vein on the right. It courses over the right mainstem bronchus before terminating in the superior vena cava just above its junction with the right atrium. On the left side the origins of the hemiazygos vein are similar to those

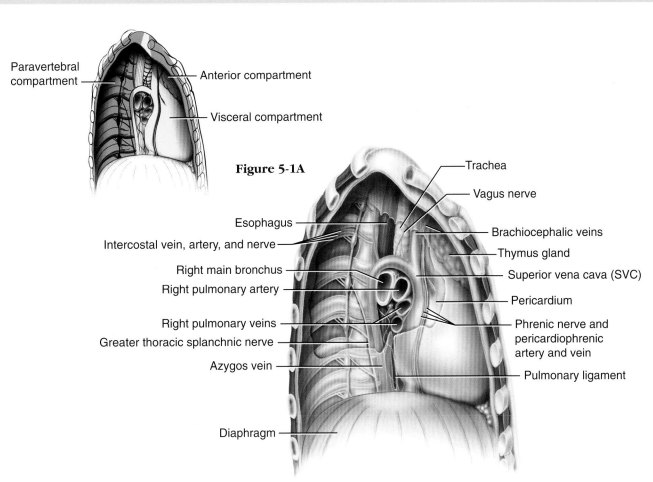

Paravertebral compartment

Anterior compartment

Visceral compartment

Figure 5-1A

Trachea

Vagus nerve

Esophagus

Intercostal vein, artery, and nerve

Brachiocephalic veins

Thymus gland

Right main bronchus

Right pulmonary artery

Superior vena cava (SVC)

Pericardium

Right pulmonary veins

Greater thoracic splanchnic nerve

Phrenic nerve and pericardiophrenic artery and vein

Azygos vein

Pulmonary ligament

Diaphragm

of the azygos vein (Fig. 5-1B), and the hemiazygos similarly accepts draining intercostal veins at each vertebral level. The hemiazygos sends communicating branches to the azygos vein posterior to the aorta at the levels of the eighth and sometimes the sixth thoracic vertebrae. Usually a small branch of the hemiazygos vein (accessory hemiazygos vein) continues superiorly for a variable distance, usually anastomosing with the left superior intercostal vein and ultimately with the left subclavian vein.

The anatomy of the thoracic duct is quite variable. It arises from the confluence of lumber lymph trunks or the cysterna chyli at the level of the second lumbar vertebra and extends to the lower neck. Embryologically it originates as paired vessels, and in 15% of patients a left lymphatic vessel can be found. The thoracic duct ascends through the aortic hiatus and in the thorax is initially located between the descending aorta and the azygos vein. At the level of the fifth or sixth thoracic vertebra the duct crosses posterior to the aorta and ascends to the base of the neck posterior to the left subclavian artery along the left lateral wall of the esophagus. It is illustrated in more detail in Chapter 7.

The most posterior aspect of the visceral compartment is occupied by the esophagus, which lies medial and slightly anterior to the azygos vein directly anterior and sometimes slightly to the left of the vertebral bodies. It extends from the thoracic inlet to the esophageal hiatus. Its anterior surface is associated with the membranous portion of the trachea superiorly and the left atrium inferiorly. See Chapter 6 for a more detailed description of the anatomy of the esophagus.

Also in the visceral compartment are the airways. A thorough description of the anatomy of the airway and lungs is provided in Chapter 3. Briefly, the trachea descends anterior to the vertebral bodies and esophagus and divides into the right and left mainstem bronchi at the level of the fifth or sixth thoracic vertebra, depending on the degree of inspiration. The right mainstem bronchus is related superiorly to the arch of the azygos vein and anteriorly to the right pulmonary artery. The left mainstem bronchus is related superiorly to the aortic arch medially and laterally to the left pulmonary artery. Anteriorly the left mainstem bronchus is related to the main pulmonary artery.

The vagus nerves (tenth cranial nerves) supply important innervation to the visceral compartment structures. They pass through the jugular foramen of the skull and descend in the carotid sheath between the jugular vein and the internal carotid artery. The right vagus nerve crosses anterior to the subclavian artery and enters the thorax, whereas the left vagus nerve enters the thorax between the left common carotid artery and the internal jugular vein, passing behind the left subclavian vein. In its course in the neck the vagus nerve gives off meningeal, auricular, pharyngeal, and carotid body branches as well as the superior laryngeal nerve. The

recurrent laryngeal nerves are of some importance. The right recurrent laryngeal nerve arises from the vagus nerve anterior to the subclavian artery and then ascends behind the subclavian artery to lie adjacent to the trachea and posterior to the common carotid artery. The left recurrent laryngeal nerve arises on the left of the aorta and immediately curves beneath it, ascending to the neck along the trachea. Once in the neck the recurrent laryngeal nerves lie in or near to the tracheoesophageal groove before being associated with the thyroid gland more superiorly, and then disappear beneath the inferior pharyngeal constrictor.

The phrenic nerve arises primarily from the fourth cervical ramus but has contributions from the third and fifth rami as well. It originates on the lateral border of the anterior scalene muscle and descends along its anterior surface. In this position it is posterior to the sternocleidomastoid and omohyoid muscles as well as the internal jugular vein and thoracic duct (on the left). The nerve enters the thorax anterior to the internal thoracic artery.

On the right side, the phrenic nerve courses lateral to the right subclavian vein and continues on the lateral surface of the superior vena cava (SVC). It lies anterior to the pulmonary hilum, continues along the inferior vena cava, and divides just above the level of the diaphragm. On the left side, the phrenic nerve has a somewhat less straight course. It crosses anterior to the left subclavian artery, lies anterior to the left internal thoracic artery, and descends in the groove between the left common carotid artery and the subclavian artery. It transverses anterior to the left vagus nerve just above the aortic arch and lies posterior to the left brachiocephalic vein, then descends anterior to the pulmonary hilum on the surface of the pericardium. The diaphragmatic portion of the phrenic nerves is described in Chapter 9.

The pericardium encases the heart and is lined by a serosal membrane that apposes the epicardium. It is continuous with the adventitia of the great vessels (aorta, pulmonary artery, pulmonary veins, superior vena cava) and superiorly with the pretracheal fascia. Inferiorly it attaches to the central tendon of the diaphragm and to a portion of the muscular diaphragm on the left. Inferiorly the pericardium is attached to the sternum by sternopericardial ligaments; similar superior ligaments are also sometimes present. Anterior relations are the chest wall (on the lower left), lungs, thymus, and pericardial fat. Posterior relations are the mainstem bronchi, esophagus, thoracic aorta, and spine. Lateral relations are the lung and phrenic nerve.

The great vessels include the aorta, pulmonary artery, pulmonary veins, and venae cavae. The ascending aorta arises at the base of the left ventricle at the level of the third costal cartilage. The relations of the ascending aorta are the thymus anteriorly, the pulmonary artery

Figure 5-1B

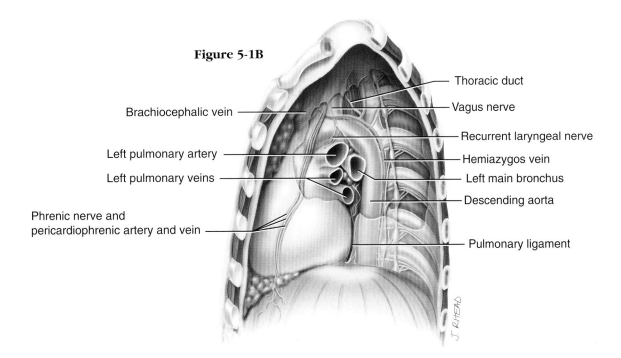

Brachiocephalic vein

Left pulmonary artery

Left pulmonary veins

Phrenic nerve and
pericardiophrenic artery and vein

Thoracic duct

Vagus nerve

Recurrent laryngeal nerve

Hemiazygos vein

Left main bronchus

Descending aorta

Pulmonary ligament

and superior vena cava laterally, and the left atrium, right pulmonary artery, and mainstem bronchi posteriorly. The ascending aorta gives rise to the aortic arch, which ascends to the level of the middle of the manubrium, and courses posteriorly and to the left over the left mainstem bronchus, and then gives rise to the descending thoracic aorta. The aortic arch gives off three major branches in order: the brachiocephalic trunk (innominate artery), the left common carotid artery, and the left subclavian artery. The relations of the aortic arch, which lies entirely in the superior mediastinum, are the trachea and esophagus posteriorly, the pulmonary artery bifurcation and left mainstem bronchus inferiorly, the thymus and pleura anteriorly, the left phrenic nerve, left vagus nerve, and pleura left laterally, and the SVC and trachea right laterally. The aortic arch becomes the descending aorta at the level of the inferior border of the fourth thoracic vertebra, which translates to the second costal cartilage anteriorly. It courses parallel to and along the left side of the spinal column in the posterior mediastinum, gradually rotating more anterior until it traverses the aortic diaphragmatic hiatus almost anterior to the spine. It is related to the left hilum, left atrium, esophagus, azygos vein, thoracic duct, vertebral column, and pleura.

The pulmonary artery arises at the level of the base of the right ventricle and is the most anterior of the great vessels. It courses entirely within the pericardium, bifurcating after 5 cm into the right and left pulmonary arteries. The latter vessels are described in detail in Chapter 3.

The superior vena cava forms at the confluence of the innominate vein, the right subclavian vein, and the right internal jugular vein, or at the confluence of the brachiocephalic veins if the right subclavian vein and right internal jugular vein coalesce before joining the SVC. The SVC extends inferiorly for about 7 cm to its junction with the right atrium. The phrenic nerve courses anterolaterally along the SVC, and the right vagus nerve is found along its posteromedial edge. Other relations are the trachea posteromedially, the pleura anterolaterally, the right pulmonary hilum posteriorly, and the aortic arch and brachiocephalic artery medially.

The inferior vena cava passes through a hiatus in the central tendon of the diaphragm on the right of and anterolateral to the spinal column at the level of the eighth and ninth thoracic vertebrae. Its inferior portion is extrapericardial, and the more cephalad half is intrapericardial; it is superior to and drains into the inferoposterior right atrium. The right phrenic nerve courses along its lateral border. Other relations include the pericardium medially and the pleura laterally.

The thymus gland is located primarily in the anterosuperior mediastinum; portions typically extend as high as the lower poles of the thyroid gland, and sometimes as low as the diaphragm. The gland comprises paired upper and lower poles, and there is usually considerable asymmetry between the paired poles. The upper poles are related to the deep strap muscles anteriorly and to the carotid vessels and trachea posteriorly and medially. The thymic isthmus lies just superior to the innominate vein. The lower poles usually descend anterior to the innominate vein, but sometimes wrap posterior to the vein as well. The lower poles of the gland are related to the manubrium anteriorly and to mediastinal fat and pleura laterally. Microscopic rests of ectopic thymic tissue may be found anywhere in the anterior mediastinum and in the neck anterior to the trachea. The arterial blood supply to the thymus is from small direct branches of the thyrocervical trunk, especially the inferior thyroid arteries, and the internal thoracic arteries. The venous drainage is primarily through two or three short branches to the innominate vein, and small draining veins sometimes connect to the internal thoracic and inferior thyroid veins.

The internal mammary arteries arise from the proximal subclavian arteries above the sternal ends of the clavicles. They descend posterior to the first six costal cartilages, and then give off a musculophrenic branch before anastomosing with the superior epigastric arteries. The internal mammary veins are venae comitantes that course parallel to the internal thoracic arteries to the level of the third costal cartilage, at which point they coalesce and ascend medial to the artery, draining into the ipsilateral brachiocephalic vein.

The anatomy of the diaphragm is described in greater detail in Chapter 9 and is not summarized here.

The three-dimensional relationships within the mediastinum are sometimes difficult to visualize but are nevertheless extremely important to understand. At each vertical level of the mediastinum different structures are encountered at different depths within it. Approaching the mediastinum anteriorly, the most superficial structures include the pleura and lungs, the inferior portions of the anterior pericardium, and the thymus gland, and deeper lie the brachiocephalic vein and then the brachiocephalic artery (Fig. 5-1C). At a level slightly more inferior than the thymus gland, beyond the pleura and lungs lie the ascending portion of the aortic arch and SVC, and deep to these structures are the trachea, esophagus, and descending portion of the aortic arch (Fig. 5-1D). More inferior than this, one first encounters the ascending aorta and main pulmonary artery as the first structures deep to the lungs and pleura. Beyond these structures lie the pulmonary veins, airways, right and left pulmonary arteries, azygos vein, thoracic duct, and esophagus (Fig. 5-1E).

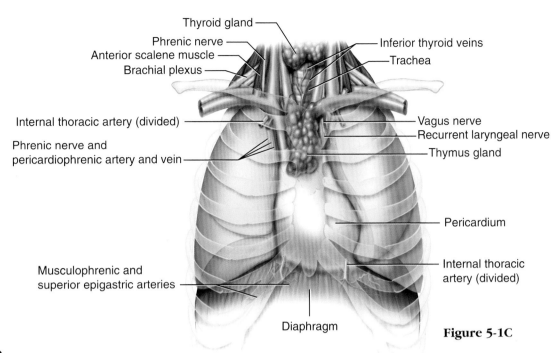

Thyroid gland

Phrenic nerve

Anterior scalene muscle

Brachial plexus

Inferior thyroid veins

Trachea

Internal thoracic artery (divided)

Phrenic nerve and
pericardiophrenic artery and vein

Vagus nerve

Recurrent laryngeal nerve

Thymus gland

Pericardium

Internal thoracic
artery (divided)

Musculophrenic and
superior epigastric arteries

Diaphragm

Figure 5-1C

Figure 5-1D

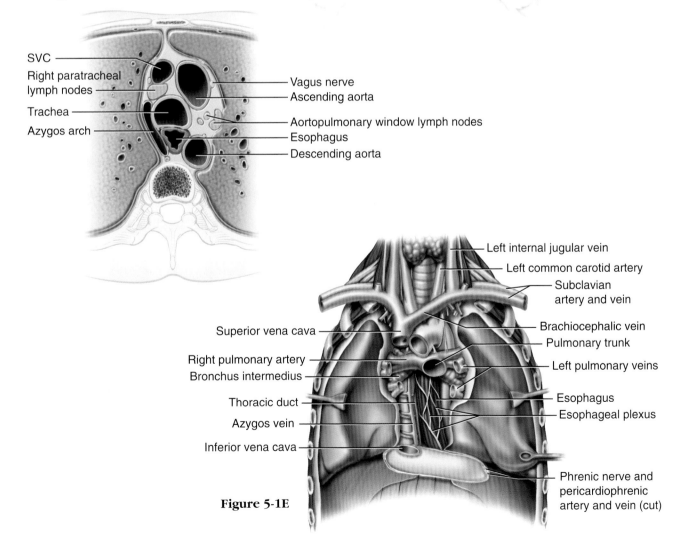

SVC

Right paratracheal
lymph nodes

Trachea

Azygos arch

Vagus nerve

Ascending aorta

Aortopulmonary window lymph nodes

Esophagus

Descending aorta

Left internal jugular vein

Left common carotid artery

Subclavian
artery and vein

Superior vena cava

Right pulmonary artery

Bronchus intermedius

Thoracic duct

Azygos vein

Inferior vena cava

Brachiocephalic vein

Pulmonary trunk

Left pulmonary veins

Esophagus

Esophageal plexus

Phrenic nerve and
pericardiophrenic
artery and vein (cut)

Figure 5-1E

5-2 Cervical Mediastinoscopy

Cervical mediastinoscopy and its sister procedure, parasternal mediastinotomy, have been used since the late 1950s for evaluating abnormalities of the mediastinum and for staging thoracic malignancies. Cervical mediastinoscopy is most commonly used for staging lung cancer. Primary indications for the procedure are evaluation of N2 and N3 lymph nodes. The primary contraindication to the use of cervical mediastinoscopy is the patient's inability to extend the neck. It was once thought that the presence of SVC syndrome was a strong contraindication to cervical mediastinoscopy, but this is in many instances an important reason to perform such a diagnostic and staging procedure. Patients who have previously undergone cervical mediastinoscopy are also candidates for repeat cervical mediastinoscopy, although the operation is technically more difficult and the yield is not as good as when a primary procedure is performed.

Patients are sometimes referred inappropriately for cervical mediastinoscopy. It is important to recognize that, under most circumstances, only the pretracheal, paratracheal, and subcarinal spaces are accessible to biopsy using this technique. As is evident in Figure 5-2A, abnormalities of the anterior mediastinum are not amenable to biopsy through cervical mediastinoscopy. Such masses may be appropriately biopsied using a parasternal mediastinotomy technique, which is illustrated in Figures 5-3A–D.

Cervical mediastinoscopy is typically performed as an outpatient procedure. The operation is performed with the patient under a general anesthetic with the patient positioned supine and with the neck extended. The head is stabilized on a circular foam pad. There is disagreement about the need to monitor blood pressure in the right radial artery. Some surgeons and anesthesiologists believe that excessive compression of the innominate artery may lead to compromise of cerebral circulation. However, this is an extremely unlikely event, and routine monitoring of this type is not necessary. Because of a remote possibility of injury to the major mediastinal blood vessels, the preparation area extends down to the umbilicus to permit emergency sternotomy should such be necessary.

An incision site is chosen above the level of the sternal notch and below the level of the cricoid cartilage (see Fig. 5-2B inset). The region is palpated and the inferior extent of the thyroid gland is assessed. Ideally, an area in which the tracheal rings can be palpated is selected. It is important to keep in mind that the initial access for mediastinoscopy is performed by dissecting directly perpendicular from the skin toward the trachea, rather than attempting to dissect inferiorly into the medi-

astinum. The inferior dissection is performed only after the pretracheal space has been reached. The skin incision measures about 3 cm in length, which is sufficient for the surgeon to insert an index finger for palpation and dissection. A larger incision provides no additional access for mediastinoscopy. Unless there is a middle thyroid vein present, it is unusual to have to divide vascular structures in the neck to access the pretracheal space. The strap muscles are separated in the midline, the inferior poles of the thyroid gland are retracted superiorly, and the pretracheal fascia is divided. The pretracheal space is bluntly dissected deep into the mediastinum, first with a cotton dissector and then with the surgeon's index finger (Fig. 5-2B). The innominate artery and aorta are routinely palpable during mediastinoscopy. It is sometimes possible to palpate paratracheal lymph nodes distal to the innominate artery. Palpation of the precarinal space is not usually possible because of the distance from the incision to this space.

The mediastinoscope is inserted and the tip of the scope is used to gently dissect the plane between the trachea and the mediastinal tissues (Fig. 5-2C). Regardless of whether the surgeon is using a standard mediastinoscope or a videomediastinoscope, it is essential that the surgeon be able to visualize the anterior leading tip of the scope to avoid injury to mediastinal structures. Dissection is facilitated with a cotton dissector or with the tip of a long suction device. The scope is typically inserted to the level of the carina (Fig. 5-2D), where the pulmonary artery is evident anterior to the precarinal lymph nodes. Target lymph node areas for biopsy are often indicated by abnormalities on the CT scan. During mediastinal staging for lung cancer, it is appropriate to routinely biopsy additional lymph node regions to provide complete staging information. Appropriate labeling of such biopsies is essential to ensure accurate mediastinal staging.

It is often easiest to begin in the precarinal area and then work more superiorly to perform additional biopsies. Dissection with the tip of a cotton dissector or the tip of a long suction device is used to break through the pretracheal fascia and enter the plane of the lymph nodes. Unless the outline of a lymph node is obvious, it is wise to aspirate the tissue with a long needle to ensure that there is no blood vessel in the region. Sufficient biopsies are taken to obtain diagnostic tissue. If there is any doubt, it is wise to obtain a frozen section before completing the mediastinoscopy. Hemostasis is achieved with a suction-cautery device or using pledgets soaked in dilute epinephrine. The superficial strap muscles are reapproximated with a running suture. The platysma and skin are closed separately with running sutures. It is usually not necessary to obtain a chest radiograph prior to the patient's discharge.

Figure 5-2A

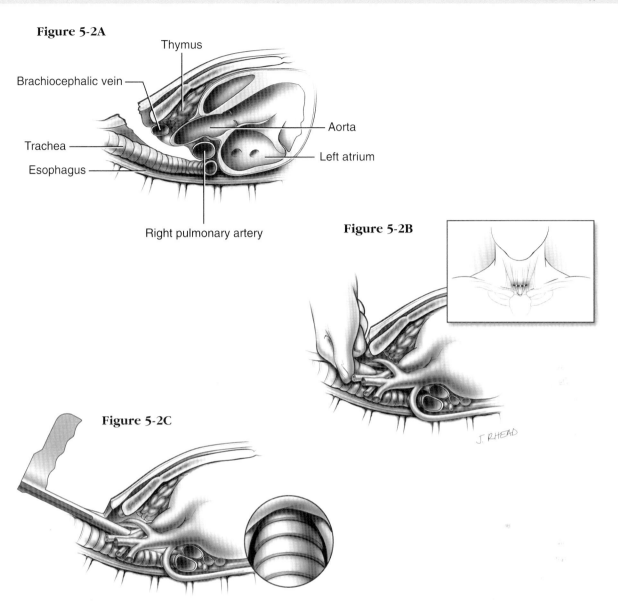

Thymus

Brachiocephalic vein

Trachea

Esophagus

Aorta

Left atrium

Right pulmonary artery

Figure 5-2B

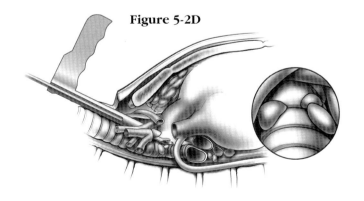

J. RHEAD

Figure 5-2C

Figure 5-2D

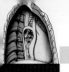

5-3 Parasternal Mediastinotomy

Parasternal mediastinotomy is most often used to biopsy hilar lymph nodes, anterior mediastinal tissues, or lymph nodes in the level 5 and 6 nodal regions. The procedure is performed under a general anesthetic using a single lumen endotracheal tube for the airway and is usually performed on an outpatient basis. There are no specific contraindications to performing parasternal mediastinotomy, although patients who have undergone high-dose mediastinal irradiation may have sufficient fibrosis to obliterate typical mediastinal tissue planes.

The patient is positioned supine and the arms are aligned alongside the torso. Either right or left parasternal mediastinotomy may be performed, although it is most commonly accomplished on the left side (see Fig. 5-3A inset). The side is selected based on the position of the tissue abnormality being biopsied. A 3-to-4-cm incision is created over the second intercostal space or over the second costal cartilage (Fig. 5-3A). Whether a costal cartilage is removed is determined by the amount of exposure provided by the intercostal space. Creating a vertical incision enables the surgeon to extend the incision to a different interspace if necessary. Dissection is carried down through the pectoralis muscle with electrocautery (see Fig. 5-3A). If costal cartilage resection is performed, the perichondrium is scored longitudinally and is bluntly dissected from the costal cartilage (Fig. 5-3B). The cartilage is disarticulated from the rib and then from the sternum. The posterior perichondrium is entered. The parietal pleura may be swept laterally to limit entry to the mediastinal space or is divided to permit entry into the mediastinal and pleural spaces. It is often possible to sweep the internal thoracic vessels medially, but occasionally it is necessary to ligate and divide these vessels to provide adequate exposure (Fig. 5-3C).

Once the incision is opened, with entry either into the mediastinal or pleural spaces, anterior mediastinal masses are usually immediately evident and can be biopsied. For nodal disease a standard or videomediastinoscope is inserted. On the left side, the mediastinoscope will enter easily to the level of the aortopulmonary window (Fig. 5-3D). On the right side, the mediastinoscope will enter to the plane adjacent to the superior vena cava. Blunt dissection with a cotton dissector or the tip of a cautery device is usually sufficient to identify the abnormal lymph nodes. As when cervical mediastinoscopy is performed, it is usually wise to aspirate tissues with a long needle prior to performing any biopsies.

Once the biopsies are completed, the pectoralis fascia is reapproximated with a running suture. Prior to tying the last suture, the incision is flooded with saline and the anesthesiologist is instructed to provide a deep inspiration to force air from the pleural space. This eliminates most of any intrapleural air that might be present and obviates the need for chest tube drainage postoperatively.

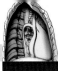

Figure 5-3A

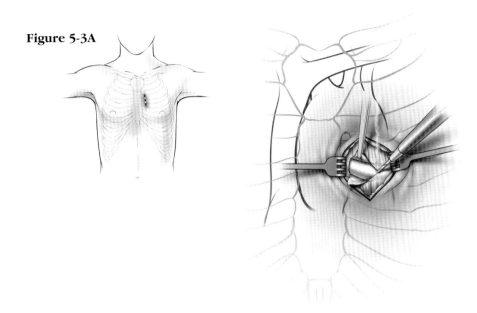

Figure 5-3B

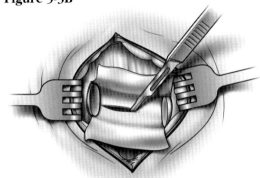

Figure 5-3C

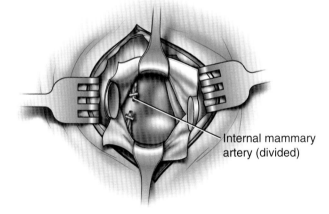

Internal mammary
artery (divided)

Figure 5-3D

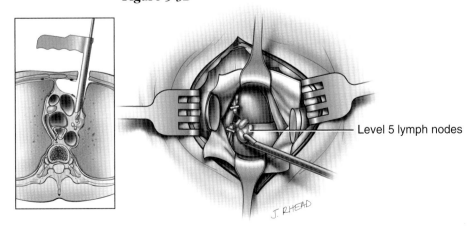

Level 5 lymph nodes

J. R. HEAD

5-4 Transcervical Thymectomy

Procedures involving the thymus gland are performed primarily for management of myasthenia gravis and for thymic tumors. Transcervical thymectomy is reserved for management of myasthenia gravis in the absence of thymoma. It is generally applicable to patients who are younger and who have not been on long-term steroid management for their myasthenia gravis; both older age and prolonged steroid use cause involution of the gland, making dissection using this technique difficult. Other contraindications to transcervical thymectomy for management of myasthenia gravis include the inability of patients to extend their necks, the presence of a thymoma, and mediastinal fibrosis secondary to prior radiation therapy.

Thymectomy for management of myasthenia gravis should not be performed unless the patient has been adequately prepared medically. This includes administration of sufficient medication (cholinesterase inhibitors, steroids, other immune system suppressants) to substantially control myasthenic symptoms. If necessary, modulation of the immune system with infusion of immune globulin or plasmapheresis should be considered prior to instituting surgical management. The beneficial effects of thymectomy are usually not fully evident for months or years, indicating that thymectomy rarely needs to be performed urgently.

The correct anesthetic conduct of an operation for myasthenia gravis is essential to its success. Patients are generally managed without use of muscle relaxants. If a muscle relaxant is vital to the contact of the operation, a short-acting nondepolarizing agent should be selected. Cholinesterase inhibitors should be withheld immediately prior to the operation because patients often become hypersensitive to their effects in the immediate postoperative period. A postoperative cholinesterase inhibitor overdose mimics the effects of myasthenic crisis and management then becomes very difficult.

The patient is positioned supine with the arms alongside the torso. In contrast to the incision used for cervical mediastinoscopy, a 4-cm curvilinear incision is positioned at the level of the clavicular heads so that access to the manubrium for placement of a retractor later in the operation is possible (see Fig. 5-4A inset). Dissection is carried down between the strap muscles. Beginning on one side, the strap muscles are elevated laterally and the superior pole of the thymus gland is dissected bluntly from the surrounding tissues. There are no major arteries or veins in this region that need to be ligated. The thymo-thyroid ligament is divided once the upper pole is completely dissected (Fig. 5-4A). The contralateral pole is similarly dissected. Both poles are elevated inferiorly and the dissection is carried down on the surface of the gland to the level of the thoracic inlet. The poles are retracted superiorly and dissection is carried down laterally and anteriorly into the mediastinum.

An angled retractor suspended from the operating table is placed under the manubrium and is used to elevate the manubrium from the soft tissues of the anterior mediastinum (Fig. 5-4B). The surgeon stands above the patient's head, facing the patient's feet, and the remainder of the operation is performed from this perspective. As one pole of the thymus gland is retracted from the wound, the dissection is carried immediately on the capsule of the thymus gland laterally and anteriorly. A similar procedure is performed while retracting the other pole of the thymus gland superiorly. The body of the thymus gland, including the lower polls, gradually is retracted from the incision. Once this is accomplished, the gland is reflected inferiorly so that the veins draining directly from the thymus gland into the innominate vein are identified (Fig. 5-4C). They are dissected individually, ligated, and divided. At this point the gland is almost free from the mediastinum. As it is retracted further from the mediastinum, the inferior margins of the lower polls are identified. They are taken with a generous margin of surrounding mediastinal fat to ensure an adequate thymectomy has been performed. Inspection of the wound demonstrates a clean innominate vein and intact parietal pleural surfaces (Fig. 5-4D). No wound drain is necessary. The strap muscles are reapproximated with a running suture. The platysma and skin are closed in separate layers. The patient is extubated once adequate respiratory function is demonstrated. Monitoring in the postoperative recovery area with assessment of forced vital capacity and of global neurologic function is appropriate.

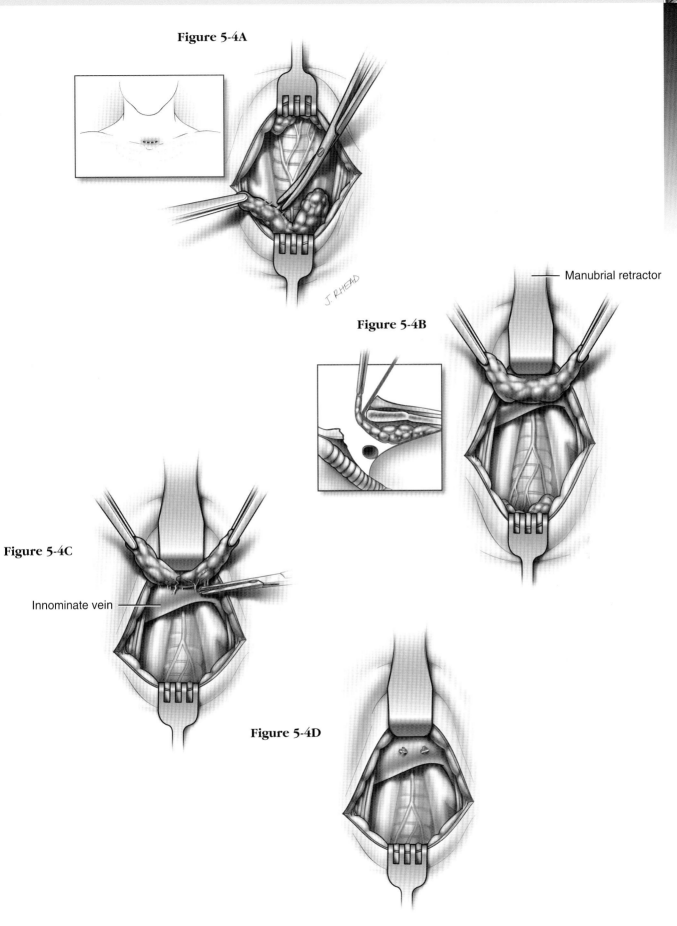

Figure 5-4A

J. R.HEAD

Figure 5-4B

Manubrial retractor

Figure 5-4C

Innominate vein

Figure 5-4D

5-5 Transsternal Thymectomy

Transsternal thymectomy is the most common technique for performing a thymectomy operation. Indications include the presence of a thymoma or myasthenia gravis. The transsternal approach is thought to provide a more complete thymectomy than the transcervical approach, and some surgeons believe that this results in better control of symptoms for myasthenia gravis. Although small encapsulated thymomas may be resected using a transcervical or minimally invasive approach, larger thymomas or those that extend outside of the capsule of the thymus gland are best removed through an open approach.

Patient preparation in the presence of myasthenia gravis is similar to that described previously in Section 5-4. The operation is performed under general anesthetic with the patient supine and the arms are tucked alongside the torso. It is sometimes useful to put a small pack along the spine to elevate the sternum and provide better exposure. The operation can be performed through a complete sternotomy or through a partial sternotomy, including the manubrium and the upper portion of the sternum proper, T-ing the incision at the level of the second or third intercostal space (Fig. 5-5A). In either case, it is important to extend the skin incision to the level of the sternal notch to provide access for excision of the upper poles of the thymus gland in the neck (see Fig. 5-5A inset). Prior to dividing the sternum, the substernal space is digitally palpated through the sternal notch to ensure that there is no encroachment of the thymoma, if present, on the bone.

After the sternum is divided, the plural reflections are swept laterally to expose the pericardial fat. The dissection is begun by grasping the pericardial fat and dissecting it from the pericardial surface (see Fig. 5-5A). If there is any suspicion that a thymoma invades the pleura or pericardium, an appropriate section of these tissues is taken with the specimen. As the pericardial fat extends laterally toward the hila of the lungs, the dissection also extends laterally. The phrenic nerves are preserved unless there is direct invasion by a thymoma. The fat, along with the right inferior pole of the thymus gland, is grasped and, under gentle traction, is dissected from the right phrenic nerve just anterior to the right hilum of the lung (Fig. 5-5B). The dissection extends along the phrenic nerve to the point where the internal thoracic veins reflect off of the chest wall and drain into the brachiocephalic vein. The dissection is carried medially toward the root of the aorta to the midline. A similar dissection is carried out on the left side, although additional tissues often are found posterolateral to the pulmonary trunk (Fig. 5-5C).

The pericardial fat and inferior poles of the thymus gland are reflected superiorly, exposing the draining vein branches from the thymus to the brachiocephalic artery. These are individually controlled and divided (Fig. 5-5D). The gland is dissected laterally across the anterior surface of the brachiocephalic vein such that all the soft tissue anterior to the vein is encompassed in the dissection. The dissection then proceeds cephalad, isolating the superior poles of the gland and dissecting them upward until the thymothyroid ligaments are reached and are divided.

An alternative to open thymectomy is a minimally invasive thymectomy. Several approaches for this technique have been described, including an exclusive left approach, an exclusive right approach, and a subxiphoid approach. As a prelude to performing a minimally invasive thymectomy, some authors recommend insufflation of air into the anterior mediastinum prior to the operation, using a needle or catheter inserted into the substernal notch, to begin dissection of the soft tissues from the retrosternal space. Regardless of which approach is chosen for a minimally invasive thymectomy, the general principles of the operation are similar. They include preservation of the phrenic nerves when possible, wide excision of soft tissues if they are invaded by a thymoma, and complete thymectomy, including dissection of the upper poles of the gland. To accomplish this latter aspect when a minimally invasive thymectomy is performed, some authors find that a cervical counter incision is still necessary.

Figure 5-5A

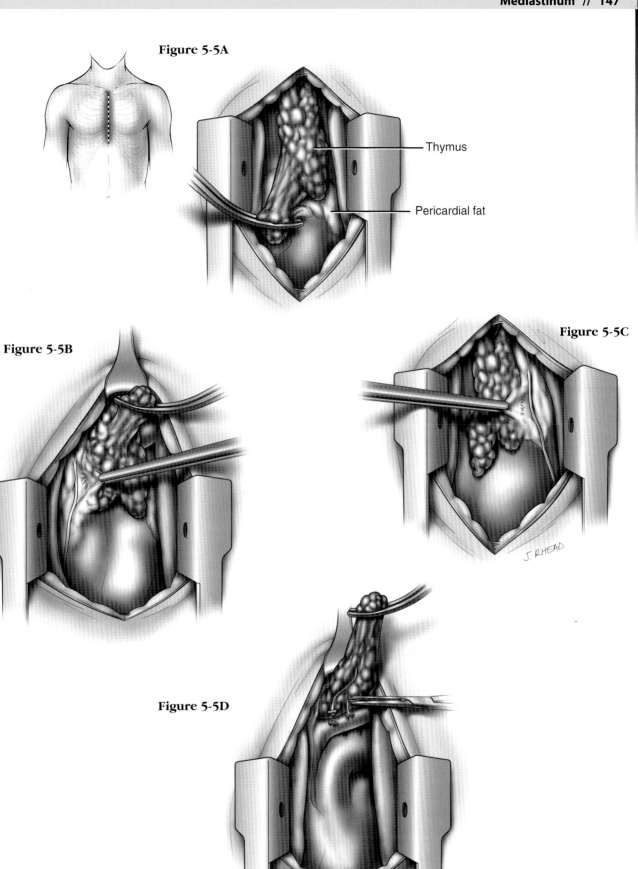

Thymus

Pericardial fat

Figure 5-5B

Figure 5-5C

J. R. HEAD

Figure 5-5D

5-6 Subxiphoid Pericardiotomy

Subxiphoid pericardiotomy is performed most often for management of a pericardial effusion or for exploration to determine if trauma has caused intrapericardial bleeding due to myocardial injury. As such, it is often performed in patients who are somewhat unstable. Fortunately, it can be performed using just local anesthetic under some circumstances, avoiding the hemodynamic consequences of general anesthesia. The patient is positioned supine and the arms can be positioned alongside the torso or out to the side. If additional hemodynamic monitoring is necessary, leaving at least one arm out to the side facilitates this. The patient's entire chest and abdomen are prepared in case and a sternotomy is necessary.

A vertical incision measuring 6 to 8 cm is centered over the xiphoid process and upper abdomen (see Fig. 5-6A inset). This positions the incision over the dome of the diaphragm, giving access to the lower anterior and base of the pericardium (Fig. 5-6A). The linea alba is divided to the level of the xiphoid process. The preperitoneal tissues are left intact. Under most circumstances, it is advantageous to excise the xiphoid process to provide better access to the pericardium (Fig. 5-6B). The pericardium is cleaned of surrounding fibrofatty tissue. It is grasped with a Kocher clamp and pulled into the incision.

If there is a question about possible cardiac tamponade physiology, an angiocatheter can be inserted through the pericardium and intrapericardial pressures can be measured prior to drainage of the pericardium. A small window of pericardium is excised to permit drainage of any pericardial fluid (Fig. 5-6C). Digital palpation of the pericardial surface and epicardium of the heart may reveal tumor implants in patients with malignant pericardial effusions. In some instances pericardioscopy, using a mediastinoscope or flexible videobronchoscope, may be appropriate to further explore these surfaces. If a traumatic hemopericardium is identified, further open exploration is appropriate to determine the cause and repair it.

Patients with malignant pericardial effusions require external drainage for a sufficient period of time to permit symphysis of the epicardial and pericardial surfaces to prevent recurrence of the effusion. To accomplish this, one or two drains are placed, one anterior to the heart and the other angled on the inferior surface of the heart, and are brought out through separate stab incisions inferior to the incision so that the linea alba may be closed over the tubes (Fig. 5-6D). The concept of creating a "window" communicating between the pericardial space and the abdominal cavity is unfounded; even if both cavities communicate with each other at the time of performing a pericardial drainage procedure, this communication closes within hours of suturing the incision. Similar misconceptions surround the creation of a "window" between the pericardial and pleural spaces.

Figure 5-6A

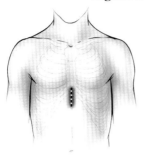

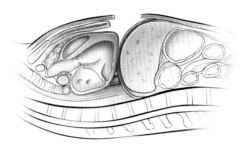

Figure 5-6B

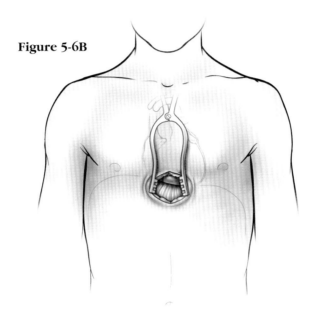

Figure 5-6C

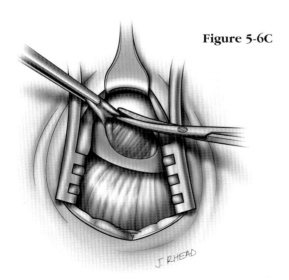

Figure 5-6D

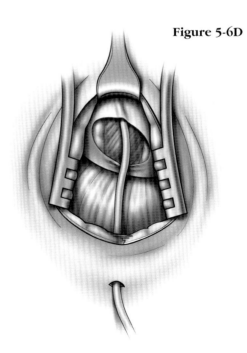

5-7 Mediastinal Cyst Excision

Typical mediastinal cysts include bronchogenic, esophageal duplication, pericardial, and thymic cysts. Resection is indicated when symptoms are present, when the diagnosis is uncertain, or for cysts related to the esophagus or airway that are at risk for becoming infected. There is controversy as to whether the risk of a carcinoma developing in such a cyst is sufficient to warrant routine resection of most mediastinal cysts. Although historically cyst resection was performed through an open thoracotomy, most such cysts now are resected using minimally invasive techniques.

Resection of a typical bronchogenic cyst is illustrated in Figures 5-7A–D. Cysts in other locations require alternate placements of thoracic ports to provide optimal access to the region of the cyst. The patient is placed in a true lateral position with the surgeon standing at the patient's back. The ipsilateral lung is isolated. The camera port is placed inferiorly, a lung retraction port displaced anteriorly, and the operating ports are placed posteriorly (see Fig. 5-7A inset). The mediastinal pleura overlying the cyst is incised, and any investing fascia that typically covers such a cyst is divided to expose the surface of the cyst (Fig. 5-7A). Cysts that are small and can be removed intact through an access incision are excised intact. Most cysts are too large to be removed intact through thoracoscopic techniques. In such instances, it is appropriate to aspirate the fluid contents of the cyst to collapse the wall of the cyst; this prevents spillage of the contents into the pleural space should accidental entry into the cyst occur during dissection (Fig. 5-7B).

In most instances cysts should be removed entirely, leaving no mucosal remnants behind. This is accomplished by careful dissection of the cyst wall from the surrounding investing fascia (Fig. 5-7C). However, in some instances, the tissue of origin of the cyst is at risk for injury, leading to serious complications, or the dissection is technically difficult because of previous inflammation or infection of the cyst. In such instances, the base of the cyst may be left intact, and any mucosal lining that remains present is cauterized to eliminate it (Fig. 5-7D).

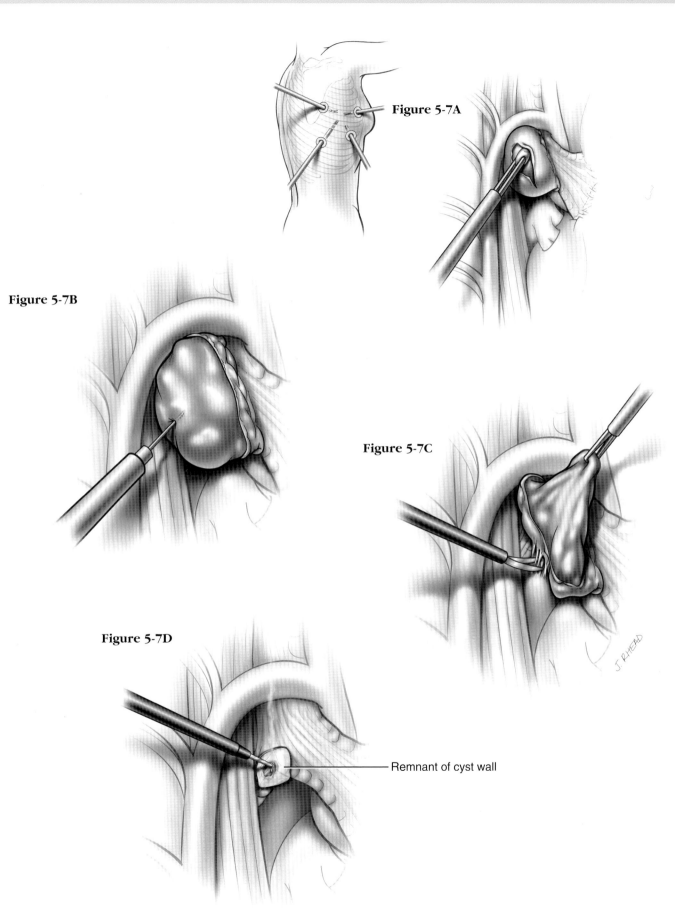

Figure 5-7A

Figure 5-7B

Figure 5-7C

Figure 5-7D

Remnant of cyst wall

5-8 Neurogenic Tumor Excision

Neurogenic tumors are typically found in the paravertebral sulcus and arise from peripheral nerves or sympathetic ganglia. In adults, the most common neurogenic tumors are schwannomas and neurofibromas. Almost all of these tumors are slow-growing and benign, and wide resection is not necessary. Resection is usually indicated to achieve a diagnosis and treat the abnormality before it becomes large and symptomatic. Historically, most neurogenic tumors were excised using open techniques. In some instances a dumbbell configuration requires a posterior laminectomy, in addition to a lateral thoracotomy, to enable complete excision. With the advent of minimally invasive techniques for excision of neurogenic tumors, this can be performed in combination with posterior laminectomy if a dumbbell configuration exists. Otherwise, complete excision is usually feasible with minimally invasive techniques. If a posterior laminectomy is necessary to free the portion of the tumor that is within the spinal canal or a neural foramen, performing the laminectomy as the first phase of the operation permits the remainder of the tumor to be excised with minimally invasive techniques.

The patient is placed in a true lateral position and the ipsilateral lung is isolated. The surgeon can stand either at the patient's front or back. The camera port is posterior, the surgeon and the operating ports are anterior, and the lung retraction port is superior and anterior (Fig. 5-8A). The pleura overlying the neurogenic tumor is divided and separated from the surface of the tumor. The investing fascial layer is similarly separated from the surface of the tumor (Fig. 5-8B). At this point the typical neurogenic tumor is quite mobile. Careful and gentle dissection frees it from its attachments to the chest wall. Individual small arteries and veins feeding the tumor are clipped and divided (Fig. 5-8C). At this point the tumor is typically hanging by a small stalk, its attachment of neural origin. This is carefully isolated and clipped before being divided (Fig. 5-8D). The tumor is placed in a specimen bag and removed through the largest port site. The surgical site is inspected to ensure there is no spinal fluid leakage. Use of a pleural drain is appropriate for 24 hours following the operation.

Figure 5-8A

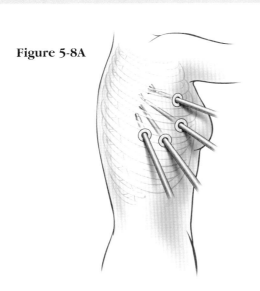

Figure 5-8B

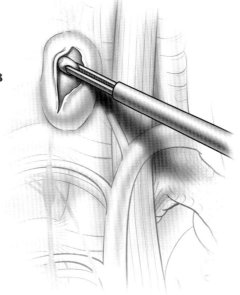

Figure 5-8C

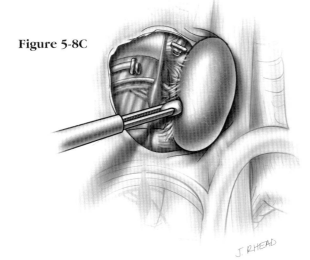

J. R. HEAD

Figure 5-8D

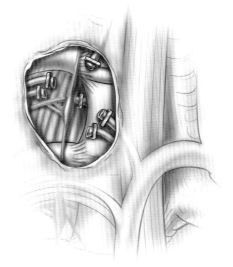

Chapter 6

Esophagus

6-1 Anatomy

The esophagus is a muscular tube that originates at the level of the cricoid cartilage (sixth cervical vertebra) and extends caudad to the esophagogastric junction, a distance of about 25 cm. In the neck it lies posterior to the trachea and is adjacent to the left lobe of the thyroid gland, primarily because it is situated more on the left in the cervical region prior to returning to the midline in the upper thorax. The recurrent laryngeal nerves extend cephalad in or near the tracheoesophageal groove (Fig. 6-1A). The superior and middle thyroid arteries typically lie superior to the main portion of the cervical esophagus. However, a middle thyroid vein often crosses from the thyroid gland to the internal jugular vein in the region in which the cervical esophagus is usually dissected. The esophagus is related laterally to the carotid artery, particularly on the left side. The blood supply to the cervical esophagus is the inferior thyroid artery, and the primary site of venous drainage is the inferior thyroid vein. The primary innervation of the cervical and upper thoracic esophagus is via branches of the recurrent laryngeal nerves and by postganglionic sympathetic fibers.

From a posterior perspective the esophagus is seen arising at the level of the cricopharyngeus muscle, which inserts on the cricoid cartilage posterolaterally. Immediately superior to this are the inferior pharyngeal constrictor muscles, and extending cephalad are the middle and superior pharyngeal constrictor muscles (Fig. 6-1B). The circular (inner) esophageal muscle fibers originate at the inferior margin of the cricopharyngeal muscle. They are surrounded by the longitudinal esophageal muscle fibers that decussate into anterolateral bundles that ascend deep to the inferior pharyngeal constrictor and insert on the cricoid cartilage. This often leaves an area somewhat devoid of muscle investment immediately superior to the cricopharyngeus muscle, known as Killian's triangle, which is the site of development of pharyngoesophageal diverticula. The external muscle layers of the esophagus comprise striated (skeletal) muscle in the upper third of the esophagus.

The esophagus crosses the thoracic inlet posterior to the trachea and anterior to the vertebra column, coursing behind and to the right of the aortic arch. It descends to the right of the thoracic aorta, slightly shifting anteriorly and laterally as it approaches the diaphragmatic hiatus (Fig. 6-1C). After the esophagus passes posterior to the carina, it is related to the left atrium. The arterial supply to the thoracic esophagus consists of four or five branches that extend directly from the aorta and form a plexus on the wall of the esophagus that communicates superiorly with branches of the inferior thyroid artery and inferiorly with branches of the left phrenic and left gastric arteries. The venous drainage of the thoracic esophagus is primarily into the azygos vein, but some drainage is also provided by the hemiazygos system. The thoracic duct is found just to the right of the esophagus below the level of the sixth thoracic vertebra, and is just medial to the azygos vein. It crosses posterior to the esophagus and rises along its left side above the level of the fifth thoracic vertebra.

At the level of the distal trachea and carina, the right and left vagus nerves decussate into a plexus that encircles the esophagus and gives off branches to the mainstem bronchi. The plexus gives rise to the anterior and posterior vagus nerves, which continue down the esophagus and through the esophageal hiatus. The innervation of the thoracic esophagus is primarily from the vagus nerves for sensory fibers, secretory control, and motor fibers for the smooth muscle of the lower thoracic esophagus. The striated muscle in the middle thoracic esophagus, which is mixed with smooth muscle in this region, is innervated by sympathetic fibers from the upper four to six thoracic spinal cord segments.

Figure 6-1A

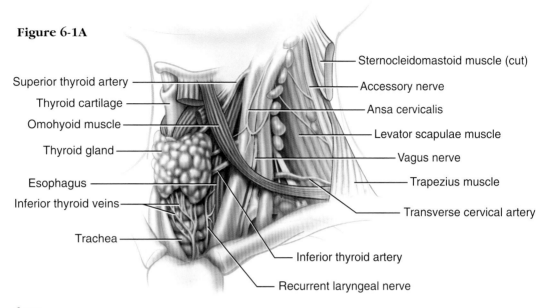

Superior thyroid artery

Thyroid cartilage

Omohyoid muscle

Thyroid gland

Esophagus

Inferior thyroid veins

Trachea

Sternocleidomastoid muscle (cut)

Accessory nerve

Ansa cervicalis

Levator scapulae muscle

Vagus nerve

Trapezius muscle

Transverse cervical artery

Inferior thyroid artery

Recurrent laryngeal nerve

Figure 6-1B

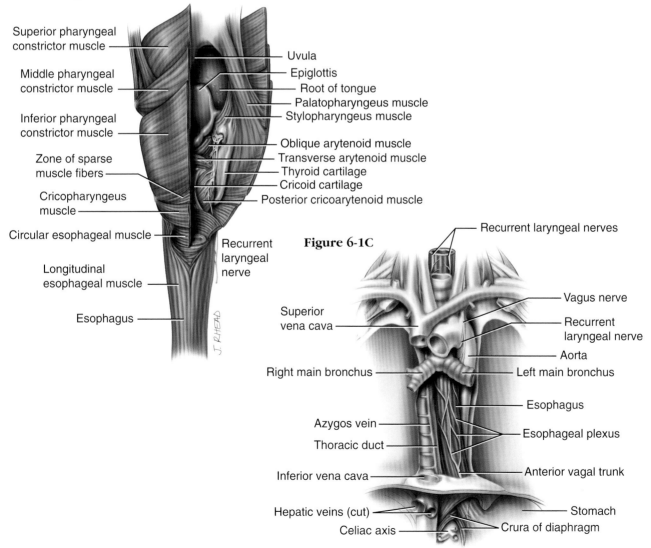

Superior pharyngeal
constrictor muscle

Middle pharyngeal
constrictor muscle

Inferior pharyngeal
constrictor muscle

Zone of sparse
muscle fibers

Cricopharyngeus
muscle

Circular esophageal muscle

Longitudinal
esophageal muscle

Esophagus

Uvula

Epiglottis

Root of tongue

Palatopharyngeus muscle

Stylopharyngeus muscle

Oblique arytenoid muscle

Transverse arytenoid muscle

Thyroid cartilage

Cricoid cartilage

Posterior cricoarytenoid muscle

Recurrent
laryngeal
nerve

J. RHEAD

Figure 6-1C

Recurrent laryngeal nerves

Superior
vena cava

Right main bronchus

Azygos vein

Thoracic duct

Inferior vena cava

Hepatic veins (cut)

Celiac axis

Vagus nerve

Recurrent
laryngeal nerve

Aorta

Left main bronchus

Esophagus

Esophageal plexus

Anterior vagal trunk

Stomach

Crura of diaphragm

The relationships of the thoracic esophagus to the surrounding structures that are important from a surgical perspective are shown in Figures 6-1D and E. As the esophagus is approached through the right thorax using an open or thoracoscopic technique, the primary superior relationship is to the posterior trachea. Immediately above the azygos arch the relationships include the superior intercostal vein posteriorly and the right vagus nerve anterolaterally. Caudad to this the esophagus is in direct contact with the carina, both mainstem bronchi, and the subcarinal lymph nodes. More inferiorly the relationships anterior are to the pulmonary veins and the posterior pericardium, while posteriorly the aorta, spine, and upper portion of the azygos vein are in contact with the esophagus. As the hiatus is approached, the thoracic duct is related to the esophagus posteriorly as it wends to the left away from the azygos vein.

When approached from the left thoracic perspective, the superior thoracic esophagus is related to the spine, the left recurrent laryngeal nerve, and to some extent the thoracic duct as it ascends from posterior to the esophagus into the thoracic inlet (see Fig. 6-1D). The aortic arch and hemiazygos arch cross the esophagus in its descending course, deep to which the esophagus is related to the left mainstem bronchus and the vagal nerve plexus. More inferiorly the direct contacts are to the descending thoracic aorta, the pulmonary veins, and the posterior pericardium.

The esophageal hiatal structures are important to understand for purposes of esophageal resection as well as for surgically treating motility disorders and gastroesophageal reflux disease. The esophageal hiatus is located at the level of the tenth thoracic vertebra. It is formed from the decussation of the right diaphragmatic pillar, into which the phrenoesophageal membrane inserts, separating the abdominal and thoracic cavities at the hiatus (Fig. 6-1F). Posterior to the esophageal hiatus, the aortic hiatus is limited anteriorly by the median arcuate ligament, which is of importance in performing some fundoplications. Inferior to the aortic hiatus, the aorta gives off small inferior phrenic and esophageal branches. The first important intraabdominal branch of the aorta is the celiac axis, which gives rise to the common hepatic artery, the splenic artery, and the left gastric artery. The anterior vagus nerve descends on the anterior aspect of the esophagus, gives off gastric and hepatic branches, and continues to descend along the lesser curve of the stomach. The posterior vagus nerve is also intimately related to the esophagus, and gives off gastric branches as it descends along the lesser gastric curvature.

An understanding of gastric anatomy is vital because the stomach is intimately involved in fundoplication and esophagectomy operations (Fig. 6-1G). There are four main sources of blood supply to the stomach. The left gastric artery arises directly from the celiac axis and descends along the lesser gastric curvature, giving off five to seven small branches directly to the stomach. These direct branches end at the level of the angulus of the stomach near the border of the antrum. The right gastric artery arises from the common hepatic artery and ascends along the lesser curvature from just beyond the pylorus; it anastomoses with the left gastric artery. The common hepatic artery gives off the gastroduodenal artery, which descends posterior to the duodenum and gives rise to the right gastroepiploic artery, which courses along the greater curvature in the gastric omentum. Of note, care should be taken whenever operating in this region to search for an aberrant left hepatic artery, which can arise from the left gastric artery as the primary blood supply to the left lobe of the liver. This should be preserved if it appears that its sacrifice will lead to hepatic ischemia. The splenic artery provides blood supply to the pancreas through small perforating vessels along its length before it decussates into smaller branches that enter the splenic hilum and course cephalad along the gastric fundus as the short gastric vessels. The splenic artery gives rise to the left gastroepiploic artery, which provides a few small branches to the greater curvature of the stomach. Although many textbooks describe a communication between the left and right gastroepiploic arcades, this communication is usually quite small and is somewhat peripheral in the omentum; it should not be routinely relied upon as a means for providing blood flow to the gastric fundus.

Short gastric veins from the upper greater curvature and stomach join the splenic vein. Similarly, the left gastroepiploic vein courses along the lateral greater curvature, draining the body of the stomach and a portion of the omentum, and empties into the splenic vein. The right gastroepiploic vein drains the gastric body and omentum, passes posterior to the duodenum and empties into the superior mesenteric vein. The left gastric vein ascends along the lesser curvature, accepts tributaries from descending esophageal veins, and continues inferiorly posterior to the peritoneum of the lesser sac to empty directly into the portal vein. The right gastric vein is usually small; it accompanies the right gastric artery and empties into the portal vein at the level of the pylorus.

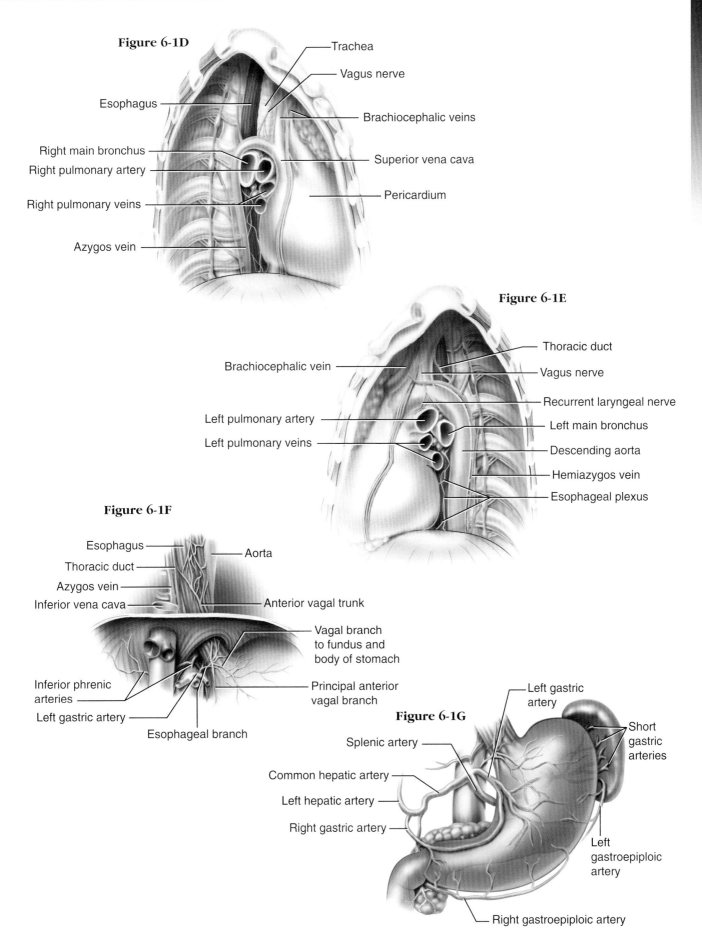

Figure 6-1D

Trachea
Vagus nerve
Esophagus
Brachiocephalic veins
Right main bronchus
Superior vena cava
Right pulmonary artery
Right pulmonary veins
Pericardium
Azygos vein

Figure 6-1E

Thoracic duct
Brachiocephalic vein
Vagus nerve
Recurrent laryngeal nerve
Left pulmonary artery
Left main bronchus
Left pulmonary veins
Descending aorta
Hemiazygos vein
Esophageal plexus

Figure 6-1F

Esophagus
Aorta
Thoracic duct
Azygos vein
Inferior vena cava
Anterior vagal trunk
Vagal branch to fundus and body of stomach
Inferior phrenic arteries
Principal anterior vagal branch
Left gastric artery
Esophageal branch

Figure 6-1G

Left gastric artery
Splenic artery
Short gastric arteries
Common hepatic artery
Left hepatic artery
Right gastric artery
Left gastroepiploic artery
Right gastroepiploic artery

6-2 Laparoscopic Total Fundoplication (Nissen)

Laparoscopic total fundoplication is one of the most common major surgical operations performed, largely because of the high frequency of uncontrolled gastroesophageal acid reflux, particularly in Western societies. Indications for this operation include: unremitting symptoms of gastroesophageal acid reflux despite maximal medical therapy; complications of reflux such as ulceration or stricture; inability or refusal to comply with medical therapy; severe acid reflux symptoms in younger patients who face a lifetime of medical therapy, even in whom symptom control is possible with medical therapy; and possibly the presence of Barrett's esophagus, particularly long segment Barrett's esophagus, in which case the indications for surgery are not primarily symptom resolution but focus on prevention of development of adenocarcinoma.

Patients are managed on maximal dosage of acid suppression in the immediate preoperative period to reduce esophageal inflammation as much as possible. Open operations are reserved for patients who have had extensive prior surgery or for some patients with very large hiatal hernia in whom hernia reduction and fundoplication cannot reliably be performed using minimally invasive techniques. Laparoscopic approaches are used for the vast majority of fundoplication operations. The operation is performed with the patient supine; the surgeon stands either between the patient's legs or to the patient's right side, and the assistants are on the patient's left. Four to five ports are placed, the first being the camera port, which is typically positioned in the left upper quadrant 6 to 8 cm from the umbilicus. It is best to use either a 30- or 45-degree telescope during this operation. A liver retractor port is placed just inferior to the xiphoid process, and the retractor is placed to permit elevation of the left lobe of the liver. Using a table fixation device to hold this retractor maintains the liver in the desired position without the need for an additional surgical assistant. Two operating ports are placed in the epigastrium and a retraction port is often placed laterally in the left upper quadrant.

The dissection is begun by dividing the right crus from the esophagus, beginning superior to the nerve of Latarjet (Fig. 6-2A). The peritoneum is grasped overlying this plane, and a cautery scissors or ultrasound shears is used to divide the tissues (Fig. 6-2B). The esophagus is bluntly dissected from the crus, taking care not to enter the right pleural space. The peritoneal division continues anterior to the esophagus, preserving the anterior vagus nerve. The telescope orientation is moved to look from the left, and the crus is dissected from the esophagus on the left side. The telescope is rotated back to provide a view from the patient's right, and the posterior dissection is begun. The esophagus, with the posterior vagus nerve attached, is elevated anteriorly and the window posterior to it is opened primarily with blunt dissection. The dissection from this side is complete when the decussation of the right crus is evident and a posterior window of at least 5 to 6 cm has been developed (Fig. 6-2C). The telescope is again oriented for a view from the patient's left. Beginning proximal to the termination of the right gastroepiploic vessels, the short gastric vessels are divided and the fundus is freed from the spleen to permit its eventual use in the fundoplication (Fig. 6-2D). The stomach is reflected to the patient's right, exposing the retroperitoneal attachments. These are divided with cautery scissors or the ultrasonic shears. The fat pad that lies anteriorly across the esophagogastric junction is dissected free and is removed, enabling accurate identification of this important anatomic landmark. Once this landmark has been adequately identified, some surgeons prefer to place a rubber drain around the esophagus for use in retracting it into the abdomen, permitting dissection of the mediastinal portion of the esophagus. The esophagus is mobilized from mediastinal tissues, taking care not to enter the left pleural space, sufficient to ensure that a segment at least 5 cm long rests comfortably within the abdomen without downward traction, ensuring a tension-free fundoplication. If this condition cannot be achieved, consideration should be given to performing a gastric lengthening procedure (see Section 6-7).

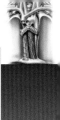

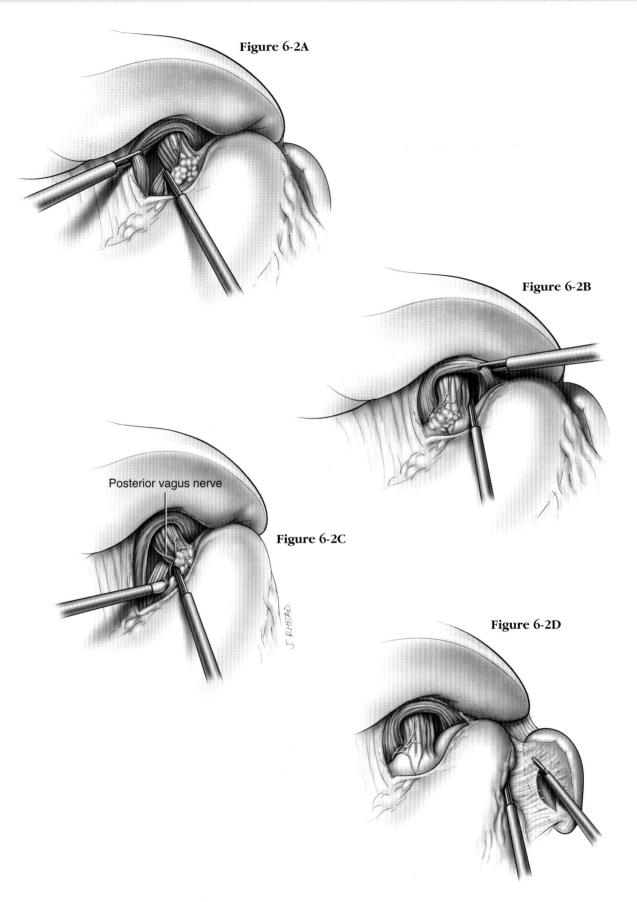

Figure 6-2A

Figure 6-2B

Posterior vagus nerve

Figure 6-2C

Figure 6-2D

The crura are closed with heavy interrupted sutures, taking care to use large bites of diaphragm tissue and achieve an adequate hiatal closure (Fig. 6-2E). Usually three or four such sutures are required. The remaining hiatal opening should not exceed 1 to 1.5 cm. The esophagus is elevated anteriorly and an instrument is passed behind it into the left upper quadrant. A point on the gastric fundus is selected for use in performing the fundoplication, and this point is handed to the instrument behind the esophagus, enabling the fundus to be pulled behind the esophagus and to the patient's right (see Fig. 6-2F inset). A delicate balance must be achieved in selecting the correct point on the fundus to use for the fundoplication. Choosing a point too close to the esophagogastric junction requires that the fundoplication sutures be placed on the right side of the esophagus rather than more anteriorly, whereas choosing a spot more distally along the greater curvature requires that too much of the stomach be located behind the esophagus, distorting the fundoplication. After the stomach has been pulled through the window behind the esophagus, the two points on it that are to be the targets for suturing are grasped and a "shoe shine" maneuver is performed, sliding the stomach back and forth behind the esophagus (Fig. 6-2F). This ensures that there is no limitation of movement and that there is adequate redundancy of the portion of the stomach to be used for fundoplication.

A large (54 Fr) mercury-weighted bougie is passed orally across the gastroesophageal junction. It is best to have pulled the stomach posterior to the esophagus prior to passing the bougie, because the stiffness of the bougie can prohibit passing of instruments posterior to the esophagus. The fundoplication is performed with the bougie in place. Sites for the sutures are chosen carefully, avoiding evident vessels on the stomach, damage to which might cause an intramural hematoma and interfere with an optimal fundoplication. The wrap should be 1 to 2 cm long, depending on the preference of the surgeon. Although it is the custom of some surgeons to

perform "U" stitches reinforced by felt pledgets, simple heavy sutures of braided nonabsorbable material are sufficient.

Two sutures are placed 1 cm apart to create a 1-cm wrap, and three such sutures are placed to create a 2-cm wrap. It is sometimes useful to mark the gastroesophageal junction with a small vascular clip to be used as a reference point for determining where each stitch should be placed. The most cephalad suture is placed first, beginning on the left portion of the fundus, taking a generous bite of the esophagus, and then passing through the wrapped portion of the fundus. Although Figure 6-2G demonstrates three sutures having been placed but not tied, this is for illustrative purposes only; when performing this operation laparoscopically, it is necessary to tie each stitch upon its completion. Each stitch includes a bite of the esophagus to firmly anchor the wrap. The most caudad stitch must be placed just superior to the gastroesophageal junction, ensuring that the wrap is performed around the esophagus. The completed wrap is evident as a symmetric collar around the distal esophagus, and sits within the peritoneal cavity without tension (Fig. 6-2H). Some surgeons further anchor the wrap to the crura with interrupted sutures, but this is unnecessary if the wrap has been performed without tension. If the wrap is under tension from inadequate mobilization of the esophagus or inadequate esophageal length, wrap herniation will result whether or not anchoring sutures are placed between the wrap and the crura.

Patients are managed postoperatively in the hospital until they demonstrate adequate bowel function and the ability to eat. Whether a nasogastric tube is necessary depends on the individual patient and the preference of the surgeon; they are not required in most patients. The diet is modified to include soft solid food in small quantities for a period of at least a week or two postoperatively, which corresponds to the minimum period of delayed gastric emptying postoperatively.

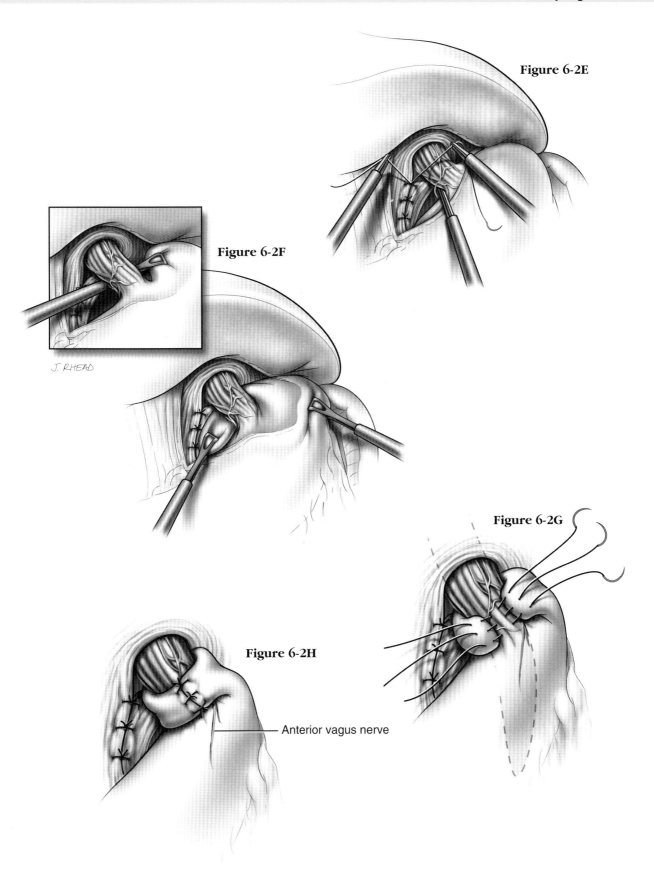

Figure 6-2E

Figure 6-2F

J. RHEAD

Figure 6-2G

Figure 6-2H

Anterior vagus nerve

6-3   Transthoracic Total Fundoplication (Nissen)

In some patients laparoscopic fundoplication for management of gastroesophageal reflux disease cannot be performed or is contraindicated, and in such situations a transthoracic approach is often the next best option. Advantages of an open transthoracic approach compared to an open abdominal approach include an improved ability to mobilize the intrathoracic esophagus, dissect adhesions between a herniated stomach and intrathoracic organs, and perform a gastroplasty if needed. In addition, the transthoracic approach avoids much of the tedious dissection necessary when performing a reoperation on a patient who has suffered a failed fundoplication or other major upper abdominal surgery.

The patient is placed in a true left lateral decubitus position; use of lung isolation techniques by the anesthesiologist is strongly recommended. A standard lateral thoracotomy is performed, dividing the latissimus dorsi but sparing the serratus anterior (see Fig. 6-3A inset). The intercostal space used to access the pleural space depends on the individual patient; more obese patients who have high-riding diaphragms are best approached through the seventh interspace, but the most common approach is through the eighth intercostal space. The latter space is also ideal if the incision needs to be extended to a thoracoabdominal approach. The esophagus is mobilized circumferentially midway between the hiatus and the inferior pulmonary vein, taking care to include both vagus nerves with the esophagus and to avoid entry into the contralateral pleura space. Once surrounded by a rubber drain to aid in countertraction, the esophagus is dissected further cephalad to above the level of the inferior pulmonary vein. The vagal plexus is encountered in this region, and can be dissected off the esophagus and left intact, permitting esophageal mobilization without disruption of the vagal nerves.

The esophagus is mobilized distally, taking particular care to avoid entry into the right pleural space inferiorly, where the pleura most closely approaches the esophagus. The most caudad portion of the dissection depends on whether a noticeable hiatal hernia exists. In the absence of a hernia, the rim of the hiatus is grasped with an Allis or Babcock clamp and the peritoneum immediately deep to the rim is divided, permitting entry into the peritoneal space (Fig. 6-3A). Once entry is confirmed, the hiatus is dissected circumferentially. Posteriorly the retroperitoneal tissues are opened, exposing the left lobe of the liver, ensuring that complete esophageal and upper gastric mobilization is performed. The only challenging aspect of this portion of the dissection is management of the posteromedial region, where inferior diaphragmatic vessels (Belsey's artery, among them) anastomose with branches of the left gastric artery.

Careful control of these tissues between clamps prior to their division helps to avoid intraabdominal bleeding, which at times can be difficult to control from the chest. The dissection is complete when the stomach can be easily brought into the chest, completely displacing the esophagogastric junction into the hemithorax. Care must also be taken to avoid injury to the inferior vena cava, which can easily be identified medial to the caudate lobe of the liver.

If a hiatal hernia exists, the dissection is usually performed more easily. The hernia sac is entered near the hiatus, and is dissected circumferentially from the rim of the hiatus. The sac is excised from the stomach and esophagus, ensuring that the vagus nerves are preserved in the process. The posterior vagus nerve, in particular, is subject to injury during dissection of a hiatal hernia because it sometimes gets separated from the wall of the esophagus. Once the hernia sac is resected, in cases of a moderate to large hiatal hernia, no further hiatal dissection is necessary. Because hiatal hernias are, by definition, associated with substantial widening of the esophageal hiatus, hiatal closure is sometimes more difficult. As an aid to hiatal closure, the pericardium may be dissected off of the medial portion of the diaphragm, freeing up a 2-to-3-cm wide swath of diaphragm, the increased mobility of which reduces tension on any subsequent crural closure.

The gastric fundus is mobilized sufficiently to permit performance of a total fundoplication wrap without tension once the wrap has been reduced into the abdomen. This requires division of several short gastric vessels. Babcock clamps are used to retract the stomach into the left hemithorax. When the first short gastric vessel comes into view, it is individually ligated and divided (Fig. 6-3B). This division permits placement of additional traction on the greater curvature of the stomach, permitting the next short gastric vessel to be exposed. The vessels are sequentially divided in this way.

The gastric fat pad is resected, exposing the region of the gastroesophageal junction. The location of this site is best assessed without any traction on the stomach or esophagus. A decision is made at this point as to whether there is a sufficient amount of intraabdominal esophagus to permit creation of a fundoplication that will reside in the abdomen without undue tension. If insufficient length exists, additional dissection of the esophagus cephalad may be sufficient to establish the needed length. If this fails, then a lengthening gastroplasty is necessary (see Section 6-7).

Beginning at the decussation of the crura posteriorly, hiatal closure stitches are placed but are left untied. Heavy braided nonabsorbable sutures are placed 1 cm apart and about 1 cm from the edge of the hiatal rim (Fig. 6-3C). Usually three to four such sutures are necessary to close the hiatus sufficiently so that after completion of the repair, the tip of only one finger can be inserted

Figure 6-3A

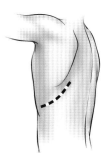

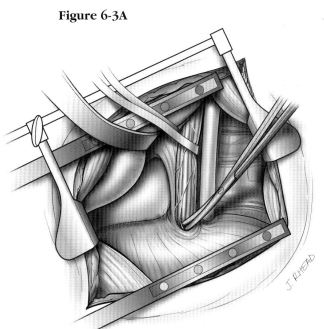

Figure 6-3B

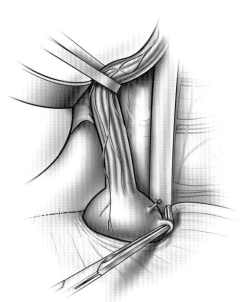

Figure 6-3C

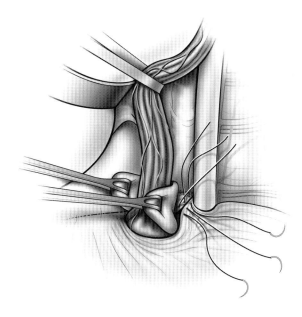

alongside the esophagus. Care must be taken to avoid injury to intraabdominal structures during this process, including the spleen, liver, omentum, and bowel. This is facilitated by use of a spoon-shaped retractor positioned on the under surface of the diaphragm.

A large (54 Fr) mercury-weighted bougie is passed orally across the esophagogastric junction. The fundus is oriented posteriorly around the esophagus, choosing sites for sutures in a manner described previously in Section 6-2. In this instance it is easiest to place the most caudad stitch first, taking healthy bites of stomach, esophagus, and then stomach. Care is taken to ensure that the most caudad suture is placed clearly above the esophagogastric junction (Fig. 6-3D). The stitches are tied as they are placed. Usually a three-stitch wrap, placing the sutures 1 cm apart to create a 2-cm fundoplication, is sufficient (Fig. 6-3E). The wrap must be loose enough to permit passage of the surgeon's finger within the wrap after removal of the bougie from the esophageal lumen.

With the wrap completed and the bougie removed, the wrap is reduced into the abdomen (Fig. 6-3F). For patients without prior hiatal hernia, this sometimes requires some finesse, as the hiatus is normally not large enough to accommodate the wrap. Gentle, persistent, evenly distributed pressure is usually successful in accomplishing this task. Again, an assessment is made to ensure that the wrap will reside within the abdomen without undue tension, thus minimizing the risk of recurrence.

Although some surgeons place anchoring sutures between the fundoplication and the rim of the hiatus, these are unnecessary if the wrap is performed without tension. Such sutures are insufficient to prevent wrap herniation or breakdown if there is tension on the wrap. If the fundoplication does not sit within the abdomen without tension, consideration should be given to undoing the wrap and performing a lengthening gastroplasty.

The crural stitches are tied, beginning with the most posterior suture. As the last one or two stitches are tied, an assessment is made of how tight the hiatal opening is becoming. Once it is sized to permit passage of the tip of a single finger, no further sutures are necessary, and any untied stitches are removed. In some instances the hiatal opening remains somewhat oversized after tying all of the originally placed hiatal stitches. In this situation, rather than trying to place additional sutures between the crura without disturbing the fundoplication, it is easiest to place a lateral suture or two to further tighten the hiatus. A nasogastric tube is placed. A single chest drain is placed and the incision is closed. Postoperative management is similar to that for patients undergoing laparoscopic fundoplication, except that return of gastrointestinal motility seems to be slower after an open operation than a miminally invasive procedure. Pain control is a more pressing issue after a thoracotomy, and administration of narcotic analgesics may contribute significantly to the difference in regaining gut motility between these two patient groups.

Figure 6-3D

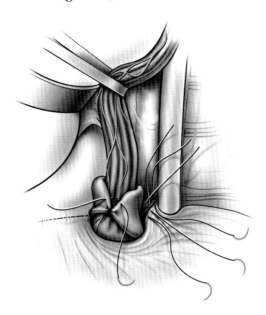

Figure 6-3E

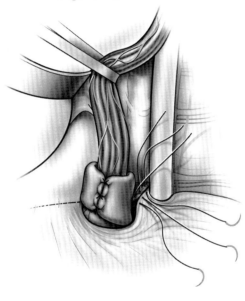

Figure 6-3F

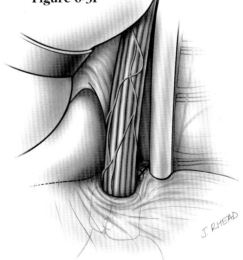

J. R. HEAD

6-4 Partial Posterior Fundoplication (Toupet)

The indications for partial fundoplication are similar to those for total fundoplication, but the short- and long-term effects of partial fundoplication are somewhat different than total fundoplication. In general, a total fundoplication provides better long-term protection against acid reflux but is associated with a higher incidence of postoperative dysphagia. Randomized studies demonstrate that patient satisfaction is similar regardless of which type of fundoplication is performed. Historically, partial fundoplication was often reserved for patients with substantial esophageal dysmotility, with the thought that a partial wrap would impair swallowing less in this patient group. More recent data suggest that the degree of dysphagia experienced after total fundoplication is not significantly different than after partial fundoplication, indicating that total fundoplication is appropriate even in patients with a substantial esophageal motility disorder. Currently, the most common indication for partial fundoplication, in addition to surgeon preference, is the existence of a primary esophageal motility disorder such as achalasia, when fundoplication is added after esophageal myotomy to help control postoperative acid reflux.

In performing a posterior partial (Toupet) fundoplication, either a laparoscopic or open abdominal approach is appropriate. It is necessary to mobilize the esophagus and gastric fundus in a manner very similar to that for total fundoplication (see Section 6-2). After mobilization is complete, the gastric fat pad is excised and the location of the esophagogastric junction is confirmed. The crura, having been dissected as described previously in Section 6-2, are approximated with interrupted heavy sutures of braided nonabsorbable material.

Sites on the gastric fundus are selected for the fundoplication that are similar to those chosen for performance of a complete fundoplication. The stomach is pulled posterior to the esophagus and a "shoe shine" maneuver is performed to ensure that adequate gastric mobilization has been accomplished. The suturing is begun on the patient's left, stitching the gastric fundus to the left side of the esophagus (Fig. 6-4A). Two additional sutures are placed, spaced 1 cm apart, to create a portion of the 2-cm wrap. It is important that the most caudad suture be placed clearly on the esophageal side of the esophagogastric junction. The right side of the fundoplication is then sutured. At a point opposite the stitches on the left side, the stomach is sutured to the right side of the esophagus to create a 2-cm wrap (Fig. 6-4B). This portion of the gastric fundus is also sutured to the right pillar of the hiatus, fixing the gastric fundus to the diaphragm (Fig. 6-4C). Postoperative management after a partial posterior fundoplication is similar to that for a laparoscopic total fundoplication.

Figure 6-4A

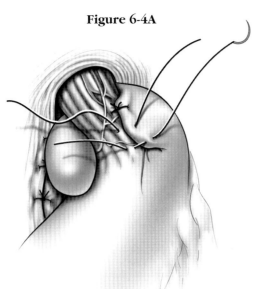

Figure 6-4B

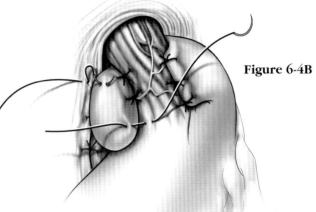

Figure 6-4C

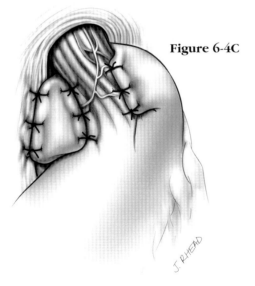

6-5 Partial Anterior Fundoplication (Dor)

Indications for performing a partial anterior fundoplication are similar to those for performing a partial posterior fundoplication. The partial anterior fundoplication is easier to perform, since, in the absence of a hiatal hernia, it is not necessary to dissect the hiatus circumferentially, and because the short gastric vessels usually do not need to be divided to provide sufficient gastric mobility to enable the wrap to be performed.

The operation may be performed either laparoscopically or using an open laparotomy. The right pillar of the crus is separated from the esophagus, and the anterior aspect of the esophagus is cleared of peritoneum. As always, the anterior vagus nerve is preserved. The esophagus is dissected on the left lateral side sufficiently to expose the left pillar of the crus. For this operation it is unlikely that the posterior vagus nerve will be clearly evident. The gastric fat pad is excised. Unlike the total fundoplication and partial posterior fundoplication, creation of a window posterior to the esophagus is not necessary, but the crura must be dissected sufficiently to place crural stitches if there is evidence that the hiatal aperture is too large. For anterior fundoplication accompanying myotomy for a motility disorder, crural repair is rarely necessary. Unless the short gastric vessels are very short and anchor the gastric fundus laterally, they need not be divided to enable a tension-free wrap to be performed.

The fundoplication is assessed by grasping the fundus near its tip and further along the greater curvature, drawing it across the stomach to assess its mobility and ensure that the wrap can easily be performed. It is sometimes necessary to adjust the locations where the gastric sutures will be placed to get the fundus to lie nicely across the esophagus. The tip of the fundus is sutured to the left lateral wall of the esophagus with a heavy braided nonabsorbable material, beginning about 2 cm above the esophagogastric junction (Fig. 6-5A). Two additional sutures are placed, spaced 1 cm apart, ending just proximal to the esophagogastric junction.

A spot more distal along the greater curvature is selected that easily reaches the right side of the esophagus, opposite the most cephalad stitch on the left. The uppermost right-sided suture is placed through the stomach at this point, through the esophagus, and through the right crus of the diaphragm, anchoring the wrap securely to both the esophagus and the diaphragm (Fig. 6-5B). Two additional sutures are placed, spaced 1 cm apart, including only stomach and the right side of the esophagus, and ending just above the esophagogastric junction (Fig. 6-5C).

The postoperative management of patients who undergo partial anterior fundoplications may be somewhat simpler than for total or partial posterior fundoplications because of the limited dissection that is necessary to perform the operation. Gastric motility is less disturbed, and placement of a nasogastric tube is almost never required. Oral intake begins with liquids on the day of the operation, and hospitalization longer than a single postoperative day is rarely necessary.

Figure 6-5A

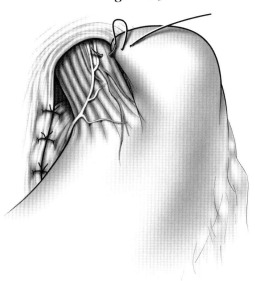

Figure 6-5B

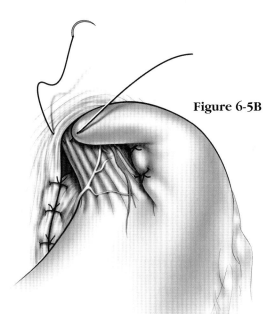

Figure 6-5C

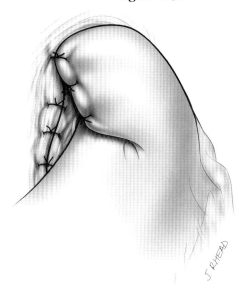

6-6   Transthoracic Partial Fundoplication (Belsey)

In the uncommon situation in which a transthoracic partial fundoplication is indicated, the Belsey fundoplication is well suited to the patient's needs. Indications include: inability to perform a laparoscopic fundoplication in patients in whom a partial fundoplication is needed; fundoplication after transthoracic lengthening gastroplasty, which is often simpler to perform using a Belsey rather than a Nissen technique; fundoplication after repair of a giant paraesophageal hernia, in which situation the Belsey wrap secures the stomach beneath the diaphragm more securely than any other type of fundoplication; and fundoplication after myotomy for motility disorders, including achalasia, diffuse esophageal spasm, and nonspecific motility disorders associated with esophageal pulsion diverticula.

The operation is performed through a standard left lateral thoracotomy, dividing the latissimus dorsi and sparing the serratus anterior. It is useful for the anesthesiologist to use a lung isolation technique for airway management. The intercostal space used for the incision depends on the individual patient; obese patients who have high-riding diaphragms are approached through the seventh interspace, but in most patients the eighth intercostal space is used. The esophagus is mobilized as described in Section 6-3, preserving the vagus nerves. The distal esophagus and proximal stomach are mobilized (also described in Section 6-3), but it is not necessary to divide more than one or two of the short gastric vessels to achieve sufficient gastric mobilization to allow a successful Belsey fundoplication. The gastric fat pad is excised and the esophagogastric junction is clearly identified. Crural sutures are placed and are left untied.

The fundoplication is initiated by pulling the gastric fundus into the hemithorax. The aim of the procedure is to create a wrap encompassing from 240 to 270 degrees of the circumference of the esophagus, which corresponds roughly to the portion of the circumference that lies between the right and left vagus nerves. Thus, the nerves are used as landmarks for placing the fundoplication sutures. The first row of sutures incorporates a generous bite of stomach 1 cm distal to the esophagogastric junction, a generous bite of esophagus 1 cm proximal to the junction, and then returns the stitch in a "U" fashion through the esophagus and stomach at a distance of about 5 mm from the initial bites. The most posterior stitch is immediately anterior to the left vagus nerve, the medial stitch is adjacent to the right vagus

nerve, and the central stitch is halfway between these two (Fig. 6-6A). These sutures are tied, creating a wrap of 1 cm of stomach onto the esophagus.

The second row of sutures incorporates bites on the esophagus that are 1 cm proximal to the sutures in the first row, with the lateral and medial sutures again placed immediately adjacent to the vagus nerves, and with the third suture centered between them. The gastric bites are taken a bit more laterally and medially, incorporating slightly more stomach in the second row than in the first row of sutures. Most importantly, each stitch is begun by bringing it through the diaphragm from the pleural surface to the peritoneal surface prior to taking the stomach bite. After the stitch has assumed its "U" configuration, with bites back through the esophagus and stomach completed, the stitch is brought back through the diaphragm from the peritoneal to the pleural surface (Fig. 6-6B). Placing the diaphragm portion of the sutures is facilitated by positioning a spoon-shaped retractor through the hiatus, separating the abdominal contents from the diaphragm, preventing injury to intraabdominal structures. The most medial and posterolateral second-row sutures pass through the diaphragm 1 to 2 cm from the closest crural suture used to close the hiatus.

The partial wrap, with the second row of sutures still untied, is delivered into the abdomen using gentle, persistent, global pressure. Once the wrap is reduced, the second-row sutures are pulled up tight, ensuring that no redundancy remains, and are tied. This results in the fundoplication being securely approximated to the adjacent esophagus, and, simultaneously, to the underside of the diaphragm (Fig. 6-6C). A cross-sectional view of the tissues incorporated in the first and second rows of sutures, with the resultant fundoplication, is shown in Figure 6-6D. The crural sutures are then tied.

Management of patients following a Belsey fundoplication is similar to management of patients after a transthoracic Nissen fundoplication. One important difference that must be stressed is that the esophageal lumen and the gastric lumen are no longer in the same axial plane following this partial fundoplication. The decision as to whether to place a nasogastric tube at the conclusion of the fundoplication, prior to chest closure, must be made carefully. It is useful to guide the nasogastric tube manually through the fundoplication to ensure that its passage does not get hung up at the level of the newly angulated esophagogastric junction. Postoperatively, if a patient requires placement of a nasogastric tube, placement of the tube should be performed by an experienced professional to minimize the risk of esophageal perforation.

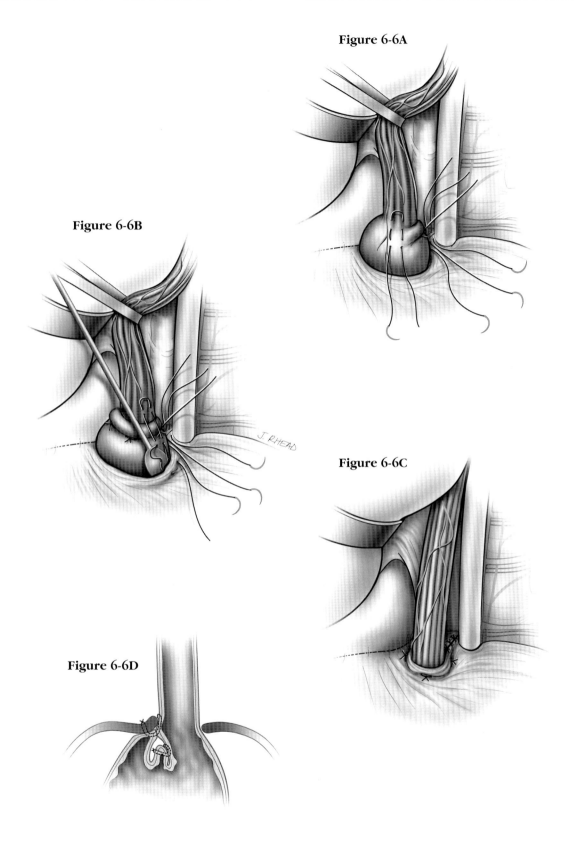

Figure 6-6A

Figure 6-6B

Figure 6-6C

Figure 6-6D

J. RHEAD

6-7 Collis Gastroplasty

A lengthening gastroplasty is created when the esophagogastric junction cannot be sufficiently reduced into the abdomen to enable an intraabdominal fundoplication to be performed without upward tension on the wrap. There is considerable controversy about the causes of so-called esophageal shortening and even about whether such a condition exists with any regularity. Exploring this controversy is not within the purview of this text. In some surgeons' hands a lengthening gastroplasty is required infrequently, whereas the technique is used commonly in other surgeons' practices. The original lengthening gastroplasty technique was described as being performed through a left thoracotomy, and this technique is described here. More recent methods for performing lengthening procedures laparoscopically are described at the conclusion of this section but are not illustrated, as they are still being refined.

The approach to performing a transthoracic Collis gastroplasty is similar to that for a transthoracic fundoplication, as described in Section 6-3. The esophagus is mobilized to the level of the aortic arch. The hiatus is dissected circumferentially. When it is judged that there is insufficient esophageal length to permit a standard intraabdominal fundoplication, the esophagus and stomach are prepared for the gastroplasty procedure. Several short gastric vessels are divided; an additional vessel or two may require division to accomplish sufficient gastric mobilization, bringing at least one third of the stomach into the thorax.

The fundus is grasped with Babcock clamps and stretched away from the lesser gastric curvature. A large mercury-weighted bougie (54 Fr) is passed orally across the esophagogastric junction so that the maximal diameter lies immediately adjacent to the lesser gastric curvature (Fig. 6-7A). A linear cutting stapler with a 5-to-6-cm-long cartridge is positioned adjacent to the dilator. Care is taken to avoid angling the stapler away from the lesser curve, which can narrow the base of the extended fundus and create ischemia. Once the correct position is confirmed, the stapler is fired to extend the tubular esophagus (Fig. 6-7B). The resulting staple line is reinforced by oversewing it with monofilament absorbable sutures (Fig. 6-7C).

When the gastroplasty is completed, a standard fundoplication is performed around the neoesophagus. Either a total (Nissen) or partial (Belsey) fundoplication is suitable in these circumstances, although a total fundoplication offers better control of acid reflux. The apex of the extended fundus forms the lead point of the wrap if a total fundoplication is performed, or serves as the midpoint of the wrap if a Belsey fundoplication is selected. In either case the fundoplication is positioned so that as much of the staple/suture line is covered, reinforcing the tissues (Fig. 6-7D). The crural sutures are tied after the fundoplication is reduced into the abdomen.

The techniques for performing a lengthening gastroplasty from an abdominal approach are numerous. The initial description consisted of using an EEA stapler to create an aperture at the point along the lesser gastric curvature where the lengthening staple line would terminate. The linear cutting stapler was then fired from this aperture, parallel to a bougie in the stomach, cephalad to the junction of the esophagus and fundus. Alternatively, the stapler was fired in the manner described earlier for creating the lengthening gastroplasty by inserting the stapler through a thoracic port, angling it down through the esophageal hiatus. This was described using both right and left chest approaches. Finally, the newest technique involves firing a linear cutting stapler from the gastric fundus at an angle toward the desired distal extent of the gastroplasty, followed by firing the linear cutting stapler cephalad parallel to the lesser gastric curvature to complete the gastroplasty. This effectively excises a wedge of gastric fundus between the fundus and the neoesophagus. It has the advantages of not requiring an initial gastric aperture or placement of a thoracic port, but the disadvantage is that a portion of the stomach is resected. This may interfere with any future operation for esophageal replacement should the patient's benign disease reach end-stage status and require esophagectomy.

Postoperative management after a Collis gastroplasty is more conservative than after standard fundoplications. Gastric distension places tension on the staple line and can cause leak or frank disruption under unusual circumstances. Nasogastric drainage is routine, and is discontinued after adequate gastric emptying is evident. The patient's diet should be limited to multiple small feedings for a period of several weeks postoperatively.

Figure 6-7A

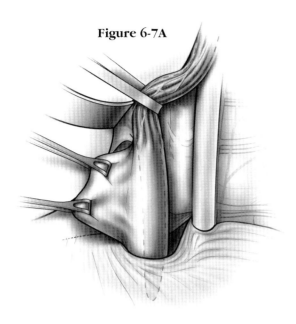

Figure 6-7B

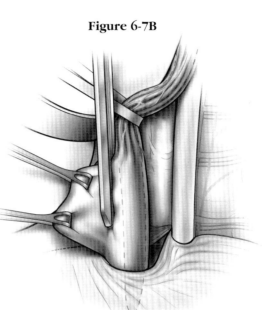

Figure 6-7C

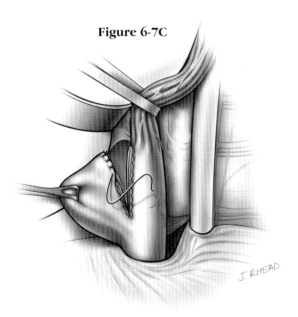

J. RHEAD

Figure 6-7D

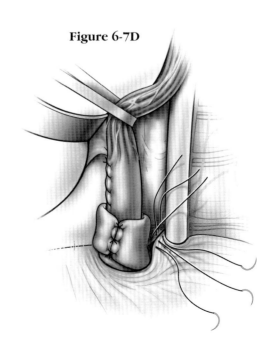

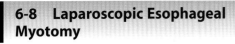

6-8 Laparoscopic Esophageal Myotomy

Esophageal myotomy is performed for management of motility disorders including achalasia, diffuse esophageal spasm, and pulsion diverticulum. The laparoscopic approach is most appropriate for treating achalasia, and low-lying pulsion diverticula may also be treated in this manner at times. More information on management of pulsion diverticula is included later in Section 6-10. This approach gives more reliable results than does a thoracoscopic approach and is much better tolerated than laparotomy or thoracotomy for performing myotomy. Any transabdominal myotomy needs to be accompanied by partial fundoplication to compensate for destruction of the lower esophageal sphincter mechanism. Total fundoplication has been used for this purpose as well, but the so-called floppy Nissen used by some surgeons in this situation is challenging to create with sufficient looseness to prevent dysphagia postoperatively.

Measures are taken to reduce the risk of aspiration during anesthetic induction. Patients are maintained on clear liquids for a period of two to three days preoperatively to ensure that no solid food is retained in the esophagus or stomach. General anesthesia is induced using a rapid sequence technique, and patients are maintained in a reverse Trendelenberg position. Esophagoscopy is performed shortly after induction of general anesthesia to evacuate any retained food. The patient is positioned supine so that the surgeon can stand at the patient's right side or between the patient's legs. After insufflation of carbon dioxide to create a pneumoperitoneum, a camera port is placed in the left upper quadrant 6 to 8 cm from the umbilicus. A liver retractor is placed just inferior to the xiphoid process and is fixed to the operating table. Two operating ports are placed in the right upper quadrant with the most medial port approaching the midline (see Fig. 6-8A inset).

The initial dissection is similar to that for performing a partial anterior (Dor) fundoplication (see Section 6-5). The anterior and lateral surfaces of the esophagus are dissected from the rim of the hiatus, and the esophagus is dissected for several centimeters into the mediasti-num. The gastric fat pad is reflected inferiorly or is excised (Fig. 6-8A). If an anterior (Dor) fundoplication is planned, no division of the short gastric vessels is necessary. For patients in whom a posterior (Toupet) fundoplication is to be performed, a window posterior to the esophagus must be created as was described in sections 6-2 and 6-4. In addition, several of the short gastric vessels must be divided from superior extending caudad.

The esophagogastric junction is clearly identified and the region for the myotomy is outlined, extending from 4 to 5 cm above the esophagogastric junction to 1 to 2 cm inferior to this spot. A dilute solution of epinephrine is injected submucosally along this line, opening the submucosal plane and helping to avoid bleeding by constricting the blood vessels lying therein. The esophageal muscle layers are divided beginning a couple of centimeters proximal to the esophagogastric junction using, at appropriate times, cautery scissors, hook cautery, or possibly ultrasonic shears (Fig. 6-8B). Once the submucosal plane is clearly identified, the muscle dissection is easily carried cephalad except possibly in patients who have undergone botulinum toxin therapy or pneumatic balloon dilation, both of which may cause fibrosis that partially obliterate this plane. After completing the cephalad portion of the myotomy, it is continued caudad across the esophagogastric junction at least 1 to 2 cm onto the stomach. The muscle layers thin somewhat when the stomach is reached, and a plexus of submucosal vessels that are largely oriented transverse to the direction of the myotomy comes into view. It may be appropriate to monitor the inferior extent of myotomy endoscopically to ensure that the lower esophageal sphincter has been completely divided. Endoscopy also can be used to insufflate air into the region of the myotomy to investigate for any possible transmural injury to the esophageal or gastric wall. If such an injury is identified, it is closed with simple interrupted sutures, and an anterior, rather than posterior, fundoplication is performed to reinforce the repair. Once the myotomy is complete (Fig. 6-8C), the muscle layer is grasped and is bluntly dissected from the underlying mucosa for a distance of at least 1 cm, further separating the cut edges of the muscle and helping to prevent the edges from healing together.

Figure 6-8A

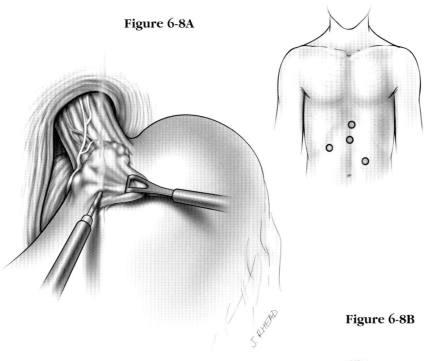

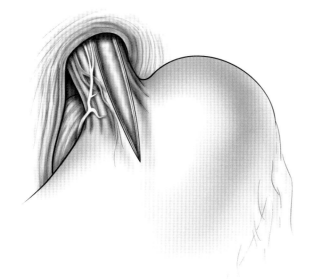

J. RHEAD

Figure 6-8B

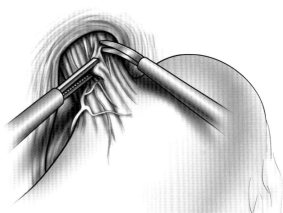

Figure 6-8C

For patients undergoing an anterior fundoplication, an appropriate site on the gastric fundus is selected to begin the wrap on the left of the esophagus, which will permit additional fundus to be folded across the myotomy to reach the right crus. The initial suture is placed through the cut edge of muscle on the left side of the esophagus about 2 cm above the esophagogastric junction. Two additional sutures are placed, 1 cm apart, extending caudad to complete the left side of the wrap. The wrap is continued with a suture placed from the fundus, through the cut edge of muscle on the right side of the esophagus, and through the right crus about 2 cm proximal to the esophagogastric junction (Fig. 6-8D). Two additional sutures are placed 1 cm apart, completing the wrap and covering the lower part of the myotomy (Fig. 6-8E).

If a posterior fundoplication is performed, it is accomplished for the most part as described in Section 6-4. The gastric fundus is grasped and is positioned posterior to the esophagus. The initial suture is placed 2 cm above the esophagogastric junction on the left side through the fundus and the cut edge of the esophagus. Two additional sutures are placed at 1-cm intervals extending caudad, ending just above the esphagogastric junction. The fundus lying to the right side of the esophagus is sutured to the cut edge of the muscle on the right side of the esophagus in a similar fashion. This portion of the fundus is also attached to the right pillar of the hiatus with interrupted sutures (Fig. 6-8F).

Postoperative management after esophageal myotomy is straightforward. No nasograstric drainage is necessary. A liquid diet is begun on the same afternoon as the operation, and patients are discharged on this diet the following day. The diet is advanced to soft solid food after a period of several days, and a regular diet, absent foods of high fiber content, is resumed within a week to 10 days.

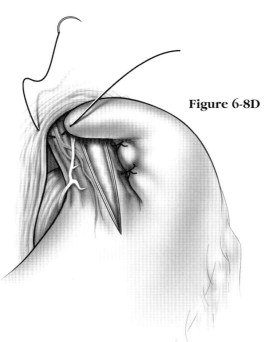

Figure 6-8D

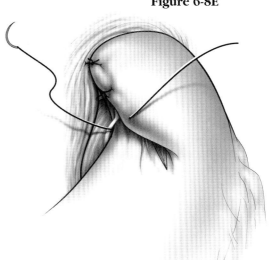

Figure 6-8E

Figure 6-8F

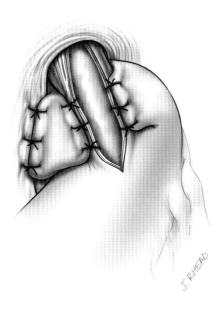

6-9 Thoracic Approaches to Esophageal Myotomy

Myotomy for management of achalasia, diffuse esophageal spasm, high amplitude peristaltic contractions of the esophagus, and nonspecific motility disorders associated with esophageal diverticulum can be performed through a left thoracotomy or via a left thoracoscopic approach. Indications for using this approach rather than an abdominal approach include prohibitive intraabdominal adhesions, the need for a myotomy that extends more cephalad than typical for an abdominal approach, and the need to manage a pulsion diverticulum that is not accessible through an abdominal approach. More information on management of pulsion diverticula is included later in Section 6-10.

Anesthetic considerations are similar to those for laparoscopic esophageal myotomy; specifically, the patient is maintained on a liquid diet for two to three days preoperatively, anesthesia is induced with the patient in mild reverse Trendelenberg position, and a rapid sequence induction is performed. A double lumen tube or bronchial blocker is placed to permit isolation of the left lung. Endoscopy is performed initially to evacuate any retained food or fluid from the posterior oropharynx and esophagus. The patient is placed in a true right lateral decubitus position (see Fig. 6-9A inset). Options for approaching the esophagus include thoracoscopy or a standard lateral thoracotomy. The thoracoscopic approach is discussed first; it is most appropriate for performance of a myotomy limited to the esophagus and lower esophageal sphincter, sparing the stomach, when no fundoplication is planned.

As with many minimally invasive operations, correct port placement is essential to success. The camera port is positioned between the mid and anterior axillary lines in about the eighth interspace. A port is placed superior and anterior to this to permit lung retraction. Two operating ports are placed in the posterior axillary line relatively low in the thorax. An additional port can be placed in the costophrenic sulcus to provide inferior displacement of the diaphragm, exposing the hiatus (see Fig. 6-9A inset; Fig. 6-9A). Sometimes this exposure can be gained by placing a heavy suture in the dome of the diaphragm, which is passed through a small access site near the costophrenic sulcus; traction on the suture exposes the hiatus, eliminating the need for an additional port.

The pulmonary ligament is divided, exposing the esophagus to the level of the inferior pulmonary vein. The myotomy is started about 5 cm proximal to the esophagogastric junction (Fig. 6-9B). A dilute solution of epinephrine is injected submucosally to reduce bleeding (and the need for cautery near the mucosa) and to help develop the plane of dissection. Using cautery scissors the muscle layers of the esophagus are divided to expose the submucosal plane. This plane is dissected bluntly for a centimeter or so at a time, after which the overlying muscle is divided. Dissection is carried caudad to the hiatus, and is extended another 1 cm or so to conclusively divide the muscles that make up the lower esophageal high-pressure zone (Fig. 6-9C) as the esophagus is retracted superiorly. The myotomy deliberately ends prior to division of the muscular layers of the stomach, and no dissection of the hiatus is performed. This leaves most of the antireflux mechanisms intact, and thus no fundoplication is required. Using blunt dissection, the muscle layers are dissected from the underlying mucosa (see Fig. 6-9C inset).

The proximal extent of myotomy depends on the underlying pathology. For managing achalasia, a short myotomy is usually sufficient. However, patients with vigorous achalasia who have pain as a prominent symptom component, may benefit from extending the myotomy at least to the level of the inferior pulmonary vein, especially if the muscular layers are thickened to this level. Patients with diffuse spasm should also have a longer myotomy performed.

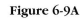

Figure 6-9A

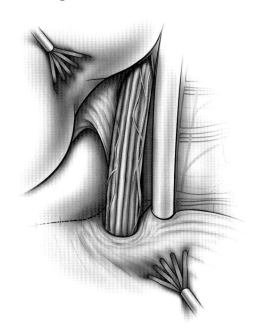

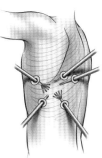

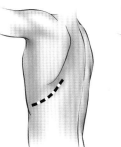

Figure 6-9B

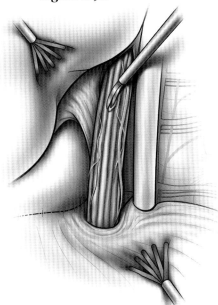

Figure 6-9C

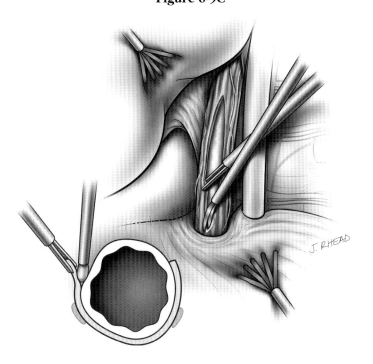

J. RHEAD

An open transthoracic myotomy is performed in a somewhat similar manner. The anesthetic management of these patients is exactly the same as for thoracoscopic myotomy. The operation is performed through a standard lateral thoracotomy, dividing the latissimus dorsi and sparing the serratus anterior, and entering the eighth intercostal space (see Fig. 6-9D inset). The pulmonary ligament is divided. The esophagus is mobilized circumferentially from distal to the inferior pulmonary vein to the hiatus, taking care to preserve the vagus nerves and keep them with the esophagus during retraction. The hiatus is dissected circumferentially, as described in Section 6-3, to permit performance of a partial fundoplication after completing the myotomy. This dissection must be sufficiently complete to permit drawing the gastric fundus and esophagogastric junction into the thoracic cavity. The gastric fat pad is excised and the esophagogastric junction is clearly identified.

The region of myotomy is identified and injected submucosally with a dilute solution of epinephrine. As for thoracoscopic approaches, a limited distal myotomy (5 cm or so in length) is sufficient for managing achalasia in the absence of symptoms of vigorous achalasia (Fig. 6-9D). A myotomy extending more proximally is appropriate for patients with vigorous achalasia and diffuse esophageal spasm. The myotomy is started cephalad and is extended caudad through the lower esophageal high-pressure zone and for at least 1 cm onto the stomach (Fig. 6-9E). The edges of the cut muscle are dissected from the underlying mucosa for a distance of at least 1 cm. Crural sutures are placed and are left untied.

A partial anterior fundoplication (Belsey) is performed in a manner similar to that described in Section 6-6. After noting the exact level of the esophagogastric junction, the first row of sutures is placed from the gastric fundus 1 cm below the junction to the esophagus and 1 cm above the junction and back again in a "U" fashion. The sutures are positioned to correspond roughly to the position of the vagus nerves on the esophagus. In contrast to a standard Belsey fundoplication, the center stitch is omitted when performing this wrap over a myotomy. The sutures are tied. The second row of sutures is placed 1 cm more distal on the stomach and 1 cm more proximal on the esophagus, and the lower ends are brought through the diaphragm from the peritoneal to the pleural surface. Again, the center suture is eliminated from this row (Fig. 6-9F). The fundoplication is reduced into the abdomen and the sutures are tied, anchoring the wrap to the underside of the diaphragm. The crural sutures are tied, leaving space alongside the esophagus within the hiatus sufficient to permit passage of a fingertip only (Fig. 6-9G).

Postoperative management after transthoracic myotomy and partial fundoplication is uncomplicated. A single pleural drainage catheter is sufficient, and this is usually removed on the first postoperative day. Oral liquids are begun within the first one or two postoperative days. The patient is advanced to a soft, low residue diet after several days, and is not permitted to have a normal diet for a week or two postoperatively. The patient is discharged when the drain is removed, pain is controlled on oral analgesics, and a liquid diet is tolerated.

Figure 6-9D

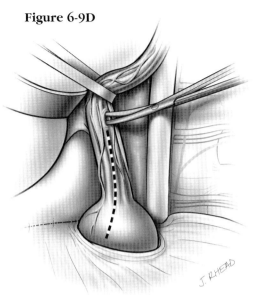

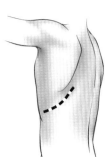

Figure 6-9E

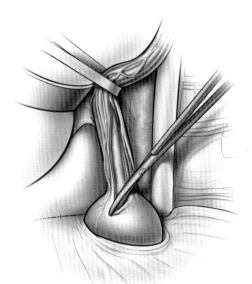

Figure 6-9F

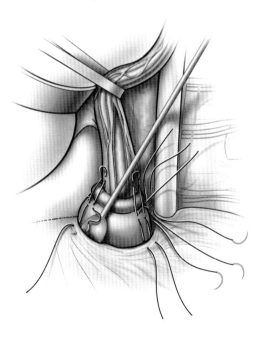

Figure 6-9G

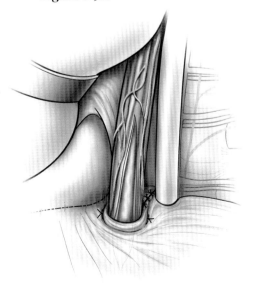

6-10 Management of Pulsion Diverticula

Pulsion diverticula are uncommon products of nonspecific esophageal motility disorders. They appear to arise through preexisting defects in the esophageal wall, perhaps associated with perforating vessels, in the setting of high-pressure segmenting contractions of the esophagus. Because the relationship between these diverticula and an underlying motility disorder is not always recognized, surgeons sometimes fail to include myotomy as an essential element of their surgical management. This results in an unacceptably high incidence of recurrent diverticulum or leakage at the resection site. Indications for treatment of pulsion diverticula include frequent regurgitation of undigested food, resulting in a risk of aspiration, and dysphagia from the underlying motility disorder. Wide-mouthed diverticula that rarely retain food and fluid often can be managed nonsurgically.

Diverticula that are located near the esophagogastric junction may be managed with resection and myotomy through a laparoscopic approach. Most diverticula, however, are best managed using an open or video-assisted transthoracic approach. Diverticula typically present posterior and to the right of the esophagus. However, the optimal approach to their management is through the left chest, which provides better access to the esophagus hiatus and permits a long myotomy when necessary. Preoperative management on a liquid diet for two to three days helps to eliminate retained food in the diverticulum. Anesthetic management should include induction in a reverse Trendelenberg position, use of a rapid sequence technique, and airway management permitting left lung isolation. Esophagoscopy following induction permits evacuation of any retained food from the diverticulum and the esophagus.

After retraction of the lung anteriorly and superiorly, the esophagus is mobilized circumferentially from the inferior pulmonary vein to the hiatus. Care is taken to preserve the vagus nerves. The diverticulum presents medially and is grasped with Babcock clamps and retracted into the pleural space after being dissected from surrounding tissues. This rotates the esophagus nearly 180 degrees (see Fig. 6-10A inset). The investing connective tissue is dissected from the surface of the diverticulum and is excised at the level of the esophagus (Fig. 6-10A). Care is taken to preserve the adjacent right vagus nerve. When the neck of the diverticulum is exposed, the diverticulum is excised with a stapler at this level or is clamped, divided, and oversewn (Fig. 6-10B). In either case, after closure of the esophageal mucosal layer, the overlying muscle layer is sutured to reinforce the closure (Fig. 6-10C).

The esophagus is rotated back to a neutral position (see Fig. 6-10D inset). A location on the esophageal wall directly opposite the diverticulectomy is identified for esophageal myotomy. Dilute epinephrine is injected submucosally to aid in the dissection in this plane. The myotomy is begun at the level of the diverticulectomy and is extended cephalad and caudad beyond the upper and lower limits of the diverticulectomy closure (Fig. 6-10D). For low-lying diverticula it may be appropriate to extend the myotomy through the lower esophageal sphincter, which then requires creation of a partial fundoplication as previously described in Section 6-9. A nasogastric tube is placed prior to completing the operation.

Postoperative management includes nasogastric drainage for a period of two or three days to eliminate undue pressure on the staple/suture line. Patients are then started on a liquid diet and are not advanced to solid food for a period of at least several days. A regular diet may be resumed after a week.

Figure 6-10A

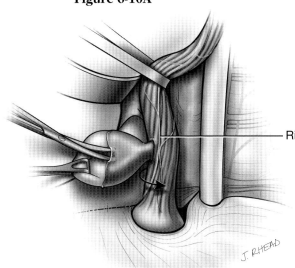

Rotated cross-sectional view

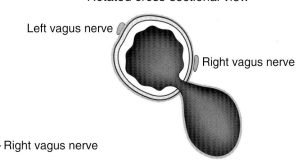

Left vagus nerve

Right vagus nerve

Right vagus nerve

J. R'HEAD

Figure 6-10B

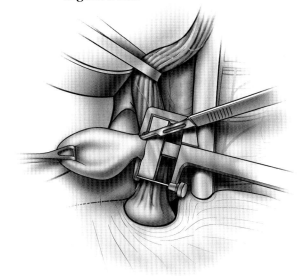

Figure 6-10C

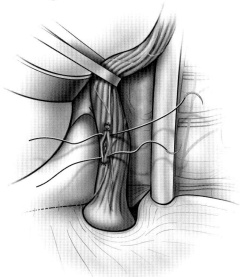

Figure 6-10D

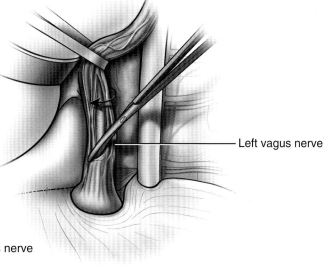

Left vagus nerve

De-rotated cross-sectional view

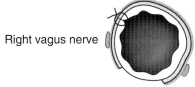

Right vagus nerve

Left vagus nerve

6-11 Management of Pharyngoesophageal Diverticulum

Pharyngoesophageal (Zenker's) diverticulum results from a lack of coordination between pharyngeal constrictor muscle contraction during deglutition and relaxation of the cricopharyngeus muscle. The resultant high segmental pressures create a pseudodiverticulum emerging through Killian's triangle, an area relatively devoid of investing musculature located posteriorly between the inferior pharyngeal constrictor and the cricopharyngeus muscle. Abbreviated expressions of this process include the presence of a cricopharyngeal bar, which is evident as a prominent indentation extending from posterior on lateral views of an esophagram. Intervention is appropriate in the presence of frequent regurgitation, moderate to severe dysphagia, or aspiration pneumonia. The traditional approach to treating a pharyngoesophageal diverticulum is transcervical cricopharyngeal myotomy followed by appropriate management of the diverticulum. An alternative approach is transoral division of the septum between the esophagus and diverticulum, creating a common cavity. The open approach is described first.

For open cricopharyngeal myotomy, the patient is instructed to take liquids for a period of two to three days preoperatively to help eliminate any solid material that might be retained in the diverticulum. General anesthesia is induced with the patient in reverse Trendelenberg position using a rapid sequence induction to help prevent aspiration. Esophagoscopy is performed to remove any contents of the diverticulum or esophagus that might put the patient at risk for aspiration. The patient is positioned supine with the neck neutral or slightly extended and with the head rotated slightly to the right. The diverticulum usually presents to the left, and therefore the operation is most easily performed through the left neck. The incision may be made parallel to the sternocleidomastoid muscle, but the region of interest is centered on the cricopharyngeus muscle, which lies at the level of the cricoid cartilage, and so a horizontal incision in a skin crease at this level provides excellent exposure and is superior from a cosmetic perspective (see Fig. 6-11A inset).

The strap muscles are retracted medially and a plane is developed medial to the sternocleidomastoid muscle and medial to the carotid sheath. It is sometimes necessary to divide a middle thyroid vein, but encountering other important vessels in this plane is rare. Care is taken to avoid injury to the recurrent laryngeal nerve. The prevertebral plane is developed posterior to the esopha-

gus. At this point the diverticulum is evident extending in the direction of the mediastinum. Gentle traction with Babcock clamps is usually sufficient to elevate the diverticulum into the incision (Fig. 6-11A). Using blunt dissection, the tip of the diverticulum is easily dissected from any loose mediastinal attachments. The investing fascia is dissected from the diverticulum to the level of the neck of the diverticulum. Careful delineation of the true diverticulum at this level makes the subsequent myotomy straightforward.

Using scissors or a right angle to dissect submucosally beneath the cricopharyngeus, while simultaneously retracting the diverticulum cephalad, the plane of dissection is easily identified. The muscle layers are divided completely as the myotomy is extended completely through the cricopharyngeus muscle and onto the esophagus for a distance of 4 to 5 cm (Fig. 6-11B). The edges of the muscle are bluntly dissected from the underlying mucosa for a distance of at least 1 cm. The mucosa should bulge out from between the cut edges without evident hindrance at this point in the operation.

Having completed the myotomy, arguably the key portion of the operation, management of the diverticulum may take one of several forms. If the patient only has a cricopharyngeal bar or has a small (1 to 2 cm) diverticulum, no further therapy is necessary. Larger diverticula require definitive therapy. One option is to invert the diverticulum such that it lies upside down relative to its normal position. The diverticulum is then flattened against the prevertebral fascia posterior to the inferior pharyngeal constrictor and is sutured to the prevertebral fascia with interrupted mattress sutures (Fig. 6-11C). It is best to place all of the sutures through the fascia first, because once the diverticulum is positioned in this relatively small space there is little room to permit suture placement. Alternatively, the diverticulum is excised by stapling it shut across its neck and excising the sac (Fig. 6-11D). This exposes the patient to a small risk of suture line leak, which is not present if diverticulopexy is performed.

An alternative to traditional open methods of managing cricopharyngeal diverticulum is transoral stapling to create a common cavity between the esophagus and diverticulum. This procedure has been described in many forms since the early 20th century, but the introduction of the linear cutting stapler has greatly improved the safety of this technique. The procedure gives results that are similar to but perhaps not quite as good as a more traditional open approach. The transoral technique is best used in patients who have good neck extension, whose diverticula are between 2 and 4 cm in length, and who are not optimal candidates for an open approach.

Figure 6-11A

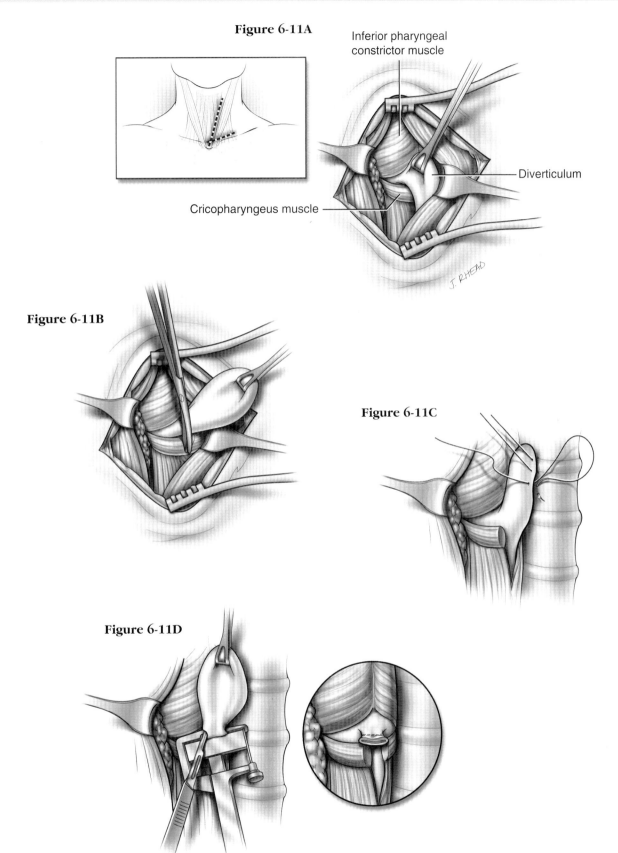

Inferior pharyngeal
constrictor muscle

Diverticulum

Cricopharyngeus muscle

J. R. HEAD

Figure 6-11B

Figure 6-11C

Figure 6-11D

The procedure is performed under general endotracheal anesthesia, and the attendant considerations are similar to those for the open procedure. The patient is positioned supine with the neck extended. Standing at the patient's head, a special laryngoscope is inserted with one blade in the esophagus and the second blade in the diverticulum, exposing the muscle wall of the esophagus and the wall of the diverticulum between the two blades (Fig. 6-11E). The diverticulum is suctioned clear to prevent aspiration during the procedure. A modified linear cutting stapler, with the typical 1-cm blunt terminal end considerably shortened, is inserted with the stapler cartridge in the esophagus and the anvil in the diverticulum (Fig. 6-11F). When the stapler is inserted maximally such that there will be minimal residual diverticulum at the conclusion of the procedure, it is closed and fired, creating a common cavity between the esophagus and diverticulum (Fig. 6-11G). Although food will continue to pass into the diverticulum, the absence of a barrier between the esophagus and diverticulum permits immediate emptying of the cavity and passage down the esophagus (Fig. 6-11H). Over time it is expected that the diverticulum tissues will retract, making the passage of food more linear in orientation.

Patients are permitted to take liquids by mouth immediately after cricopharyngeal myotomy, and discharge is usually possible on the first postoperative day. Patients do not resume a normal diet until at least one week postoperatively, and are instructed to eat slowly and chew carefully to avoid aspiration while they regain coordination and muscle strength in their deglutitive mechanisms.

Figure 6-11E

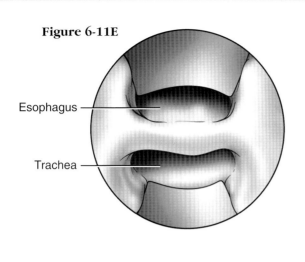

Esophagus

Trachea

Figure 6-11F

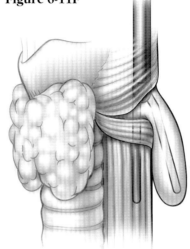

Figure 6-11G

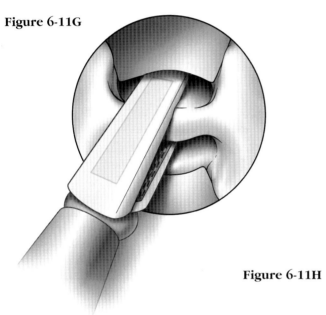

Figure 6-11H

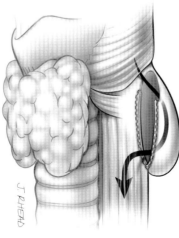

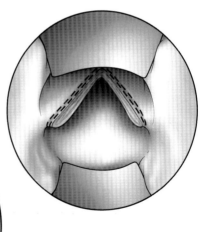

J. RHEAD

6-12 Transhiatal Esophagectomy

Transhiatal esophagectomy is a common approach for managing both benign and malignant disease. Indications for using this technique rather than open esophagectomy include carcinoma limited to the esophageal mucosa, end-stage acid reflux disease or motility disorders not requiring nodal dissection, and gastroesophageal junction tumors for which a standard regional nodal dissection can be performed without performing a thoracotomy. Relative contraindications include reoperative esophageal surgery in which there has been extensive mobilization of the thoracic esophagus, primary esophageal cancer extending beyond the esophageal wall or associated with extensive adenopathy, and, in some cases, tumors of the middle and upper thoracic esophagus that cannot be visualized using this approach. As with most esophageal surgical approaches, the training and preference of the surgeon are important determinants of the appropriate technique for an individual patient.

The patient is positioned supine, and the arms are positioned alongside the patient's torso. Careful positioning and padding help avoid pressure on monitoring lines, compression injuries to nerves, and inadequate access to the rails on the sides of the operating table, which are used to mount self-retaining retractors. Epidural analgesia is usually insufficient to cover the extent of dissection required for this operation, but may be used to provide analgesia for the laparotomy portion. Central pressure monitoring is not usually required unless the patient has a history of cardiovascular problems. A single lumen endotracheal tube is sufficient for airway management.

The initial approach is through a laparotomy, consisting of either an upper midline incision or an inverted "V" (chevron) incision (see Fig. 6-12A inset). Exploration of the abdomen is performed to eliminate the possibility of associated pathology that would change the conduct of the operation. It is often useful to mobilize the left lobe of the liver to provide adequate access to the hiatus. Self-retaining retractors are placed to keep the wound open and elevate the liver. Assuming that the stomach is to be used as the reconstructive organ, the gastric dissection is performed after the ability to accomplish a complete resection is confirmed. The greater curve is mobilized preserving the right gastroepiploic vessels. The left gastric and short gastric vessels are sacrificed. The gastrohepatic ligament is divided, taking care to ensure that an aberrant left hepatic artery is not sacrificed. The left gastric vessels are divided at their bases. In the case of cancer, an appropriate lymph node dissection is performed, depending on the location of the cancer and on the oncologic philosophy of the surgeon.

The peritoneum overlying the esophagus is divided, freeing the esophagus from the crura bilaterally (Fig. 6-12A). The attachments of the esophagus to the retroperitoneum are divided and the esophagus is encircled with an umbilical tape or Penrose drain to permit downward traction on the esophagus during subsequent dissection. If necessary, the hiatus is widened by dividing it anteriorly to permit more access to the lower mediastinum. The attachments to the esophagus that are visible are divided. It is best to divide the vagus nerves at this point in the operation as high in the mediastinum as is feasible.

Although some authors state that dissection under direct vision can be performed to the level of the carina, this is not typically the case. When no further attachments are accessible under direct vision, manual dissection is performed. This is begun posteriorly on the wall of the esophagus, where there is the least risk of injury to surrounding structures, separating the esophagus from the prevertebral fascia. Straying into periesophageal tissues risks additional bleeding and can lead to entry into inappropriate planes of dissection and subsequent complications. The posterior dissection is performed bluntly by extending one or two fingers gently in a stepwise manner to the level of the carina (Fig. 6-12B). When this has been accomplished, a similar dissection is performed anteriorly. The dissecting fingers are swept from side to side after the anterior dissection is accomplished, freeing a portion of the lateral attachments of the esophagus (Fig. 6-12C). When the vagal plexus is reached between the level of the inferior pulmonary vein and the carina, dissection beneath the plexus preserves the bronchial branches, lessening the risk of postoperative pulmonary complications. Particular care is taken to stay on the esophageal wall when the periaortic tissues are dissected. Avulsion of just one of the four or five arteries leading directly from the aorta to the esophagus may lead to bleeding requiring a thoracotomy to control. This is avoided by keeping the dissection plane close to the esophageal wall, where the aortic branches have arborized into end vessels that spasm sufficiently to stop bleeding in a short period of time. The dissection is complete when the esophagus has been circumferentially mobilized to the level of the carina.

The neck is opened using a transverse incision in a skin crease at or below the level of the cricoid cartilage or using an incision parallel to the medial edge of the sternocleidomastoid muscle. Anatomic studies suggest that approaching the esophagus from the left neck rather than the right neck reduces the risk of recurrent laryngeal nerve injury. Dissection is carried between the carotid sheath and strap muscles to the prevertebral plane. The prevertebral plane is dissected medially to the contralateral side and inferiorly as far as the dissecting finger reaches. Taking care to avoid injury to the

Figure 6-12A

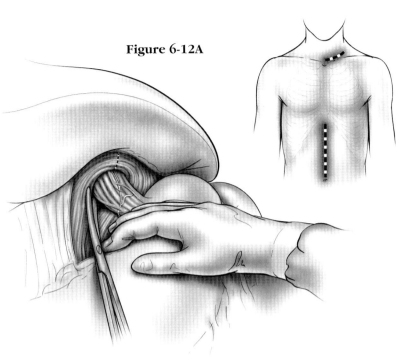

Figure 6-12B

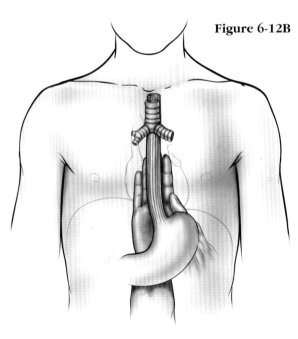

Figure 6-12C

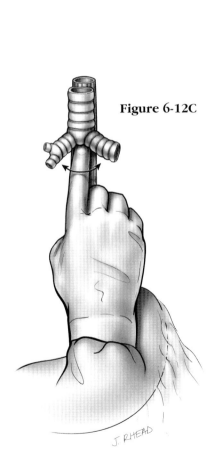

recurrent laryngeal nerve, the plane between the esophagus and trachea is developed. Finger dissection is used to free the contralateral margin of the esophagus to the prevertebral plane, completing the circumferential dissection (Fig. 6-12D). An umbilical tape is passed around the esophagus to facilitate distal dissection.

Placing traction on the proximal tape, the esophagus is bluntly dissected circumferentially to the level of the carina. It is often necessary to work from below and above alternately to enable sufficient traction on the remaining attachments to localize and divide them (Fig. 6-12E). When the esophagus has been completely mobilized it moves freely up and down within the mediastinum as traction is placed on one or the other traction tape. As much esophagus as possible is retracted out of the cervical incision and a point for transection is selected, optimizing the length of esophagus resected in the case of a cancer, but preserving more of the esophagus when surgery is performed for benign disease.

A long umbilical tape is placed lengthwise on the anterior surface of the esophagus and is included in the staple line of the transection, which is performed with a linear cutting stapler (Fig. 6-12F). The short proximal end of the umbilical tape marks the anterior surface of the cervical esophagus, enabling it to be identified for purposes of a subsequent anastomosis. The long end, which is attached to the distal cut end of the cervical esophagus, is also sutured to the esophagus to prevent its being dislodged as the esophagus is drawn into the abdomen. The end of the umbilical tape that is not attached to the esophagus is retained with a hemostat to prevent its being drawn into the mediastinum. The tape thus provides a guide to the esophageal bed in the posterior mediastinum, which will form the route for future reconstruction (Fig. 6-12G). Once the esophagus is in the abdomen, it is transected, including the lesser curvature of the stomach, creating a gastric tube for reconstruction. Alternatively, the entire stomach is preserved and a different method of reconstruction is performed, such as long segment colon interposition.

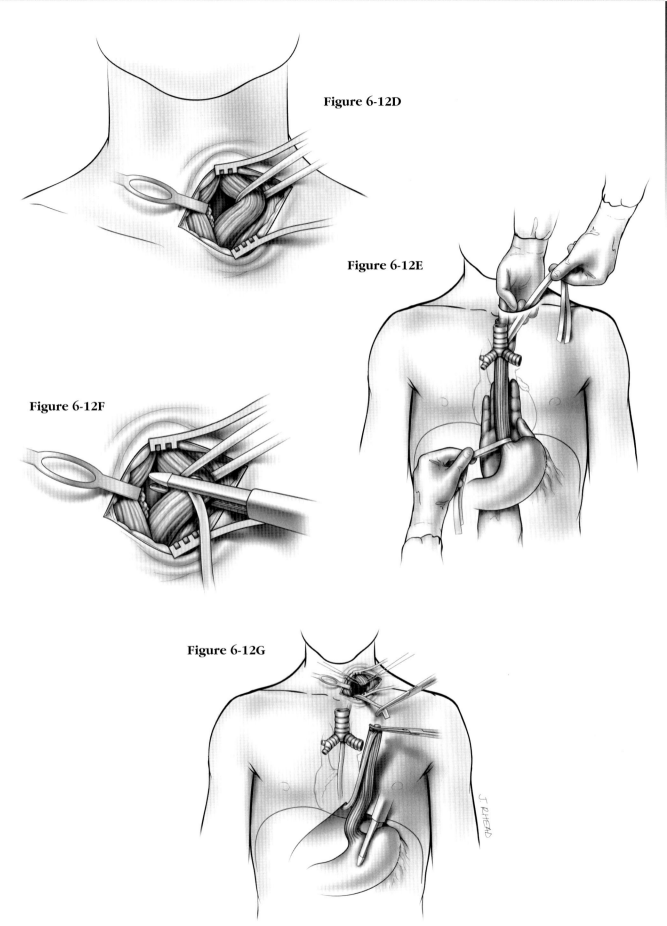

Figure 6-12D

Figure 6-12E

Figure 6-12F

Figure 6-12G

6-13   Ivor Lewis Esophagectomy

The most common approach to esophagectomy is the Ivor Lewis technique, which can be performed open or using minimally invasive surgery. When done using an open technique, it can be performed through a laparotomy and thoracotomy with a high intrathoracic anastomosis (2-hole approach) or adding a cervical incision to permit a cervical anastomosis (3-hole esophagectomy). This technique can be used for virtually any esophagectomy, although exposure to the hiatus is not as good as when a low left thoracotomy is used (see Section 6-14). However, the exposure to the remaining thoracic esophagus, associated lymph nodes, azygos vein, and thoracic duct is ideal. There are no specific contraindications to this operation, although the number and location of the incisions no doubt contribute to a higher risk of pulmonary complications postoperatively, thus making this operative approach less than optimal for patients with compromised performance status or pulmonary dysfunction.

The operation may be performed with the patient in a modified lateral position, exposing the abdomen, chest, and neck simultaneously (Fig. 6-13A). The need to perform an anterolateral thoracotomy is somewhat limiting in providing access to intrathoracic structures, and a right neck incision is frequently used if a cervical anastomosis is performed, which is not as ideal as a left neck incision. Simultaneous exposure of this sort, however, avoids the need to break the sterile field and reposition the patient, and permits a full exploration of the two main body cavities before committing to a resection if contraindications to esophagectomy are identified. Alternatively, and most commonly, the patient is positioned supine for the abdominal portion of the operation and in a true lateral position for the thoracic portion, using a standard lateral or a posterolateral thoracotomy (see Fig. 6-13A). This gives optimal exposure to both the abdomen and the chest. In which position to begin the operation is sometimes controversial, since findings in either body cavity can lead to inoperability, and a full exploration cannot be completed until the dissection is completed in the first body cavity that is opened.

The operation will be described using the supine and subsequently the lateral position, with performance of a high intrathoracic anastomosis. This is a useful approach for both open and minimally invasive techniques. Use of an epidural catheter is appropriate for postoperative analgesia if an open approach is selected, but this is not necessary when a minimally invasive technique is employed. Use of a double lumen tube for lung isolation is critical, particularly for a minimally invasive approach. Central pressure monitoring is not required unless patients have underlying cardiovascular impairment.

The abdominal approach is similar to that described for a transhiatal esophagectomy. The stomach is mobilized and prepared for use as a reconstructive organ. The omentum is divided from the greater curvature, preserving the right gastroepiploic arcade. The left gastroepiploic and short gastric vessels are divided. The gastrohepatic ligament is divided and the left gastric vessels are divided near their bases. The extent of lymph node dissection is determined by the preferences of the surgeon. The peritoneum is divided along the right crus, anteriorly across the esophagus, and along the left crus. The retroperitoneal attachments to the stomach are divided. The low attachments to the esophagus in the mediastinum are divided. If a minimally invasive approach is used for the operation, a Penrose drain is placed around the low intrathoracic esophagus to facilitate the thoracoscopic dissection. If desired, a gastric emptying procedure is performed (pyloromyotomy or pyloroplasty).

The chest is opened through the fifth or sixth interspace, depending on the location of the tumor and the habitus of the patient. In obese patients the diaphragm is elevated, and a higher interspace gives better access. After an exploration has been completed, esophageal mobilization begins. The pulmonary ligament is divided. The pleura is divided posterior and anterior to the esophagus from the diaphragm to the azygos arch (Fig. 6-13B). For a standard esophagectomy the azygos vein and thoracic duct are left intact. A radical en bloc esophagectomy often includes resection of one or both of these structures. The esophagus is mobilized from its bed including all soft tissue extending to the lung, pericardium, aorta, and opposite pleura. If not already accomplished, the hiatus is opened circumferentially to complete the mobilization of the esophagus and stomach to the level of the azygos vein (Fig. 6-13C). All associated lymph nodes are resected and are labeled according to their stations. Care is taken in dissecting the subcarinal region to avoid thermal injury to the membranous left mainstem bronchus, which is distended by the bronchial cuff of the double lumen tube (Fig. 6-13D).

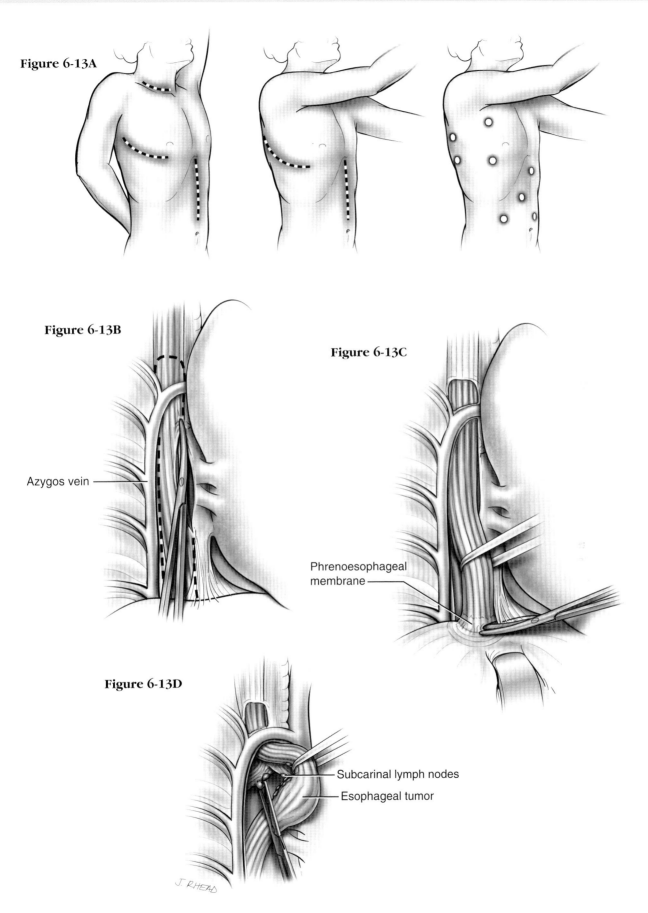

Figure 6-13A

Figure 6-13B

Azygos vein

Figure 6-13C

Phrenoesophageal membrane

Figure 6-13D

Subcarinal lymph nodes

Esophageal tumor

J. RHEAD

The pleura is divided superior to the azygos vein and the vein is dissected. It is transected and ligated or is divided with a linear vascular stapler. If the esophageal tumor is adjacent to the vein, a segment of the vein is resected en bloc with the specimen (Fig. 6-13E). The esophagus is mobilized superiorly to the desired level. Lymph nodes are dissected from the recurrent laryngeal nerve stations without injuring the nerves (Fig. 6-13F).

It is usually appropriate to prophylactically ligate the thoracic duct to prevent the development of a chylo-thorax postoperatively. This is accomplished by in situ ligation rather than requiring formal identification and dissection of the duct. The pleura is opened immediately medial to the azygos vein a few centimeters superior to the diaphragm. A right angle clamp is passed against the underlying prevertebral fascia, encompassing all soft tissues lateral to the aorta (Fig. 6-13G). A heavy ligature is passed around the tissue, which includes the thoracic duct, and is tied (see Fig. 6-13G inset).

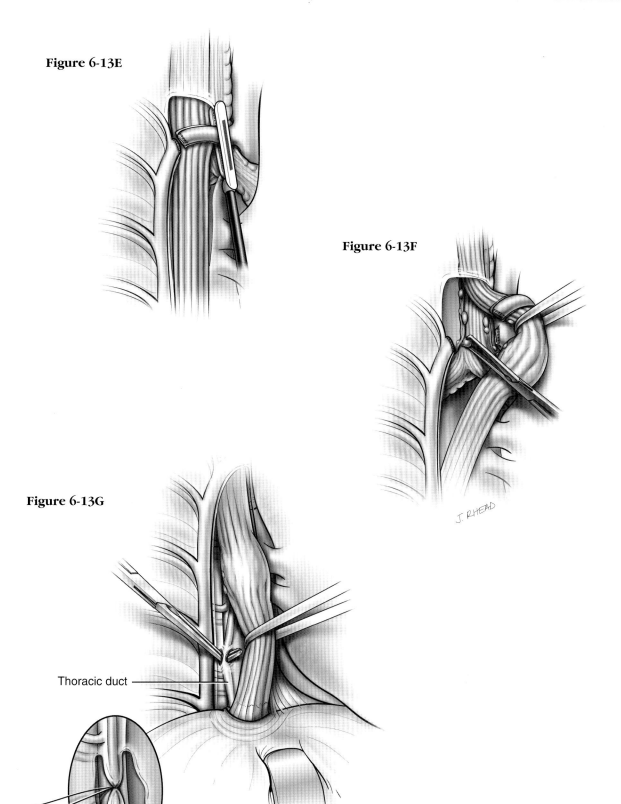

Figure 6-13E

Figure 6-13F

J. RHEAD

Figure 6-13G

Thoracic duct

6-14 Esophagectomy via Left Thoracotomy

Use of a so-called exclusive left thoracotomy for esophagectomy is most appropriate for benign disease and for tumors of the distal third of the esophagus and the esophagogastric junction. The approach, including a peripheral diaphragm incision, provides excellent access to the upper abdominal organs including the stomach, spleen, pancreas, transverse colon, and gallbladder. This exposure, while excellent, does take some practice to adjust to. The approach offers the possibility of extending the incision across the costal margin into the upper abdomen (thoracoabdominal incision), providing even greater access to the upper abdomen. The primary contraindication to use of this technique is a tumor lying at the level of or proximal to the aortic arch.

The operation is performed with the patient in a full lateral position (see Fig. 6-14A inset). If it is anticipated that a thoracoabdominal approach might be necessary, the patient's hips are rolled slightly open to provide more abdominal exposure. Use of an epidural catheter for postoperative analgesia is appropriate, and a double lumen tube or bronchial blocker is placed to facilitate ipsilateral lung isolation. There is no need for central venous pressure monitoring unless the patient has underlying cardiovascular disease. A standard lateral or posterolateral incision is performed in the seventh or eighth intercostal space to provide optimal access to the distal esophagus and proximal abdomen.

The pleura anterior and posterior to the esophagus is divided from the hiatus to the arch of the aorta (Fig. 6-14A). The esophagus is mobilized, taking with it all surrounding soft tissue excluding the pericardium and contralateral pleura. Posterolaterally there are usually three to five small direct branches from the aorta to the esophagus that require specific control, but the remainder of the dissection can be performed sharply or with electrocautery. Medially, the pericardium is grasped with an Allis clamp or Kocher clamp and is elevated, exposing the mediastinum to aid in the dissection. This permits visualization of the contralateral pleura, which is bluntly dissected from the tissues being resected and is left intact. Although it is feasible to include the azygos vein and/or thoracic duct in the resection through this approach, en bloc esophagectomy is not ideally suited to the approach and is best reserved for performing through a right thoracotomy.

The vagus nerves are divided below the level of the aortic arch. The pleura is opened superior to the aortic arch (Fig. 6-14B) and the esophagus is dissected circumferentially, taking care to avoid injury to the recurrent laryngeal nerve, the hemiazygos vein, and the left subclavian artery. The esophagus is surrounded with an umbilical tape or Penrose drain both above and below the arch. Using these to retract, the segment of esophagus passing medial to the arch is dissected circumferentially (Fig. 6-14C). Some of this dissection is performed bluntly within the vagal plexus to avoid denervation of the airways.

The esophagus is dissected from the hiatus. The peritoneum is grasped and divided, and the peritoneal cavity is entered. The peritoneum is divided circumferentially around the esophagus, separating it from the hiatal structures. There is often a small branch of an inferior phrenic artery that joins with a branch of the left gastric artery posteriorly (Belsey's artery) that requires ligation. The retroperitoneal portion of the dissection is complete when the left lobe of the liver is visible posterolaterally through the hiatus.

Figure 6-14A

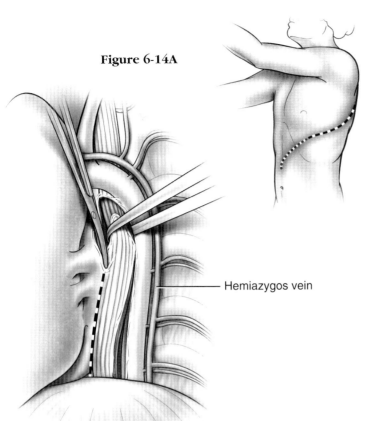

Hemiazygos vein

Figure 6-14B

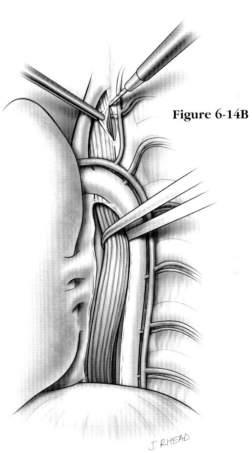

Figure 6-14C

J. RHEAD

The abdominal portion of the operation is begun by dividing the diaphragm from the sternum to the tip of the spleen (see Fig. 6-14D inset). The incision is performed so that at minimum a 2-cm rim of diaphragm is left on the chest wall to permit subsequent closure of the diaphragm. Electrocautery is used to divide the muscle and leave the peritoneum intact until complete hemostasis is accomplished. The peritoneal cavity is then entered. An exploration is undertaken to ensure that there is no contraindication to proceeding with esophagectomy.

The stomach is retracted into the wound, putting the omentum on stretch (Fig. 6-14D). The omentum is divided from the greater curvature of the stomach, leaving the right gastroepiploic arcade intact. The left gastroepiploic and short gastric vessels are divided. The gastrohepatic omentum is divided. The peritoneum overlying the proximal esophagus is opened, exposing the mobilized esophagus. Retroperitoneal attachments to the stomach are divided. The left gastric vessels are divided near their bases. Access to these vessels is somewhat limited from this approach, and extra care should be taken to secure them, since bleeding from this site is difficult to control when operating through the left chest (Fig. 6-14E). A gastric emptying procedure (pyloroplasty, pyloromyotomy) is performed.

The reconstructive conduit is prepared according to the needs of the individual patient. For purely benign disease affecting only the distal esophagus, it is feasible to resect only a short segment of the organ and perform an anastomosis at the level of the inferior pulmonary vein. This would not require dissection of the esophagus proximal to the aortic arch. Care must be taken in making this decision, and it is advisable that a reconstructive organ with reliable peristaltic characteristics be selected to avoid constant reflux from the conduit into the esophagus proximal to the anastomosis.

Figure 6-14D

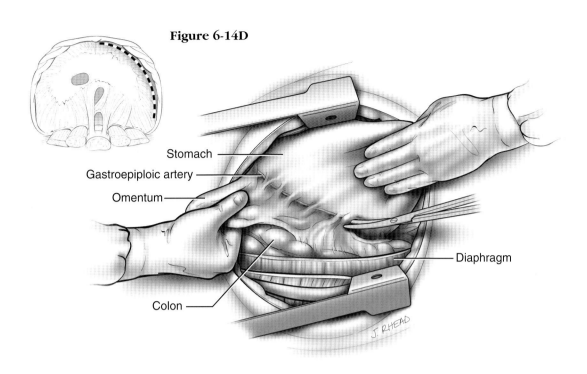

Stomach

Gastroepiploic artery

Omentum

Diaphragm

Colon

J. RHEAD

Figure 6-14E

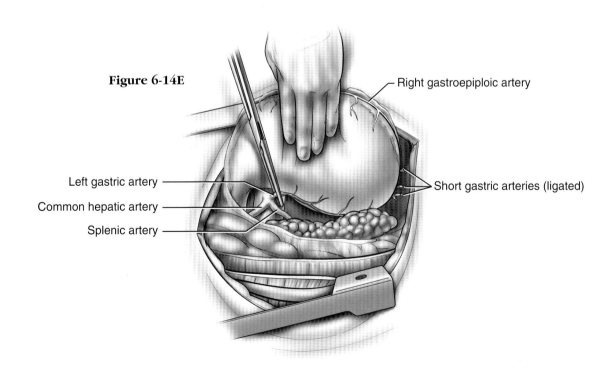

Right gastroepiploic artery

Left gastric artery

Short gastric arteries (ligated)

Common hepatic artery

Splenic artery

Under most circumstances a high intrathoracic anastomosis or a cervical anastomosis is performed, requiring division of the esophagus at an appropriate level (aortic arch for the former, apex of the hemithorax for the latter). The latter procedure is undertaken with the patient supine, requiring that the reconstructive conduit be positioned medial to the aortic arch with sufficient length to reach to the neck. The hiatus is sutured to the conduit with interrupted stitches to prevent herniation of abdominal contents into the left hemithorax.

It is more challenging to create an anastomosis proximal to the arch. The reconstructive conduit is passed medial to the aortic arch and, along with the stump of the esophagus, is brought through the previously created pleural window into the hemithorax. An end-to-side anastomosis is performed with a circular stapler or using a suture technique (Fig. 6-14F). The reconstructive organ is pulled caudad to align the organs axially, leaving the anastomosis medial to the aortic arch. Having thus eliminated intrathoracic redundancy in the reconstructive organ, the hiatus is sutured to the organ with interrupted stitches.

Appropriate closure of the diaphragm is vital to ensuring that breakdown of the suture line is prevented, avoiding herniation of abdominal contents into the left hemithorax. The edges are carefully aligned, making up for redundancy of the medial portion in comparison to the chest wall portion caused by stretching during retraction to facilitate the abdominal part of the operation. Figure-of-eight stitches are placed using heavy nonabsorbable sutures, taking bites at least 1 cm from the edges of the incision and 1 cm apart, making certain that both pleural and peritoneal fascial edges are included in each bite (Fig. 6-14G). A chest tube is placed. The incision is closed in a standard fashion.

Figure 6-14F

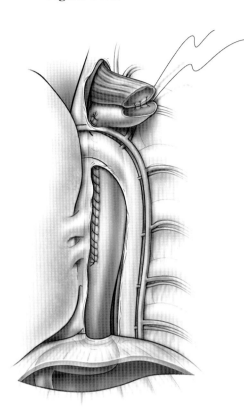

Figure 6-14G

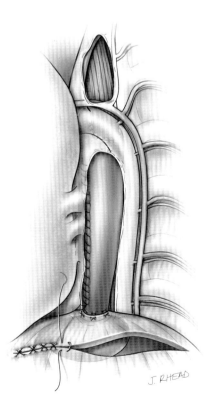

J. RHEAD

6-15   Three Field Lymphadenectomy

The standard two field lymphadenectomy for esophageal cancer encompasses proximal perigastric lymph nodes, including left gastric artery nodes and celiac axis nodes, and extends to the subcarinal region. Metastases to other nodal stations in the abdomen are known to occur, as are metastases to cervical lymph nodes, regardless of the tumor cell type and location. For this reason, an extended, or three field, lymphadenectomy is recommended by some surgeons as a means for maximally clearing involved tissues at the time of esophagectomy. Advantages include improved staging and possibly improved overall survival. The latter advantage is claimed by some surgeons and is a generally accepted premise in Japan, but clear proof of this principle has not been established. Indications for a three field lymphadenectomy include an intrathoracic cancer, evidence for technical respectability (R0 resection), and the likelihood of nodal involvement by the tumor (tumor more advanced than T1a; abnormal lymph nodes on endoscopic ultrasonography [EUS] or positron emission tomography [PET]). Contraindications include advanced age, poor performance status, cardiopulmonary dysfunction, and inability to resect all evident tumor, including the presence of a T4 tumor. The incidence of unilateral or bilateral recurrent laryngeal nerve dysfunction after this operation is high, and patients with preexisting, compromised pulmonary function are at high risk for important pulmonary complications as a result.

The abdominal portion of the operation is begun in a manner similar to that for a standard esophagectomy. After exploration reveals no evidence for nonresectability, the greater omentum is separated from the transverse colon. The omentum is divided 2 to 3 cm from the right gastroepiploic arcade and is removed as a separate specimen. The left gastroepiploic and short gastric vessels are divided. The stomach is reflected superiorly. The dissection includes all retroperitoneal nodes from the celiac axis, and extends along the splenic artery to the splenic hilum, during which the nodes are swept along with their accompanying soft tissues toward the esophageal hiatus (Fig. 6-15A). To the right of the celiac axis, the nodes and soft tissues proximal to the common hepatic artery are similarly swept cephalad, with the medial limit of the dissection being the inferior vena cava. The left gastric artery is divided at its origin with the celiac axis. As with a standard nodal dissection, the gastrohepatic omentum and lesser curvature lymph nodes are included with the specimen.

The thoracic portion of the dissection is not too dissimilar to the standard two field dissection. The pleura is incised anterior to the esophagus at the pulmonary margin and posterior to the esophagus adjacent to the aorta. The soft tissues included with the esophageal mobilization consist of the thoracic duct, contralateral pleura, and all adjacent lymph nodes inferior to the inferior pulmonary vein. The thoracic duct is ligated near the diaphragm and again near the aortic arch. The azygos vein is divided at either end of its arch, and the transverse segment of the vein is left with the specimen. The soft tissues are dissected with the specimen from the junction of the azygos vein and superior vena cava (SVC) posteriorly, including all nodal tissues adjacent to the right and left mainstem bronchi and all subcarinal tissues extending caudad to the level of the inferior pulmonary vein. This completes the second of the three fields being dissected.

The third field comprises nodal tissues proximal to the tracheal bifurcation extending into the neck. It is dissected both through the thoracotomy incision and through a collar incision. Beginning at the level of the resected azygos arch, right vagus lymph nodes are dissected using a no-touch technique along the nerve (Fig. 6-15B). The retrocaval (pretracheal) space is not disturbed. The specimen is reflected anteriorly and a similar dissection is performed along the left vagus nerve. The origin of the right recurrent laryngeal nerve is identified and the lymph node package adjacent to it is dissected using a no-touch technique into the neck (Fig. 6-15C). Similarly, left recurrent laryngeal nerve lymph nodes are dissected into the neck.

The neck is opened using a collar incision to permit completion of the third field dissection. The recurrent laryngeal node packages are identified bilaterally and the dissection of these cervicothoracic nodes is completed superiorly (Fig. 6-15D). Careful preservation of the recurrent laryngeal nerves is essential in minimizing injury to these important structures. Additional regions that are also dissected bilaterally include inferior deep cervical nodes, which are identified lateral and deep to the carotid sheath. Care is taken to preserve the accessory nerve.

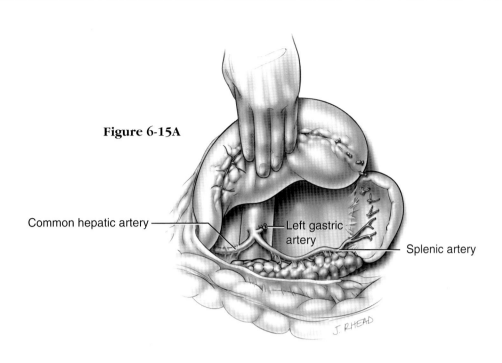

Figure 6-15A

Common hepatic artery

Left gastric artery

Splenic artery

J. RHEAD

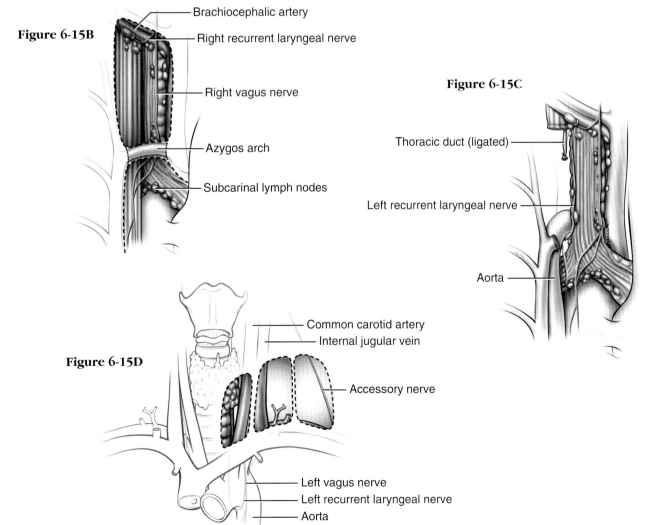

Figure 6-15B

Brachiocephalic artery

Right recurrent laryngeal nerve

Right vagus nerve

Azygos arch

Subcarinal lymph nodes

Figure 6-15C

Thoracic duct (ligated)

Left recurrent laryngeal nerve

Aorta

Common carotid artery

Internal jugular vein

Figure 6-15D

Accessory nerve

Left vagus nerve

Left recurrent laryngeal nerve

Aorta

6-16   Vagal-Sparing Esophagectomy

Performing an esophagectomy that spares the vagus nerves is a relatively new technique developed to facilitate gastric emptying, which is normally impaired by the usual mandatory vagotomy that accompanies esophagectomy. The technique is not suitable for the majority of patients who require esophagectomy, but may be considered for carefully selected patients who might benefit from the potential advantages of the operation. Because the technique of necessity does not permit removal of any tissues adjacent to the esophagus, this approach is not suitable for any except the earliest stage cancers. Reconstruction is usually performed using a segment of colon interposed between the stomach and cervical esophagus, and the additional risks associated with this must be taken into account when selecting this operation. Specific indications include benign disease such as end-stage achalasia and oncologic problems such as high-grade dysplasia and carefully staged T1a cancers without evidence for nodal involvement.

The general approach to the operation is initially similar to that for a transhiatal esophagectomy. The patient is positioned supine with the arms alongside the torso. Central venous pressure monitoring is not routinely necessary, and single lung ventilation is not necessary. The abdomen is opened using a midline or chevron incision, and an exploration is performed to ensure that there is no contraindication to resection. The esophagus is dissected from the crura bilaterally by dividing the peritoneum over the right crus, extending the division across the anterior surface of the esophagus, and continuing caudad along the left crus. Care is taken to preserve the vagus nerves, both of which are elevated from the esophagus, surrounded with vessel loops, and retracted to the patient's right. The gastric fat pad is dissected from left to right, preserving the anterior vagus nerve. Beginning at the crow's foot at the gastric angulus, a selective vagotomy is performed staying directly on the lesser gastric curvature and extending proximally. When this dissection joins the nerve trunks that were dissected from the esophagus, all branches of the vagus nerves other than direct branches to the gastric body are preserved. This helps to reduce gastric acid production while preserving antral function.

The hiatus has been completely dissected at this point. One or two proximal short gastric vessels are divided. If a colon interposition is performed, the greater omentum is separated from the transverse colon and an aperture is made into the lesser sac. This will facilitate bringing the colon graft posterior to the stomach and through the esophageal hiatus. The colon interposition segment is prepared as described in Section 6-18.

A cervical incision is performed and the cervical esophagus is mobilized. Blunt finger dissection directly on the wall of the esophagus extends the plane of dissection into the upper mediastinum. The esophagogastric junction is divided partially from the stomach with a linear vascular stapler and the lateral 2 cm of the staple line is opened to permit access to the esophagus (Fig. 6-16A). A red rubber catheter is passed up the esophagus and the lumen is washed with dilute iodine solution.

The esophagus is divided in the neck. A standard vein stripper wire is passed from below and brought out the cervical esophagus, where the large blunt tip is attached (Fig. 6-16B). The distal cervical esophagus is ligated securely below the blunt tip with a heavy suture, taking care to ensure that the ligatures do not pull off the esophagus or vein stripper, thus aborting the stripping process. An umbilical tape is tied to the large head of the vein stripper to mark the tract in the posterior mediastinum, facilitating passage of the reconstructive organ after completing the esophagectomy. An eversion esophagectomy is performed by pulling the vein stripper down into the abdomen (Fig. 6-16C). The esophagus should invert and extract with little force. The need to apply force is a sign that conversion to a transhiatal esophagectomy should be considered. After the esophagus is completely inverted, the staple line separating the esophagogastric junction from the stomach is completed and the specimen is removed (Fig. 6-16D).

Prior to bringing the reconstructive organ through the mediastinal tract, the tract is dilated to avoid constriction of the organ. This is most easily performed with a Foley catheter with an oversized (90 mL) balloon, gradually adding more saline to the balloon as the catheter is passed up and down the tract with the use of the umbilical tape marking the tract.

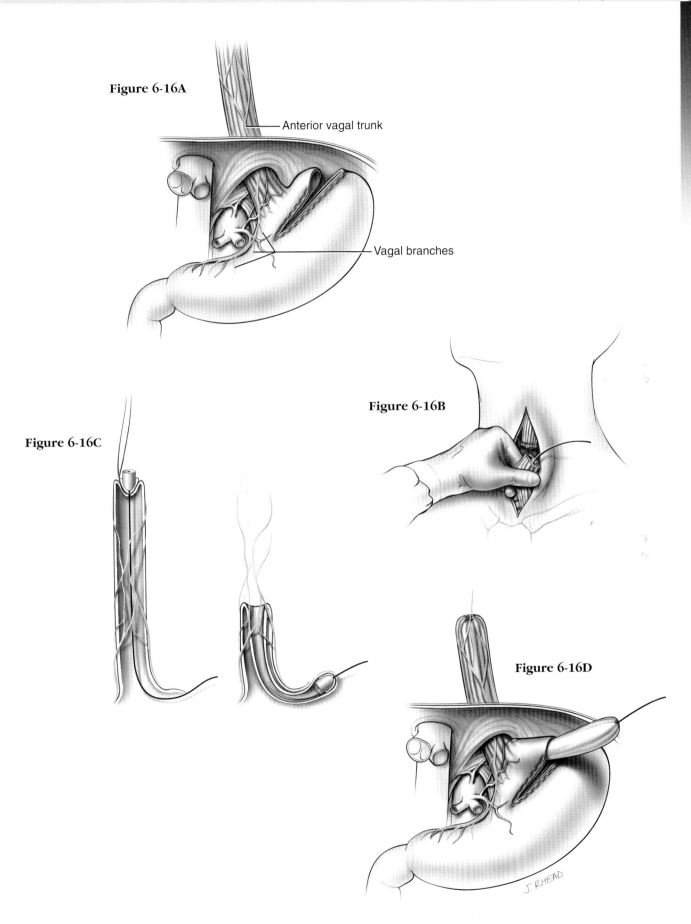

Figure 6-16A

Anterior vagal trunk

Vagal branches

Figure 6-16B

Figure 6-16C

Figure 6-16D

J. R.HEAD

6-17   Stomach Pull-up

The stomach is the organ most commonly used to reconstruct the esophagus after resection. Advantages to using the stomach include ease of preparation, reliability of the blood supply, and the need for only a single anastomosis. The dissection required to create a stomach suitable for esophageal replacement usually entails removal of lymph node stations that are frequently involved in the early dissemination of esophageal cancer, making this an integral part of the operation when performed for cancer. Disadvantages include the absence of peristaltic activity in the interposed stomach, the persistence of acid-producing mucosa in close proximity to the esophagus, and the lack of reservoir capacity. Despite these disadvantages, little superiority regarding long-term quality of life issues can be demonstrated for alternative reconstruction techniques. Most patients undergoing esophagectomy are candidates for gastric reconstruction. Contraindications to use of the stomach include prior gastric resection, prior fundoplication surgery that has compromised the integrity of the proximal stomach, and the plan for a low intraabdominal anastomosis, which, if the stomach is used for reconstructive purposes, creates a model for acid reflux possibly leading to the development of Barrett's esophagus.

There are a variety of ways that the stomach can be used as an esophageal substitute. Most often the esophagus is tailored into a tube, the diameter of which is slightly larger than the native esophagus. This has the advantage of improved gastric emptying (leaving little residual contents in the intrathoracic portion of the stomach, the presence of which makes patients prone to regurgitation and aspiration), less immediate postoperative compromise of cardiopulmonary function, and a reduction in the amount of acid-producing mucosa. Whole stomach can also be used as a substitute, which has the advantages of improved blood supply, no need for a long staple line to "tubularize" the stomach, and improved reservoir capacity. The primary alternative to these techniques, which is not discussed in this chapter, is the reverse gastric tube described by Roux, which is created from the greater curvature of the stomach.

The preparation of the stomach for use as an esophageal reconstructive organ begins with dissection of the greater curvature. The omentum is usually left attached to the colon and is divided from the stomach 2 to 3 cm from the right gastroepiploic arcade, carefully preserving these vessels, upon which the blood supply to the stomach will largely depend. The arcade terminates 15 to 20 cm from the pylorus; despite the description of communicating vessels between the right and left gastroepiploic arcardes in anatomical texts, a useful connection adjacent to the stomach is rarely identified. Thus, the dissection of the greater curvature is carried beyond the termination of the right gastroepiploic vessels directly on the wall of the stomach. The left gastroepiploic vessels and the short gastric vessels are divided to the apex of the gastric fundus. Retroperitoneal vessels are divided as the stomach is retracted medially.

The gastrohepatic omentum is divided close to the liver. If there is an aberrant left hepatic artery, it is dissected and test-clamped to determine whether it needs to be preserved. If clamping results in ischemia of the left hepatic lobe, the vessel must be preserved, which indicates the level at which the left gastric artery is divided. The dissection is carried cephalad to the hiatus and the peritoneum is divided anterior to the esophagus to meet the dissection that was performed from the greater curvature side. The right crus is grasped with an Allis clamp and elevated. The tissues connecting the esophagus to the crus are divided, permitting entry into the mediastinum. The left crus is elevated and similarly dissected. The stomach is reflected either to the left or superiorly, revealing the left gastric vessels. The artery is divided at its origin from the celiac axis. The vein is also divided at this level. Soft tissues in the retroperitoneal space are dissected to mobilize the remaining stomach in accordance with the type of lymphatic dissection dictated by the nature of the disease necessitating esophagectomy and by the preferences of the surgeon. A gastric emptying procedure (pyloromyotomy, pyloroplasty, pyloric dilation) is performed.

A standard gastric tube is constructed by excising the lesser gastric curvature and esophagogastric junction. The proximal point of division preserves the tip of the fundus, which must be carefully identified to maximize the length of the gastric tube. The line of division must begin at least 5 cm from the closest extent of palpable tumor when resection is being performed for a gastroesophageal junction cancer. The distal extent of dissection is a point just cephalad to the fifth branch of the left gastric arcade along the lesser curvature, which is near the gastric angulus. This preserves all of the gastric fundus, and encompasses 90% of lymph nodes below the diaphragm that typically drain the esophagus and gastroesophageal junction. The arcade of the left gastric artery is divided at this point, eliminating the communication between the left and right gastric arteries, and the stomach wall is bared. The division of the lesser curvature from the stomach body is performed with a linear cutting stapler, and can be approached from inferior or superior, depending on the surgeon's preference (Fig. 6-17A). When done through an open incision, either approach is fine, but an approach from the lesser curvature toward the fundus is preferable when a laparoscopic technique is used. The use of reinforcing strips or over-sewing of the staple line helps decrease the possibility of leakage from this long staple line, although the use of such strips may limit the length of the gastric tube. The diameter of the completed tube should be 6 to 8 cm.

Figure 6-17A

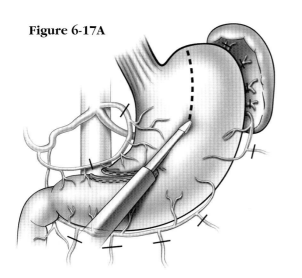

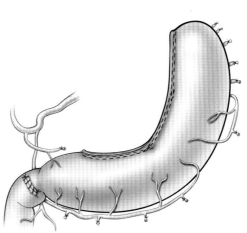

When the whole stomach is used as an esophageal reconstructive organ, the left gastric artery is divided at its origin but no division of the left gastric vascular arcade is performed, and the communication between the right and left gastric vessels is preserved (Fig. 6-17B). This provides considerable additional blood supply to the stomach. After dissecting the esophagus circumferentially and entering the mediastinum, the esophagogastric junction is identified. It is important that all squamous mucosa be excised when dividing the stomach from the esophagus; if squamous mucosa is left within the reconstructive organ, its exposure to gastric acid can lead to ulceration and possible perforation or bleeding. The staple line incorporates reinforcement strips or is oversewn to help prevent leakage. The whole stomach is ready for use.

Positioning either a gastric tube or the whole stomach preparation into the chest is sometimes challenging, particularly if the chest is not accessible to enable manual positioning of the stomach. This is usually the case when a cervical anastomosis is performed, and is always the case when a substernal route is chosen for the gastric tube. A variety of techniques have been described for pulling the stomach into the neck. The objectives are to get the stomach into position with the least amount of trauma and, at the same time, preserving its orientation so that no twisting occurs, which might substantially interfere with both the blood supply to and the performance of the stomach. One technique involves loosely suturing the stomach to a "sled" created from a malleable retractor with two holes cut in its end (Fig. 6-17C). While this functions well, it does traumatize the tip of the gastric fundus; if excessive tension is applied to the sled, the sutures can tear out of the fundus, creating a perforation that requires closure and compromises the available length of stomach. Some surgeons use a large bore chest tube for this purpose, but this does not prevent torsion of the stomach as reliably as one might wish.

A useful alternative to use of a focal traction point for getting the stomach into the neck is to use the "bag-on-suction" technique, which distributes the tension on the stomach widely, helping to prevent injury, and at the same time preserves the orientation of the stomach. After the route for reconstruction is prepared, an umbilical tape is positioned through it. A large Foley catheter is tied to the umbilical tape and drawn from the cervical incision into the abdomen. The tape is disconnected from the catheter and left in place. The stomach is placed inside of a plastic bag that is about 25 to 30 cm in length and has a diameter of about 8 to 10 cm. The tip of the Foley catheter is positioned inside of the tip of the bag, and the Foley balloon is inflated with 10 to 15 mL of saline. The bag is tied securely around the catheter proximal to the balloon (Fig. 6-17D). The draining port of the Foley catheter is attached to suction, which closely approximates the bag to the surface of the stomach. Once all air is evacuated from the bag, gentle traction is placed on the Foley catheter, while it is still on suction, gradually drawing the stomach into the chest. The Foley balloon is manually guided into the posterior mediastinal or substernal space, and the stomach easily follows this pathway. As the fundic tip reaches the neck, the bag is taken off suction and is pulled further cephalad, removing it from the mediastinum. The stomach is now ready for its anastomosis to the esophagus.

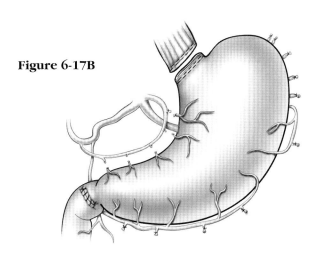

Figure 6-17B

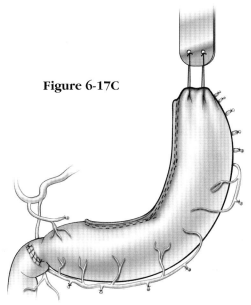

Figure 6-17C

Figure 6-17D

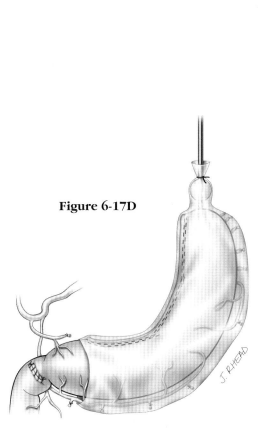

6-18   Colon Interposition

Use of the colon as an esophageal substitute has many advocates, although the technical challenges and potential complications are sometimes daunting to the infrequent esophageal surgeon. The colon has an important place in esophageal reconstructive techniques: it is ideal for long segment replacement when the stomach is unavailable, and is perfectly suited for esophageal reconstruction when a vagus-sparing esophagectomy is performed. The colon also can be used for short segment replacement, bridging the gap between esophagus and stomach when necessary. However, for this latter purpose a segment of small bowel, although more difficult to prepare and interpose, functions better because of its intrinsic peristaltic activity. Compared to use of the stomach for esophageal replacement, it has not been clearly shown that colon interposition offers substantial long-term advantages.

Prior to colon interposition, either colonoscopy or a contrast radiographic study of the colon is appropriate. In older patients an angiogram of the superior and inferior mesenteric vessels, or a multiplanar computed tomogram with vascular contrast, is performed to identify vascular abnormalities that might lead to intraoperative challenges. A mechanical and antibiotic bowel preparation is performed preoperatively.

The left and transverse colon are most commonly used for esophageal reconstruction in the adult population. The blood supply to these segments is more reliable through the marginal artery of Drummond, and there is less size discrepancy compared to the right colon. The left and transverse colon blood supply is usually based on the ascending branch of the left colic artery. In patients in whom abdominal aortic surgery has been performed, this artery may be compromised, preventing use of the left colon.

The greater omentum is divided from the colon in the avascular plane and the left and transverse colon are completely mobilized, taking care not to injure the colon mesentery. The length of colon needed for reconstruction is measured and an additional 5 to 8 cm of length is added to ensure that there will be sufficient length to use. The ascending branch of the left colic artery, itself a branch of the inferior mesenteric artery, is identified. The mesentery is transilluminated and the marginal artery (Riolan's arch) and middle colic vessels are identified. A window is created in the mesocolon preserving these vessels. The necessary length of colon is measured along the mesenteric border beginning distal to the left colic artery and extending proximally. The sites of potential division are marked with sutures, using different sutures to denote the proximal and distal margins.

At this point it is necessary to determine whether the middle colic vessels need to be included in the interposition graft. If the length of colon is relatively short, the middle colic vessels are spared. If a longer segment of colon is necessary, requiring inclusion of the middle colic vessels, the vessels are dissected to near their base to ensure that when they are divided, the continuity of the blood supply to the proximal portion of the interposition segment is not compromised. The colon is skeletonized at each proposed site of division (Fig. 6-18A). Small vascular clamps are placed on the marginal artery distal to the left colic artery, at the point of division proximally, and at the base of the middle colic vessels if they are to be included in the graft. The viability of the graft is assessed, ensuring that all segments appear well perfused. If ischemia develops, the clamps are removed and the segment is left in a warm environment to permit any vascular spasm to resolve. The use of topical vasodilators is sometimes helpful. If ischemia continues to develop during reclamping, the identified segment should not be used unless anastomosis of the vessels to donor vessels in the chest or neck is planned (supercharging). If there is no problem with ischemia, the clamped vessels are divided, and the colon is divided proximal and distal with a linear stapler.

After positioning the colon segment, the proximal anastomosis is done first, when feasible, to permit subsequent adjustment of the interposition length prior to completing the distal anastomosis. The proximal anastomosis is performed in an end-to-end fashion, or if there is a substantial size mismatch, using an end-to-side technique (see Fig. 6-18A). The graft is pulled gently in a caudad direction to eliminate any redundancy. This should not place tension on the completed anastomosis. Once redundancy is eliminated, the site where the distal anastomosis is to be performed is identified. Any redundant colon at the distal end of the graft is resected without interfering with the vascular supply to the graft. The distal anastomosis is performed to the stomach (if available), being positioned on its posterior aspect if a posterior mediastinal route is used for the interposition or on its anterior surface if another route is chosen. Alternatives for the distal anastomosis if the stomach is not available include an end-to-end anastomosis to the proximal limb of a Roux-en-Y segment, to the proximal duodenal stump, or to a jejunal pouch. The first option provides the best clinical outcomes, including freedom from bile reflux into the colon interposition.

The right colon historically has been used for esophageal reconstruction most commonly in the pediatric population. Reasons for this are likely owing to personal preferences and past training rather than any particular advantage of the right colon over the left colon. Mobilization of the colon is performed in a manner similar to that described for preparation of the left colon. After freeing the right and proximal transverse colon from peritoneal attachments, the necessary length of colon needed for reconstruction is determined. The right colon graft may be based on the right colic artery if a short segment is to be used, or is based on the middle colic vessels if a longer segment is necessary (Fig. 6-18B). Basing the graft

Figure 6-18A

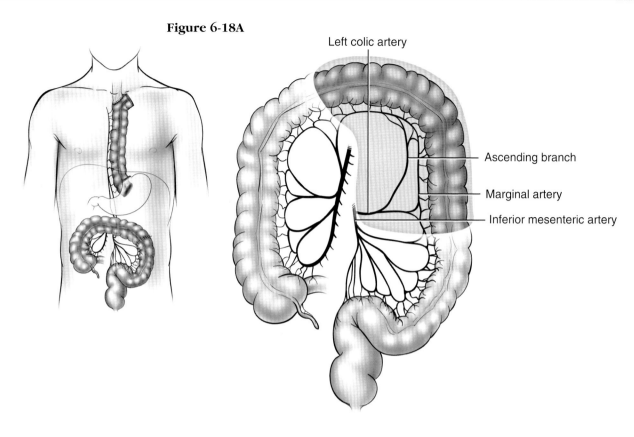

Left colic artery

Ascending branch

Marginal artery

Inferior mesenteric artery

Figure 6-18B

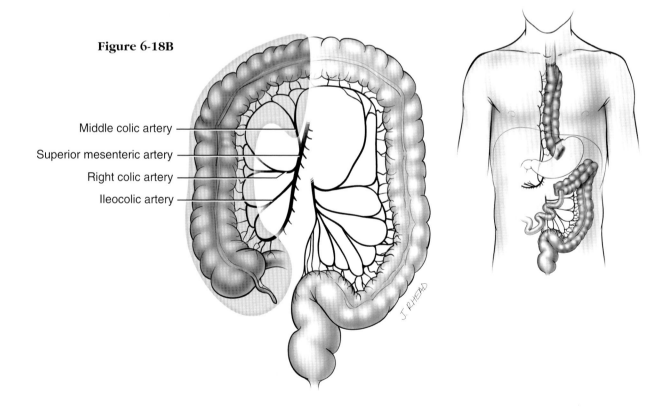

Middle colic artery

Superior mesenteric artery

Right colic artery

Ileocolic artery

on the ileocolic vessels usually necessitates placing the graft in an antiperistaltic orientation, which is best avoided if possible.

The colon is measured and marked as outlined previously. It may be tempting to preserve the terminal ileum with the right colon, permitting an anastomosis between the esophagus and terminal ileum and thereby using the ileocecal valve as an antireflux valve. However, the function of this construct is not optimal, largely because of the obstructive nature of the valve and because the bulky cecum may cause extrinsic obstruction as well. In fact, it is best to resect the cecum rather than use it for an anastomotic site because of its large size. Even after resecting the cecum, a traditional end-to-end anastomosis between the esophagus and right colon is not feasible because of the considerable size mismatch. Thus, it is advisable to use only a portion of the diameter of the colon to construct an end-to-end anastomosis. Alternatively, an end-to-side anastomosis may be created between the esophagus and one of the colonic haustra.

A short segment of colon used for reconstruction of the distal esophagus or as a free graft is most easily obtained using the transverse colon based on the middle colic vessels (Fig. 6-18C). The caliber of the transverse colon is well suited for performing an esophagocolonic anastomosis, the blood supply is reliable, and the transverse colon is easily accessed through most abdominal incisions without requiring extensive mobilization of the colon. Care must be taken, however, to isolate the middle colic vessels close enough to their origin so that the marginal arcade is left intact, preserving the blood supply to the colon segment to be used.

The procedure is started by dissecting the greater omentum from the transverse colon and entering the lesser sac. As with other types of colon interpositions, the blood supply is evaluated prior to beginning any isolation of the segment planned for use. This is best accomplished with transillumination of the transverse mesocolon. The middle colic vessels are identified, as is the marginal artery feeding the transverse colon. Based on this evaluation, a segment of transverse colon is tentatively identified for use. The length of colon necessary for reconstruction is determined, and a suitable length of transverse colon is marked with sutures, making certain that some additional length is included. The mesenteric windows on either side of the middle colic vessels are opened. The marginal artery is isolated and gently occluded at both sites of proposed colon division, ensuring that an adequate blood supply remains to the segment of transverse colon to be used for reconstruction. If all is satisfactory, the colon segment is isolated at either end by dividing the skeletonized colon and the marginal artery.

For use of a pedicled graft, the colon is brought behind the stomach and into the posterior mediastinal space for anastomosis to the esophagus. Once this end-to-end anastomosis is accomplished, the colon is gently retracted caudad to eliminate any redundancy. If too much colon has been harvested, the distal end is trimmed without sacrificing any of the blood supply. An end-to-side anastomosis is created between the colon and the back wall of the body of the stomach. As with all reconstructive tissues being brought through the diaphragm and into the chest, it is advisable to secure the interposed organ to the edges of the esophageal hiatus with 3 to 4 sutures spaced evenly, eliminating the possibility of herniation of abdominal contents into the thorax. In addition to this, a modest antireflux barrier may be created in situations in which much of the stomach is preserved but is not used for esophageal reconstruction. In such instances, the stomach body and/or fundus is sutured to the diaphragm adjacent to the esophageal hiatus in a horseshoe fashion, with the open end of the horseshoe oriented posteriorly.

Figure 6-18C

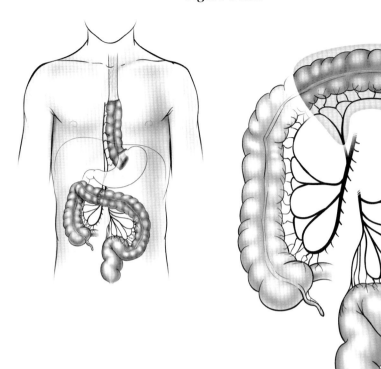

6-19 Small Bowel Interposition

The use of small bowel for esophageal reconstruction was first introduced more than a century ago, and this reconstructive technique continues to have some advantages over other methods. The diameter of the small bowel is similar to that of the esophagus, making end-to-end anastomoses more straightforward. The small bowel retains peristaltic capabilities after translocation, making it the only reconstructive tissue with this characteristic. There is sufficient redundancy to the small bowel that removal of a segment does not materially change a patient's digestive habits. However, the blood supply to the small bowel is the least reliable of the commonly used reconstructive organs, and the bowel is most easily used to replace short esophageal segments rather than the entire length of the esophagus.

Based on length restrictions, small bowel is best used for replacing a segment of the distal esophagus, typically for end-stage gastroesophageal reflux disease, or for reconstructing the cervical esophagus after resection for laryngeal and other cancers of the head and neck. The former application depends on use of a pedicled graft, whereas the latter application requires a free graft with microvascular anastomoses. It is feasible to construct a long segment small bowel interposition, but this requires preparation of a length of mesentery that includes substantial amounts of redundant small bowel, necessitating segmental resection at two or three locations along the graft to obtain an axially oriented lumen. Under these circumstances, use of the colon or stomach for reconstruction, assuming one or the other is available, is a more expeditious choice.

In creating a segment of small bowel for esophageal reconstruction it is vital to have an understanding of the vascular supply to the bowel. The jejunal blood supply originates from the superior mesenteric artery. Whereas the right colic, ileocolic, and middle colic vessels arise from the right side of this artery, the jejunal branches arise from its left side. The proximal jejunum is the most commonly used segment, and this portion of the bowel is supplied by one to five branches, most commonly three branches, arising from the superior mesenteric artery. Proximally, each branch forms an arch to an adjacent branch (primary arcade), although a few branches will fail to communicate with an adjacent branch, putting that segment of bowel at risk for ischemia if it is used for reconstruction. More distally, each branch may form two or three arches with adjacent vessels (see Fig. 6-19A inset). The first arterial branch to the jejunum commonly forms an arch to the inferior pancreaticoduodenal artery. Peripherally in the mesentery the arterial branches form secondary arcades, usually with two levels in the proximal jejunum and containing several levels more distally. The most peripheral arcade gives rise to vasa recta, which are relatively straight end-vessels that enter the bowel wall. The venous drainage runs parallel to the arterial supply and empties into the superior mesenteric vein. There is often only a single vein for every two or three artery branches.

Transillumination is used to identify the vascular arcades of the jejunum. Typically the first 15 cm of jejunum is tethered by a relatively short mesentery, making it unsuitable for use as either a pedicled or free graft. Most often the most proximal artery used to base a reconstructive segment on is the third jejunal branch from the superior mesenteric artery. The feeding vessel is selected, which is located at the aboral end of the segment, to permit adequate length while maintaining an isoperistaltic orientation to the segment. Once an adequate blood supply is identified, the required length of jejunum is determined. Care is taken to measure the jejunum on its mesenteric border, and sufficient redundancy is planned (5 to 10 cm) so that the segment will not end up being too short to bridge the gap that is created in the esophagus. The mesentery is divided from the origin of the artery on which the segment is based toward the periphery, ligating the communicating arches (Fig. 6-19A). The secondary arcades feeding the segment are preserved (Fig. 6-19B). If a longer segment of jejunum is needed than is supplied by a single artery, the arches

Inferior
pancreaticoduodenal
artery

Middle colic artery

Primary arcade

Secondary arcade

Figure 6-19A

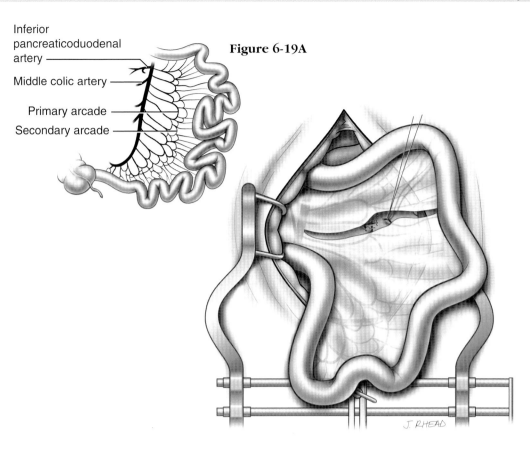

J. RHEAD

Figure 6-19B

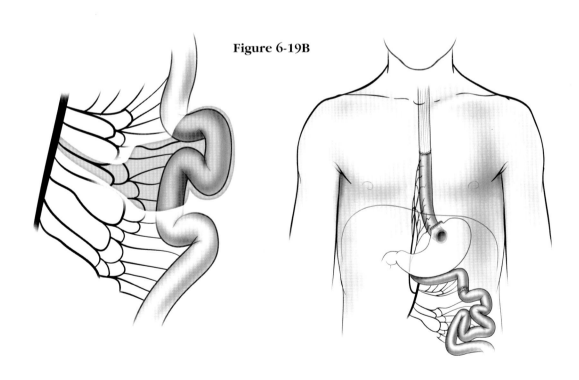

to adjacent arteries are preserved to gain greater vascularized length (Fig. 6-19C). For longer segments it is even more important that the artery and vein upon which the segment is based are located toward the aboral end of the segment. The adjacent arteries are test-clamped close to their origins to ensure the adequacy of the communicating arches. If the blood supply is sufficient, the adjacent arteries are divided close to their origins from the superior mesenteric artery.

Once the vascular supply has been isolated and the mesentery is divided, the jejunum is transected at either end of the segment using a linear cutting stapler. If the bowel is to be used as a pedicled segment, it is brought through a window in the transverse mesocolon, posterior to the stomach, and is positioned in the posterior mediastinum in an isoperistaltic orientation. The proximal anastomosis is performed first. Ideally an end-to-end anastomosis is created (see Fig. 6-19B), but in many instances the jejunal mesentery prevents complete straightening of the bowel segment. This necessitates creation of an end-to-side anastomosis. Care must be taken to avoid leaving a redundant blind end of jejunum, and any extra length of jejunum that extends beyond the anastomosis is trimmed to within 1 to 2 cm of the anastomosis. The graft is retracted caudad to prevent any extra length from being left in the thorax. A site on the stomach is selected for performing the distal anastomosis. If necessary, the distal portion of the interposition is trimmed without damaging the blood supply. The distal anastomosis is performed to the back wall of the stomach. The graft is loosely sutured to the hiatus and to the transverse mesocolon to prevent herniation through these potential sites.

When the jejunal segment is used as a free graft, its preparation is similar to that described above. Typically these segments are relatively short (20 cm or less) and are based on a single feeding artery and draining vein (Fig. 6-19D). It is important to select a segment that has a clearly defined draining vein that is in close proximity to the feeding artery for purposes of microvascular reconstruction. Whether the segment is developed with the vessels at its oral or aboral end depends on where the microvascular anastomoses are to be performed. The recipient bed for the graft is prepared; all resections are performed, hemostasis is obtained, and the donor vessels are selected and prepared. Most often branches of the ipsilateral external carotid artery or transverse cervical artery are used for arterial inflow, and venous outflow is through the external jugular vein, internal jugular vein, or posterior facial vein. The segmental vessels for the jejunal graft are divided close to their origins after the bowel has been transected at either end with a linear cutting stapler. The bowel ends are marked to ensure that the graft is interposed in an isoperistaltic orientation.

The proximal and distal bowel anastomoses are performed first; performing the vascular anastomoses first exposes them to the possibility of undue tension as the subsequent bowel anastomoses are performed. The size match between the distal end of the jejunal segment and the esophagus is usually very close, permitting an end-to-end anastomosis (see Fig. 6-19D). Some tailoring is necessary when the proximal end of the jejunum is anastomosed to the pharynx after esophagolaryngectomy. It is sometimes useful to fillet open the jejunum on its antimesenteric border for a distance of several centimeters to provide an adequate lumen for a wide anastomosis to the pharynx.

Figure 6-19C

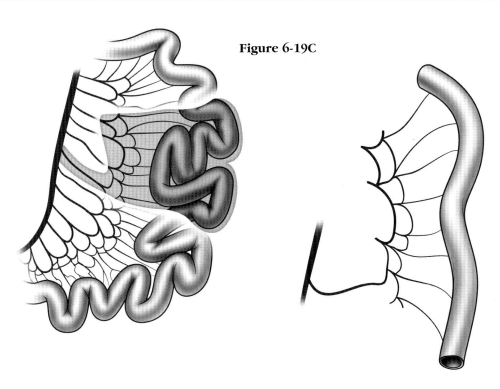

Figure 6-19D

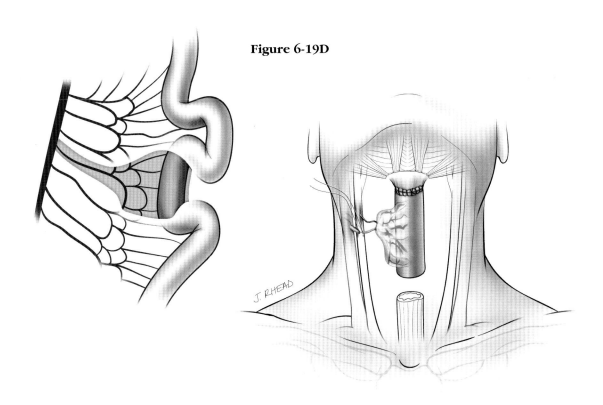

J. RHEAD

6-20   Sutured Anastomosis

Of the two methods for creating an esophageal anastomosis, suturing has historically been most popular. With the introduction of techniques using a linear cutting stapler, mechanical anastomoses are being performed with increasing frequency (see sections 6-21 and 6-22). Mechanical stapling techniques may reduce the incidence of anastomotic leak, but do not appreciably decrease the need for dilation for anastomotic stricture.

Techniques for performing a sutured esophageal anastomosis vary considerably. No single method has been proven to have overall superiority. Although the overall incidence of anastomotic leakage is similar comparing single-layer to two-layer anastomoses, use of the latter technique leads to a higher rate of anastomotic stricture. Results comparing continuous to interrupted suture techniques demonstrate no important differences, although the former technique takes less time to perform. There may be an advantage to use of a monofilament absorbable suture compared to a nonabsorbable braided suture. Surgeons should adopt the technique with which they feel most comfortable and which provides the best results in their hands.

This section describes a technique for performing an end-to-side esophagogastrostomy through a cervical incision. A similar technique may be used for an intrathoracic anastomosis between the esophagus and stomach. Variations on these techniques are appropriate for any hand-sutured esophageal anastomosis. The reconstructive organ is brought into apposition with the end of the proximal esophagus. Some surgeons recommend suturing the reconstructive organ, particularly the stomach, to a surface such as the prevertebral fascia to fix it in place and take tension off of the anastomosis. However, this technique exposes the patient to potential complications, including leakage from the stomach at the site of the anchoring suture and resultant vertebral osteomyelitis. In addition, the anastomosis cannot be performed external to the incision, requiring either a fairly large neck incision to permit access to perform the anastomosis, or redundancy of the esophagus in the neck after completion of the anastomosis. Avoiding attachments of the stomach to adjacent fascia permits the anastomosis, once completed, to be pulled slightly into the mediastinum, aligning it with the esophagus and stomach and providing an axially oriented conduit that limits dysphagia.

The esophageal stump and gastric fundus are drawn into the wound, with the tip of the gastric tube situated deep to the esophageal stump. A site on the gastric fundus is selected for the anastomosis that avoids the fundic tip and the staple/suture line along the lesser curvature, optimizing the blood supply to the anastomosis (Fig. 6-20A). This is ideally situated near the greater curvature. A 2-cm longitudinal opening is created at this point, the orientation of which avoids dividing more collateral vessels in the gastric wall supplying the tip of the fundus than a horizontal incision would. It is not necessary to remove any gastric tissue, which would have similar potentially disastrous results.

The back wall of the anastomosis is created first, using triangulation sutures to spread the tissues, thus avoiding narrowing the anastomosis by placing too much tension on the suture line (Fig. 6-20B). If a two-layer anastomosis is performed, the seromuscular layer is performed first, followed by the mucosal layer. A single-layer anastomosis incorporates both the muscular and mucosal layers; it is important to incorporate a generous (5 mm or more) width of esophageal mucosa, the submucosal layer of which provides the greatest strength of any of the layers of the esophagus. Tying knots on the inside of the esophagus, particularly if interrupted absorbable sutures are used, helps to approximate the mucosal edges, lessening the possibility of an anastomotic leak. A nasogastric tube is passed down the esophagus and across the anastomosis.

The front wall of the anastomosis is performed next. For a two-layer anastomosis, the mucosal layer is completed first, following which the seromuscular layer is sutured. For an interrupted single-layer anastomosis, the transition from tying knots on the inside to tying the knots on the outside occurs when about 80% of the anastomosis has been completed. The final sutures, being tied on the outside, are all placed before any of them is tied (Fig. 6-20C). When the anastomosis is complete and inspection reveals no obvious deficiencies, it is sometimes desirable to test its competence by distending the region of the anastomosis with air while it is submerged under saline. This can be accomplished by injecting air through the nasogastric tube after positioning the holes in the region of the anastomosis, or by performing flexible endoscopy and insufflating air. In either situation, if possible, the distal portion of the stomach tube should be occluded so that some tension develops across the anastomosis, providing an adequate assessment of its mechanical soundness. Viability is determined by inspection but, unfortunately, the test of time is sometimes the most accurate determinant of viability. Once the surgeon is satisfied that the anastomosis is as healthy and airtight as possible, it is positioned in the posterior neck or upper mediastinum by gently placed traction on the gastric tube, placing the esophagus and stomach into axial alignment. This transitions the anastomosis from an anterior to a posterior location and places it in a more caudad site than where it was performed (Fig. 6-20D).

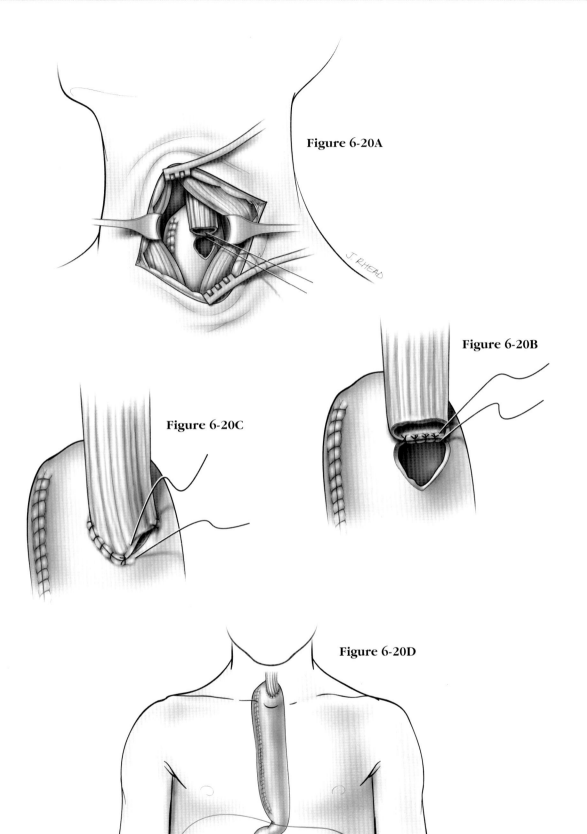

Figure 6-20A

Figure 6-20B

Figure 6-20C

Figure 6-20D

6-21   Linear Stapled Anastomosis

Developed originally in the late 1970s, this technique provides a wide anastomotic lumen and is very secure mechanically. It is applicable primarily to esophagogastric anastomoses, and generally is not used for anastomosing the esophagus to colon or jejunum. The technique has the advantage of being the quickest anastomosis to perform. However, unless the stapler is positioned carefully before being fired, this method increases the risk of gastric fundic tip necrosis because it, of necessity, divides more of the collateral circulation to the stomach than other sutured or stapled techniques. In addition, because the size of the anastomosis is larger than that of most esophageal anastomoses, use of this method for a low intrathoracic esophagogastrostomy is less than optimal owing to the large amount of gastroesophageal reflux that can result.

The esophagus and stomach are positioned as described earlier in Section 6-20, with the gastric fundic tip lying deep to the esophagus. Because the diameter of the anastomosis to be created is larger than that of most sutured anastomoses, a greater length of the gastric fundic tip is brought up posterior to the esophagus prior to creating the anastomosis. Stay sutures are placed at opposite sides of the open esophagus and are brought through the stomach at an appropriate site away from the lesser curvature. The stomach is opened to a diameter sufficient to permit one arm of a linear cutting stapler to be inserted into it (Fig. 6-21A). The stapler is posi-tioned with one arm in the esophagus and the other in the stomach. Care is taken to ensure that the stapler does not approach the lesser curvature staple line or the tip of the gastric fundus, and that the mucosal edges are closely approximated as the stapler is shut (Fig. 6-21B). Typically a single firing of a 5-cm or 6-cm stapler cartridge is sufficient to create a wide posterior portion of the anastomosis (Fig. 6-21C). If necessary, a second firing can be performed to ensure an adequate anastomotic lumen. A nasogastric tube is passed down the esophagus and across the anastomosis into the stomach. Some surgeons reinforce the staple line with interrupted sutures. Inspection of the gastric fundus posterior to the esophagus ensures that the blood supply to this portion of the stomach remains adequate prior to completing the anastomosis.

The anterior part of the anastomosis is closed in one of two ways. An interrupted or continuous suture technique is the most commonly used technique, the only caveat being that the corners of the posterior staple line should be carefully inverted into the lumen to ensure a secure closure (Fig. 6-21D). Alternatively, the edges of the stomach and esophageal margins are grasped with Babcock or Allis clamps (usually four clamps are necessary) and the clamped margin is excised with a linear cutting stapler, completing the anterior portion of the anastomosis. This is the fastest closure technique and is possibly the most secure method, but it does necessitate excision of additional tissue and should not be used if there is any concern about the size of the residual anastomotic lumen that would result.

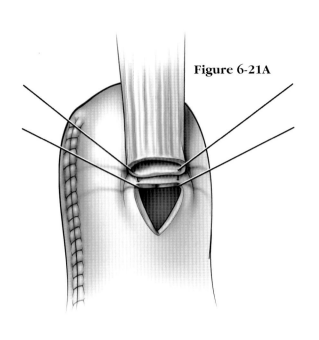

Figure 6-21A

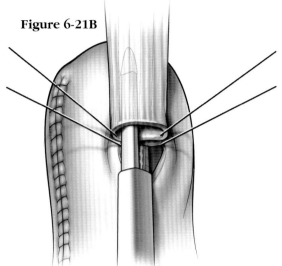

Figure 6-21B

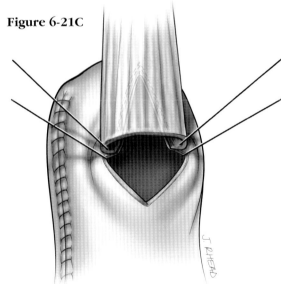

Figure 6-21C

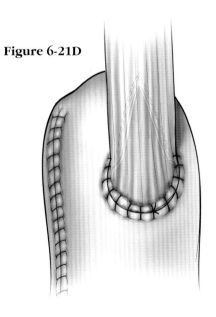

Figure 6-21D

6-22 Circular Stapled Anastomosis

The circular stapled anastomosis is historically the most common mechanical technique for creating an esophageal anastomosis. It is applicable to gastric as well as bowel anastomoses, is relatively quick to perform, and is mechanically strong. However, particularly with older stapler models, the incidence of anastomotic stricture is high, primarily because the diameter of the anastomosis is somewhat limited by mechanical factors imposed by the stapler cartridge. Dilation of the resulting strictures is less successful than dilation of strictures that result from other anastomotic techniques.

Current circular stapling techniques require that the stapling device be brought through an aperture into the lumen of the organ to be stapled, requiring closure of that aperture. This causes additional compromise to the circulation of that organ. The technique described herein avoids that problem to some extent by placing the insertion aperture in an area through which little, if any, collateral circulation passes. The technique described also works well for performing an end-to-side esophagojejunostomy. For the creation of very proximal esophageal anastomoses in the future, it will be possible to pass a device orally and fashion an anastomosis without having to compromise the interposed organ at all.

The stomach or other organ is brought into position adjacent to the esophagus. It is important that no undue tension be placed on the organs during creation of the anastomosis. Even though the mechanical holding power of the circular stapled anastomosis is quite strong, tension will undoubtedly lead to ischemia and stricture or dehiscence. A heavy purse string suture is placed in the cut end of the esophagus and the anvil is placed within the esophagus. It is sometimes necessary to dilate the esophagus slightly to permit the cartridge to be positioned correctly with its orientation perpendicular to the long axis of the esophagus. The purse string is tied (Fig. 6-22A).

A site on the gastric wall is selected for creating an opening for the stapler. It is possible to excise a portion of the lesser curvature suture line for this purpose. Another option is to excise the very tip of the fundus and to use that aperture for inserting the stapler. The stapler is inserted and a site for the anastomosis is selected that is well vascularized and is distant from the lesser curvature staple line and from the fundic tip. The stapler spike is extended and passes through the selected site. It is inserted into the anvil after removal of the spike from the anvil (Fig. 6-22B). The esophagus and stomach are brought into apposition by tightening the stapler to an appropriate tension using the guide provided by the manufacturer for the brand and model of stapler that is being used (Fig. 6-22C).

The stapler is fired and then the anvil is separated from the stapler. By angulating the stapler, the anvil is extracted from within the esophagus and the stapler with the anvil attached is removed from the stomach. The anastomosis is inspected to ensure that it is complete and that the circulation to the region is satisfactory. The tissue from the stapler is removed and the surgeon verifies that two complete rings are present. If portions of one or both rings are missing, the anastomosis must be reinforced with sutures, or consideration is given to removing the stapled tissues and performing a sutured anastomosis. The aperture in the stomach or other interposed organ is closed with a linear cutting stapler after a nasogastric tube has been passed across the anastomosis (Fig. 6-22D).

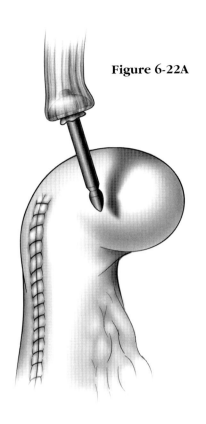

Figure 6-22A

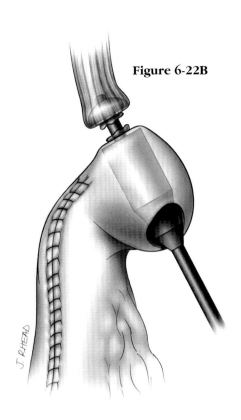

Figure 6-22B

J. R. HEAD

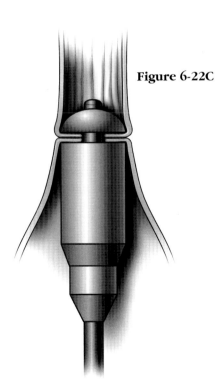

Figure 6-22C

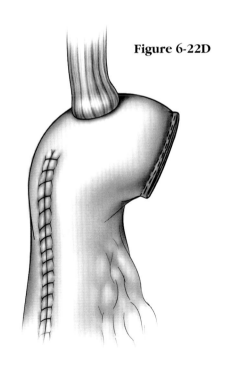

Figure 6-22D

6-23   Esophageal Exclusion

Esophageal exclusion is performed as a temporary or permanent measure, depending on the clinical circumstances. In patients suffering from malignant esophago-respiratory fistula in whom other management such as stenting is unsuccessful, esophageal exclusion and gastric bypass provide excellent palliation. Such aggressive therapy for a rapidly terminal situation should be used judiciously. The operative procedure is straightforward. The cervical esophagus is divided and the stapled distal end of the cervical esophagus is allowed to retract into the mediastinum. The esophagogastric junction is divided and the stomach is brought through a retrosternal route to the neck. A standard cervical esophagogastrostomy is performed. The communication between the esophagus and the airway drains any mucus that is produced by the excluded esophagus.

Temporary esophageal exclusion is a lifesaving technique applicable to highly selected patients suffering from esophageal perforation in whom primary repair is unsuccessful and there is ongoing, poorly controlled drainage from the site. In this situation, exclusion prevents salivary and gastric juices from further contaminating the mediastinum and/or the pleural cavities. In rare instances this technique might be applied to problems of anastomotic leakage, particularly when the anastomosis is located distally. In such instances, however, control of cephalad flow of contaminating fluids is difficult if not impossible, obviating much of the advantages provided by proximal esophageal exclusion.

There are three issues that must be addressed when an esophageal exclusion operation is considered. First, is the proximal esophagus to be completely or partially excluded, and can it be done in a manner that permits easy surgical reversal of the process when warranted? Performing a side esophagostomy incompletely excludes the esophagus, as does a double-barreled esophagostomy because of the risk of reflux of saliva into the distal segment. For these reasons it is usually appropriate to consider an end cervical esophagostomy. When performing this procedure, it is wise to keep the distal end of the divided esophagus in proximity to the esophagostomy to enable easy identification when take-down of the esophagostomy is deemed appropriate. To accomplish this, the distal end of the esophagus is stapled closed as the esophagus is divided to create the esophagostomy. The distal end is mobilized into the mediastinum as far as possible to provide length, and is sutured to the side wall of the proximal esophagus (Fig. 6-23A).

The ends of the nonabsorbable sutures are left somewhat long so that they can be easily identified during the subsequent reoperation.

The second issue of importance in the management of patients undergoing temporary esophageal exclusion is how to best manage mucus production by the esophageal body. Some manner of egress is necessary to decompress the excluded esophagus. This is particularly true for patients in whom the esophagogastric junction is ligated to prevent reflux of gastric fluids into the esophagus. If the leak heals and the segment of esophagus is excluded for a long time, a mucocele can develop. Alternatively, the pressure that builds up in the esophagus owing to persistent intrinsic contractions may lead to a blow out of the distal closure, obviating the potential benefit of total exclusion. When the communication between the distal esophagus and stomach is interrupted, it is appropriate to place a drainage catheter into the mediastinal esophagus to decompress and drain this segment. This can be placed through the staple line closure or through a purse string suture in the side of the esophagus. The catheter is brought out through a stab incision in the neck on the side opposite to the esophagostomy to avoid problems with placement of a drainage appliance over the stoma (Fig. 6-23B).

Finally, a decision must be made as to whether to partially or completely divert gastric juices. Several techniques of complete diversion have been described, including ligation of the gastroesophageal junction with umbilical tape, stapling of the junction, etc. Most reports suggest that the natural peristaltic activity of the esophagus will eventually overcome these mechanical obstructions and restore the communication between the esophagus and stomach, usually in a time frame of four to eight weeks. Although this may be an attractive way to "automatically" restore continuity, the surgeon has no control over when the communication is restored. Moreover, the technique often results in the formation of an intractable stricture in this region, which obviously complicates the process of restoring normal swallowing ability. As an alternative to complete diversion, many surgeons elect to place a gastrostomy tube to effect near-total diversion of gastric juices. This leaves the esophagogastric junction untouched. A feeding jejunostomy is placed at the time of gastrostomy tube placement to provide a means for enteral alimentation during the period the patient cannot eat (Fig. 6-23C). The presence of a gastrostomy tube combined with a patent esophagogastric junction permits retrograde contrast radiographic study of the esophageal leak to assess healing prior to taking down the cervical esophagostomy.

Figure 6-23A

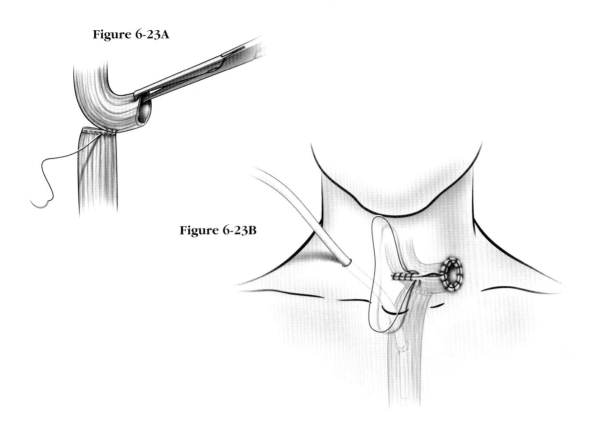

Figure 6-23B

Figure 6-23C

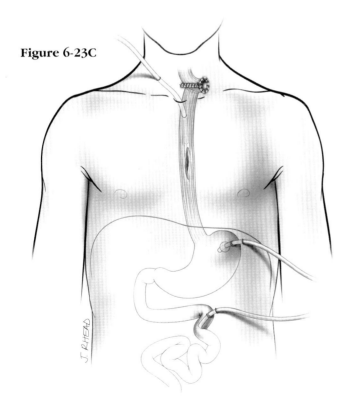

6-24 Primary Repair of Esophageal Perforation

Repair of an esophageal perforation is appropriate in patients without esophageal malignancy in whom resumption of relatively normal esophageal function can be expected once a perforation has healed. Contraindications to repair include perforated intractable stricture, perforation in the setting of an end-stage motility disorder, and perforated cancer. Patients undergoing repair should be clinically stable; repair in the presence of severe sepsis is not generally indicated because of uncertainty about the reliability of healing in this situation and the possible contribution of ongoing leakage to confusion of the clinical picture. Management of esophageal perforation has changed considerably since the 1970s. At that time primary repair was indicated only for patients in whom perforation was diagnosed early, within 12 to 24 hours, and who were otherwise healthy and in clinically stable condition. Since that period many reports have described successful results with delayed primary repair of esophageal perforation. Currently primary repair is indicated for most patients suffering from benign esophageal perforation.

An investigation is performed preoperatively to determine the site of the perforation and the hemithorax that is most affected. Spontaneous (barogenic) perforations occur most often in the distal esophagus and ruptures into the left chest. Iatrogenic perforations resulting from endoscopy usually occur at the site of an obstructing lesion such as a dense stricture. It is important to avoid approaching a high thoracic perforation through the left chest because the aortic arch limits access to the site of the perforation. It is appropriate to operate through the hemithorax that is most contaminated to permit adequate decortication and drainage; this is most often the left hemithorax (see Fig. 6-24A inset). The side of the esophagus on which the perforation occurs is not a primary determinant of the side through which the problem is approached; the esophagus is rotated easily and sufficiently to access a perforation that is on the contralateral side.

Once the chest is opened, the site of perforation is identified. Sometimes this requires intraoperative endoscopy because, especially when recognized and treated early, the intraoperative signs of perforation can be subtle. Once identified, the esophageal muscle overlying the mucosal defect is divided longitudinally to clearly expose the proximal and distal extent of mucosal disruption (Fig. 6-24A). Failure to do so will result in continued leakage. The mucosa is closed with running or interrupted suture using an absorbable monofilament or braided suture; monofilament sutures glide more easily through the mucosa and incite less local reaction than do braided sutures (Fig. 6-24B). The overlying muscle layers are reapproximated with a second layer of sutures (Fig. 6-24C).

It is often appropriate to reinforce the closure of an esophageal perforation with a vascularized flap of surrounding tissue. This is particularly apropos when recognition and treatment of the perforation is delayed. Available flaps include pleura, intercostal muscle, pericardial fat pad, diaphragm, and pericardium. Use of the diaphragm or pericardium opens a new cavity that is then exposed to the potential for infection, and so these options must be selected with caution. Pleura as a reinforcing tissue is especially useful in patients who have undergone delayed repair, in that the pleura in such instances has become thickened and hypervascular (Fig. 6-24D). Use of a thin, relatively avascular pleural flap in patients with little or no contamination and inflammation is unlikely to provide much benefit.

The esophagus and stomach are decompressed with a nasogastric tube. If there is any concern about proper healing of the perforation, a jejunostomy feeding tube is placed operatively. The hemithorax is decorticated if necessary and is generously irrigated. Appropriate drains are placed, including a soft flexible drain overlying the site of repair. A contrast study subsequently is performed when the patient is sufficiently recovered to ensure proper healing of the repair prior to instituting oral intake.

Figure 6-24A

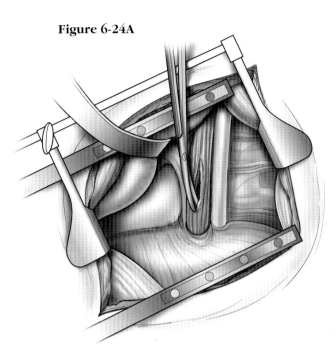

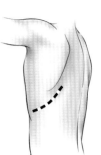

Figure 6-24B

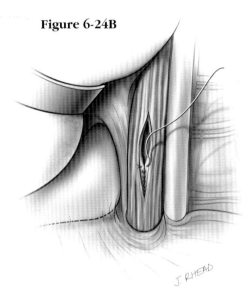

J. RHEAD

Figure 6-24C

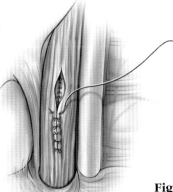

Figure 6-24D

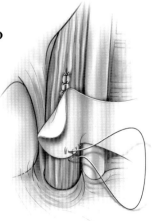

Thoracic Duct

7-1   Anatomy

The thoracic duct is a structure into which lymph is collected from bodily tissues and subsequently is discharged into the venous system. Embryologically, the lymphatic system arises by budding from paired jugular lymph sacs, paired iliac sacs, a single retroperitoneal sac, and a sac that evolves into the cisterna chyli. The thoracic duct forms from caudad growth of the jugular sacs and cephalad growth of the cisterna chyli. During embryonic life the thoracic duct consists of bilaterally symmetric plexi of lymph vessels that coalesce to form two distinct ducts. During fetal maturation, the upper third of the right duct and the lower two thirds of the left duct are obliterated, leaving the somewhat convoluted configuration of the adult thoracic duct. The manner in which the thoracic duct forms underscores the potential for developmental anomalies and anatomic variations.

There are two main divisions to the human lymphatic system. Lymph from the lower extremities, abdomen, and pelvis; left upper extremity and left hemithorax; and the left side of the head flows into the left lymphatic system and ultimately into the thoracic duct. Lymph from the right upper extremity, right hemithorax, right side of the head, and liver empties into the right lymphatic system and is ultimately drained through the right lymphatic duct. The left upper lobe of the lung is drained by the left system, and the left lower lobe and right lung are drained by the right system.

The cisterna chyli is formed by the coalescence of two lumbar lymphatic trunks and the intestinal trunk at the level of the first and second lumbar vertebrae, located to the right of the aorta. The thoracic duct arises from the cisterna chyli and crosses into the right hemithorax through the aortic hiatus (Fig. 7-1A). The duct lies on the anterior surface of the vertebral column, behind the esophagus and between the aorta and azygos vein, from the eleventh through the seventh thoracic vertebrae (Fig. 7-1B). There it is in close proximity to the greater splanchnic nerve and is usually anterior to the right intercostal branches from the aorta. The duct system is bilateral at this level in about 5% of people.

The duct ascends and crosses to the left hemithorax at the level of the sixth or fifth thoracic vertebra, passes posterior to the aortic arch, and ascends along the left border of the esophagus. At the level of the aortic arch and above, the duct system is bilateral in about one third of people. The duct ascends to the base of the neck, where it lies to the left of the esophagus within the mediastinal pleura. It ascends 3 to 5 cm above the clavicle, posterior to the subclavian artery, and is located just medial to the anterior scalene muscle. The duct empties into the venous system via the left subclavian vein, or, more commonly, near the junction of the left subclavian and left internal jugular veins.

The right lymphatic duct (not shown) is the primary vessel draining the tracheobronchial lymph nodes and receives most of the lymphatic drainage from the heart. It ascends in the right posterior mediastinum in a manner analogous to that of the thoracic duct, and terminates near the junction of the right subclavian and internal jugular veins. There are frequent communications between the ducts in the lymphatic system and between the ducts and the venous system. There are numerous valves within the thoracic duct that provide for unidirectional flow. These are most commonly found above the level of the aortic arch.

Figure 7-1A

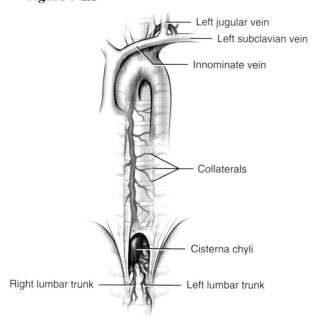

- Left jugular vein
- Left subclavian vein
- Innominate vein
- Collaterals
- Cisterna chyli
- Right lumbar trunk
- Left lumbar trunk

Figure 7-1B

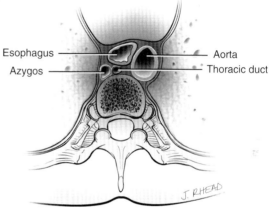

- Esophagus
- Azygos
- Aorta
- Thoracic duct

J. RHEAD

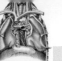
7-2 Thoracic Duct Ligation

The primary indications for surgery of the thoracic duct include prophylactic ligation during extensive mediastinal dissection, such as during esophagectomy, and therapeutic ligation for chylothorax. Under rare circumstances a thoracic duct cyst may be excised. There have also been occasional reports of surgery to anastomose the thoracic duct to an intrathoracic vein to improve lymphatic drainage in instances of lymph stasis. These latter two operations are not described here.

During esophagectomy for cancer, an operation in which the soft tissues surrounding the esophagus are widely dissected, the incidence of thoracic duct leak may be as high as 5% to 10%. Because of the morbidity of this potential complication, it is usually wise to prophylactically ligate the thoracic duct as part of the resection operation. The pleura overlying the azygos vein and thoracic duct is opened low in the right hemithorax. It is important that the dissection is performed gently, because in the previously unoperated chest the tissues of the thoracic duct are quite delicate. After the azygos vein is dissected, the thoracic duct is identified just medial to it. The duct is circumferentially dissected. As it is sometimes difficult to distinguish the thoracic duct from the surrounding fatty tissue, division of the duct with observation of clear lymph fluid flowing from it confirms the diagnosis. Both cut ends of the duct are doubly ligated. It may be helpful to place a large vascular clip across the duct as well (Fig. 7-2A).

Ligation of the thoracic duct for management of a chylothorax is more challenging. In general, thoracic duct ligation is not indicated for patients who suffer from chylothorax owing to lymphatic obstruction within the mediastinum, typically secondary to lymphoma. Chylothorax following blunt or penetrating trauma may be amenable to direct ligation of the injured lymphatic vessel, and the operation is best approached through the hemithorax that is affected by the chylothorax.

The most challenging situation arises when a patient develops a chylothorax following esophagectomy. Although a postesophagectomy chylothorax typically develops in the right hemithorax, it may be bilateral or exclusively in the left hemithorax. In the latter instance, it is appropriate to explore the patient through the left hemithorax if that was the side originally operated upon. Otherwise, it is most appropriate to explore patients through the right hemithorax. This can be performed using an open thoracotomy or using a thoracoscopic technique; the latter is difficult to use in a patient who has had a recent right thoracotomy. It is often useful to administer a heavy fat load enterally or to administer a lipophilic dye to aid in the identification of a duct leak. This should be performed within 1 to 2 hours of the planned procedure.

If a specific site of chyle leakage is identified, the duct is dissected at that level and is ligated as described above. However, this identification is often not possible in a chest recently operated on. The tissues are edematous and inflamed, and adequately identifying an injured thoracic duct is often difficult. In such situations blind ligation of the thoracic duct is appropriate. The pleura is opened in the inferior hemithorax adjacent to the azygos vein and adjacent to the descending thoracic aorta. All of the soft tissues between these two structures are encircled with a heavy ligature (Fig. 7-2B, inset). Tying this ligature successfully obliterates the duct lumen and cessation of lymph flow should follow (Fig. 7-2B). The one-way valves in the thoracic duct beyond the area of injury normally prevent backflow of chyle through the cephalad portion of the leak. Should backflow be present the proximal stump of the duct is also ligated. If there is any suspicion about an ongoing leak from a thoracic duct injury after blind ligation of the duct, it is sometimes appropriate to perform talc pleurodesis to ensure that the chylothorax is controlled.

Figure 7-2A

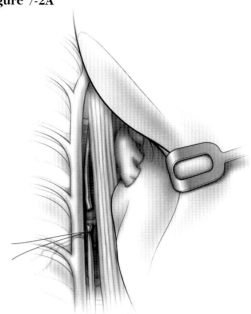

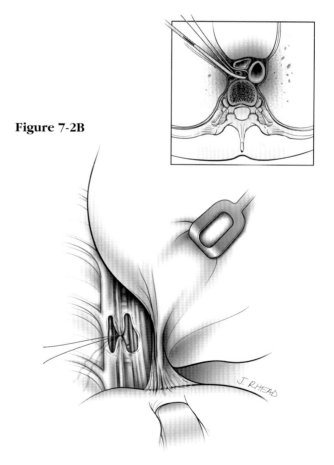

Figure 7-2B

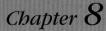

Chapter *8*

Sympathetic Chain

■ 8-1 Anatomy

The sympathetic nervous system is represented in the thorax by symmetric paired chains of nerves that extend from the thoracic inlet to the diaphragm. The nerve fibers and ganglia run vertically across the necks of the ribs, immediately adjacent to the vertbral bodies. They are covered by parietal pleura. Splanchnic branches emerge from each chain and pass medially to the abdominal sympathetic ganglia. The upper part of the system mediates pupillary dilation, the levator muscles of the upper eyelids, the eccrine sweat glands, vasoconstriction of the superficial vessels of the skin, and vasodilation of the deep arteries to striated muscles.

The specific anatomy of the first and second thoracic sympathetic ganglia is important in management of hyperhidrosis as well as vasospastic disorders and chronic pain of the upper limbs. The second thoracic ganglion is usually found at the lower border of the second rib or in the second intercostal space (Fig. 8-1A). On the right

side the superior intercostal vein is located anterior to the T2 ganglion in about 10% of patients and lies posterior to the ganglion in 40% of patients. In the remaining patients the superior intercostal vein does not involve the T2 ganglion on the right side, and in most patients the superior intercostal vein does not involve the T2 ganglion on the left side at all. The T1 and cervical ganglia are always located above the second rib. These ganglia are often fused into a common structure termed the stellate (cervicothoracic) ganglion, but in some patients these ganglia are separate. Although there are frequent communications between the first and second thoracic ganglia, these are almost always located within 8 to 10 mm lateral or medial to the ganglia and therefore are easily identified during surgery on the sympathetic chain. Communications between the second ganglia and the first and/or second intercostal nerves are also relatively frequent but again have little bearing on sympathetic surgery because of the proximity of these accessory communications to the sympathetic ganglia.

Figure 8-1A

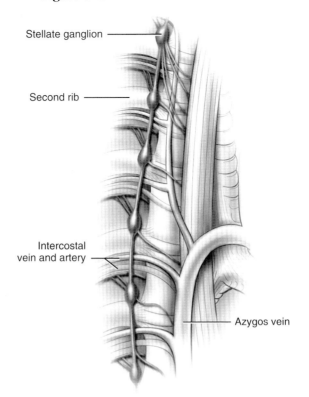

Stellate ganglion

Second rib

Intercostal
vein and artery

Azygos vein

8-2   Sympathotomy

Indications for division of the sympathetic nervous system are numerous. The most common indication is hyperhidrosis, which typically affects the palmar, plantar, and axillary regions. Other common indications for division of the sympathetic nervous system include upper extremity vascular insufficiency and chronic upper limb pain associated with reflex sympathetic dystrophy. Surgery for palmar hyperhidrosis is described here. Patients should have symptoms consistent with hyperhidrosis, including daily and often spontaneous excessive sweating of the affected surfaces, symptoms sufficiently severe to warrant surgical intervention, and absence of response to conservative medical therapy. Patients should be aware of the high incidence of compensatory sweating that accompanies this operation. If the patient is already experiencing excessive sweating of the trunk, groin, buttocks, or thighs, the risk of unacceptable compensatory sweating is substantially increased.

The sympathotomy operation is typically performed under general anesthesia on an outpatient basis. Because most patients are quite young and otherwise healthy, no specific preoperative evaluation is necessary. The patient is positioned supine with the arms placed alongside of the head. Placing the patient in mild reverse Trendelenburg assists in clearing the lung tissue from the apex of the hemithorax. A double lumen endotracheal tube is used to achieve lung isolation.

It is easiest to begin the operation on the left side, where the anatomy is usually more clear than on the right side. The ipsilateral lung is isolated from the ventilatory circuit. Small (3.5 to 5 mm) ports are placed in approximately the third and fifth intercostal spaces in the anterior axillary line (Fig. 8-2A). Infiltration of a topical anesthetic helps reduce the incidence of postoperative pain in these regions. Insufflation of carbon dioxide gas at a rapid rate to a maximum pressure of 15 mm Hg helps to achieve lung deflation quickly and is often useful in reducing operative time. Typically 10 to 20 seconds of insufflation is sufficient to achieve the desired effect. Care is taken not to expose the patient to a long interval of elevated intrapleural pressure, which can cause mediastinal shift and resultant hypoxia and hypotension.

A telescope and camera are placed through the inferior part. It is usually straightforward to identify the second rib, which is the first rib that is visible at the apex of the hemithorax. However, in patients who are very thin and in those who are quite heavy, it may not be readily apparent which rib is the second rib. In such instances use of a probe to palpate the first rib is appropriate. Ensuring that the second rib is identified accurately is important in the correct performance of the operation.

The optimal level of sympathotomy for managing palmar hyperhidrosis is controversial. Initial descriptions of the operation called for division above the T2 ganglia and often included division of the T3 and T4 ganglia as well. The recognition that a more extensive sympathotomy leads to higher rates of unacceptable compensatory sweating resulted in more limited sympathotomy operations. Randomized studies demonstrated that division of the T3 and sometimes the T4 ganglia provides therapeutic outcomes equivalent to division of the T2 ganglion but is accompanied by much lower rates of unsatisfactory compensatory sweating.

Using a hook cautery, the pleura over the sympathetic chain is divided longitudinally along the chain (Fig. 8-2B). The appropriate ganglia are identified. A hook cautery is used to mobilize the lateral and medial aspects of the ganglia; in doing so, the accessory fibers between two ganglia and between the ganglia and somatic nerve fibers are divided. Following this, the proximal margins of the ganglia are divided from the sympathetic chain (Fig. 8-2C). When the ganglia are sufficiently mobilized and divided, a 1-cm gap appears between the cut ends of the sympathetic chain. Monitoring of palmar skin temperature may provide objective evidence that a sufficient sympathotomy has been accomplished, indicated by a 1°C to 3°C rise in temperature that is usually evident within 5 to 10 minutes of the completion of the sympathotomy. Drainage catheters are placed through the operating ports and are placed under underwater seal using a specimen cup filled with saline. As the lung is re-expanded, the amount of air exiting the pleural space decreases and then ceases, indicating complete lung re-expansion. The drainage catheters are removed and the incisions are closed with adhesive. An exactly similar procedure is performed on the contralateral side if indicated. The patient is discharged after 2 to 3 hours in the postoperative care unit.

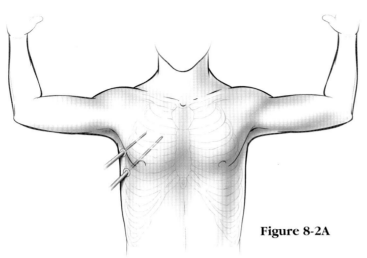

Figure 8-2A

Figure 8-2B

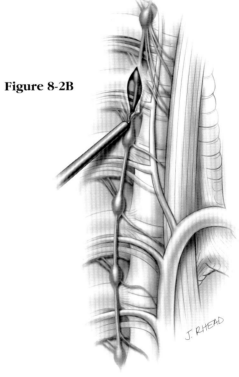

Figure 8-2C

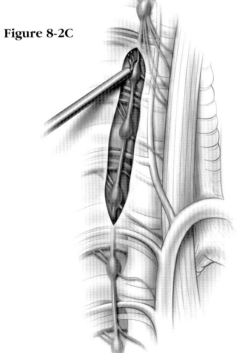

J. R. HEAD

8-3 Splanchnicectomy

The splanchnic nerves arise from the thoracic sympathetic chain and ultimately join the abdominal sympathetic ganglia. The greater splanchnic nerve comprises branches from the fifth through eighth thoracic ganglia, and courses dorsal to the azygos vein on the right side toward the costophrenic recess. On the left side the greater splanchnic nerve descends dorsal to the hemiazygos vein. The lesser splanchnic nerve comprises branches from the T9 through T11 ganglia and lies dorsolateral to the greater splanchnic nerve (Fig. 8-3A). The trunks of the splanchnic nerves penetrate the diaphragm and enter the celiac ganglia, from where branches to the celiac plexus emerge. The splanchnic nerves transmit afferent stimuli from the pancreas and other abdominal tissues to the hypothalamus, serving as the main pathway for transmission of pain. Interruption of these pathways often successfully manages chronic pancreatic and other upper abdominal pain.

Control of chronic abdominal pain, typically associated with pancreatic disorders, usually requires division of the greater and lesser nerves bilaterally. In some instances left unilateral splanchnicectomy is sufficient to provide symptomatic relief. In contrast to upper thoracic sympathotomy, a much more extensive neural division is required and the ganglia themselves are not targeted. Adequate visualization of the splanchnic nerves usually requires placing the patient in a lateral decubitus position. Ipsilateral lung isolation is achieved. Insufflation of carbon dioxide gas provides more rapid lung collapse and reduces operating time.

Two small ports are placed in approximately the eighth or ninth and sixth or seventh interspaces laterally. The pleura is opened widely over the splanchnic nerves from the level of the diaphragmatic insertion to the level of the T5 ganglion (Fig. 8-3B). To visualize the inferior extent of the splanchnic nerves, it may be necessary to insert a third port anterior and inferior to the port in the eighth or ninth interspace to permit downward retraction of the diaphragm. The pleura is peeled laterally and medially to facilitate access to all rami joining the splanchnic nerves. Using a hook cautery, the rami joining the splanchnic nerves are individually divided, completely isolating the nerves from the sympathetic chain (Fig. 8-3C). Management of the pleura space after completion of the splanchnicectomy is similar to that described for upper thoracic sympathotomy.

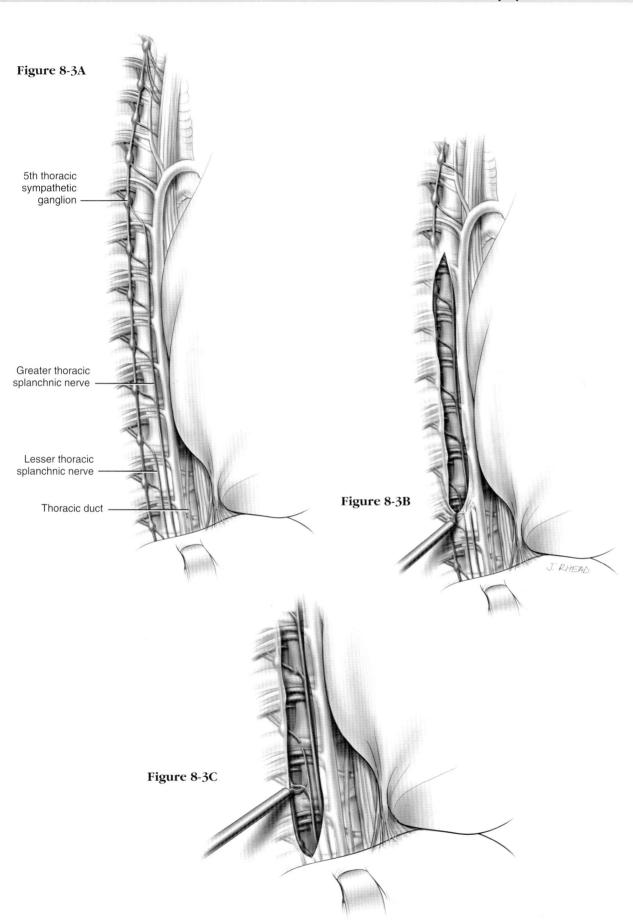

Figure 8-3A

5th thoracic
sympathetic
ganglion

Greater thoracic
splanchnic nerve

Lesser thoracic
splanchnic nerve

Thoracic duct

Figure 8-3B

Figure 8-3C

J. RHEAD

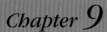

Diaphragm

9-1 Anatomy

An understanding of its embryologic development is essential in managing many of the surgical disorders of the diaphragm. The diaphragm develops from a complex and incompletely delineated process of coalescence of four entities: the septum transversum, the pleuroperitoneal membranes, the dorsal mesentery of the esophagus, and the body wall muscles (Fig. 9-1A). The septum transversum is recognizable by the third week of gestation, and by the fourth week of gestation it extends from the ventral and lateral regions of the body wall to the foregut. The septum transversum is inclined from its anteroinferior margin on the body wall to its posterior superior margin adjacent to the foregut/esophagus. It incompletely separates the pericardial and peritoneal cavities, leaving an intact pericardioperitoneal canal bilaterally. The pleuroperitoneal membranes are located dorsolateral to the pleuroperitoneal canals.

During the fifth week of gestation nerves arise from the fourth and fifth segments of the spinal cord and pass through the pleuropericardial folds into the septum transversum, forming the phrenic nerves. When the pleuropericardial folds separate from the somatopleurae to develop into the pericardium, the phrenic nerves remain attached to the folds, resulting in the phrenic nerves being located between the pericardium and the mediastinal pleura. During the sixth to eighth weeks of gestation the structures of the diaphragm, which initially are located at the level of the thoracic somites, descend to the level of first lumbar vertebra, pulling the phrenic nerves caudally to their final length.

At about the eighth week of gestation the pericardioperitoneal canals close by fusion of the edges of the pleuroperitoneal membranes from posterolateral to anteromedial, separating the pleural and peritoneal cavities. Between nine and twelve weeks of gestation the pleural cavities extend cranially and ventrally by burrowing into the body wall, forming the costodiaphragmatic recesses. In this process somatopleuric mesenchyme is separated from the dorsal body wall, developing into the muscular posterior portion of the diaphragm (see Fig. 9-1A). The latter layer receives muscle fibers from the thoracic myotomes, explaining why the outer portions of the diaphragm are innervated by the lower intercostal nerves. The right pleuroperitoneal canal closes earlier than the left, possibly explaining the higher incidence of persisting communications between the peritoneal and pleural cavities on the left.

After development of the diaphragm is complete, it is formed of muscular and tendinous portions. The muscular portions originate from the circumference of the lower thorax, including the lumbar spine (pars lumbalis), ribs (pars costalis), and sternum (pars sternalis) (Fig. 9-1B). These muscular portions are separated from each other by gaps best seen from an inferior perspective (Fig. 9-1C), and insert onto the central tendon of the diaphragm. The lumbar portion of the diaphragm, the most powerful portion, arises from the L1 through L3 lumbar vertebrae and the lateral and medial arcuate ligaments. This portion forms the right and left crura, which form the esophageal and aortic apertures. The costal portions of the diaphragm arise from the inferior six ribs and interdigitate with the transverse abdominis muscles. The potential space between the lumbar and costal muscular portions, Bochdalek's gap, is sometimes only covered by fascia and mesothelial surfaces. Failure of coverage by these tissues leads to a Bochdalek hernia, which is most commonly found on the left side. The sternal portion of the diaphragm arises from the posterior rectus sheath and from the xiphoid process, and is not always present. A space exists bilaterally between the sternal and costal parts that are known as Morgagni's or Larrey's gaps, and are the basis for Morgagni hernias, which occur most often on the right.

The tendinous portion of the diaphragm, or central tendon, is longest in its transverse plane. Its center lies immediately beneath the pericardium, with which it is partially blended. The domes of the diaphragm are quite mobile, rising as high as the fourth intercostal space on the right and the fifth intercostal space on the left at rest. The domes descend at least two interspaces during maximum inhalation.

Figure 9-1A

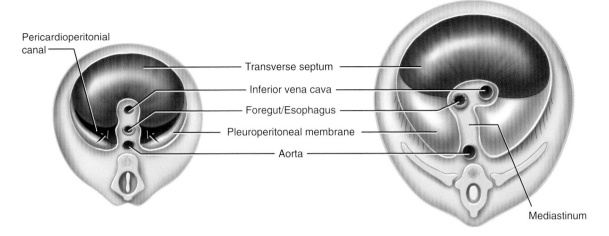

Pericardioperitonial canal

Transverse septum

Inferior vena cava

Foregut/Esophagus

Pleuroperitoneal membrane

Aorta

Mediastinum

Figure 9-1B

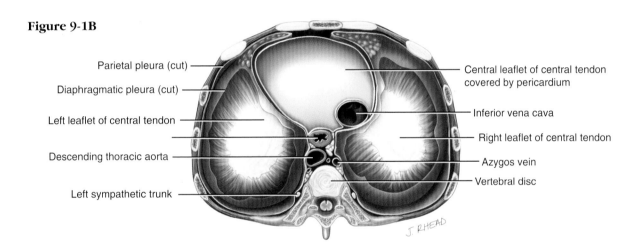

Parietal pleura (cut)

Diaphragmatic pleura (cut)

Left leaflet of central tendon

Descending thoracic aorta

Left sympathetic trunk

Central leaflet of central tendon covered by pericardium

Inferior vena cava

Right leaflet of central tendon

Azygos vein

Vertebral disc

J. RHEAD

Figure 9-1C

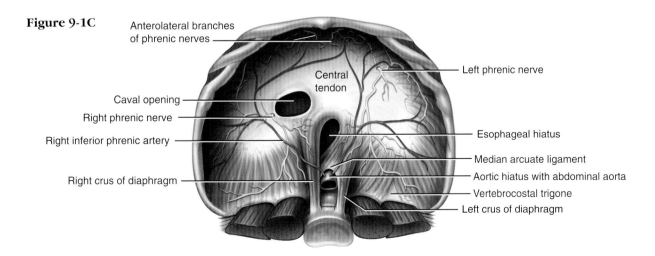

Anterolateral branches of phrenic nerves

Central tendon

Caval opening

Right phrenic nerve

Right inferior phrenic artery

Right crus of diaphragm

Left phrenic nerve

Esophageal hiatus

Median arcuate ligament

Aortic hiatus with abdominal aorta

Vertebrocostal trigone

Left crus of diaphragm

The aortic aperture is the most posterior aperture, lying slightly to the left of the midline at the level of the twelfth thoracic vertebra. It is defined by the crura laterally, the vertebral bodies posteriorly, and the diaphragm anteriorly. The esophageal aperture, located at the level of the tenth thoracic vertebra, lies anterior to and to the left of the aortic opening. It is formed from fibers of the right crus. The inferior vena cava (IVC) aperture lies between the eighth and ninth thoracic vertebrae, and is bounded by the right leaf and the central portion of the central tendon of the diaphragm.

9-2 Plication

Diaphragm plication is an appropriate consideration for patients with symptomatic diaphragm eventration or unilateral diaphragm paralysis. Causes for eventration are not well understood; the etiology appears to be related to advancing age, female gender, and obesity. Unilateral diaphragm paralysis is often a result of trauma or iatrogenic causes, such as direct intraoperative injury or prolonged exposure to cold cardioplegia. The mere existence of an elevated hemidiaphragm on a chest radiograph is not a sufficient indication for such surgery. Additional evaluation might include fluoroscopy to detect paradoxical motion during a "sniff test," pulmonary function testing documenting reduced spirometry, and possibly phrenic nerve stimulation to assess the innervation of the affected diaphragm. Absence of diaphragm contractions during phrenic nerve stimulation in the neck does not exclude the possibility that the phrenic nerve is intact distally; phrenic nerve pacing rather than diaphragm plication might be considered in patients who are very symptomatic from unilateral diaphragm paralysis.

The operation is performed through an open thoracotomy or using thoracoscopic techniques. The patient is placed in a lateral decubitus position and single lung ventilation is achieved. The most common approach is imbrication of the elevated hemidiaphragm using a series of sutures placed 2 to 3 cm apart and incorporating most of the dome of the diaphragm. Beginning either anterior or posterior, sutures are placed from lateral to medial, taking wide bites of the central tendon or muscular diaphragm (Fig. 9-2A). The suture may be placed in a mattress fashion, taking an additional series of imbrication bites back toward the lateral aspect of the diaphragm so that the final configuration is a "U" stitch. In this case the imbricating row for a single suture should not span more than 1 to 2 cm of width. Once all of the imbricating sutures are placed, they are put under tension simultaneously to avoid excess tension on a single suture, and the imbrication is accomplished as they are tied. It is helpful to reduce the dome of the diaphragm toward the diaphragm with gentle pressure. When "U" stitches are placed, the two ends of the suture are tied over the small distance of diaphragm separating them. If simple imbrication sutures are used, the two suture ends are tied over the diaphragm dome (Fig. 9-2B).

An alternative technique to the classic imbrication method is best performed through an open thoracotomy rather than thoracoscopically. The floppy section of diaphragm is grasped and elevated, creating a tent of diaphragm to be plicated. The base of this tent, where the desired dome of the diaphragm is to be situated, is grasped with Allis clamps, approximating the two sides of the tented diaphragm and excluding any abdominal tissues. Simple mattress sutures are placed, approximating the apposed tissues (Fig. 9-2C). Once all of the mattress sutures are placed, extending from one limit of the dome to the opposite limit, they are simultaneously placed under tension as the tented portion of the diaphragm is elevated with grasping clamps, and are sequentially tied. The isolated tented portion of the diaphragm is folded onto the new dome of the diaphragm and is sutured in place with mattress sutures (Fig. 9-2D).

Diaphragm plication, when performed in carefully selected patients, yields immediate improvement in respiratory symptoms and in the radiographic appearance of the thorax. Initial overcorrection of the abnormality, as evidenced by the level of the diaphragm on a plain chest radiograph, is not uncommon, and typically the overcorrection resolves over a period of several weeks. If patients fail to experience substantial symptomatic improvement, potential explanations include failure to adequately correct the defect, or the incorrect diagnosis of diaphragm dysfunction as the source of the respiratory symptoms.

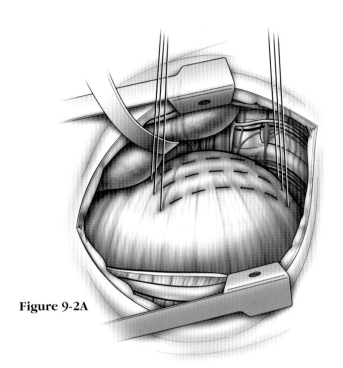

Figure 9-2A

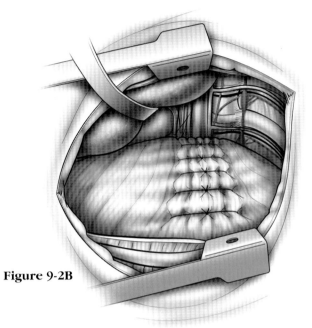

Figure 9-2B

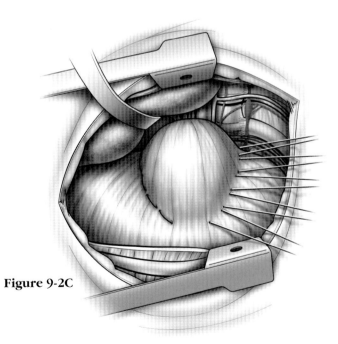

Figure 9-2C

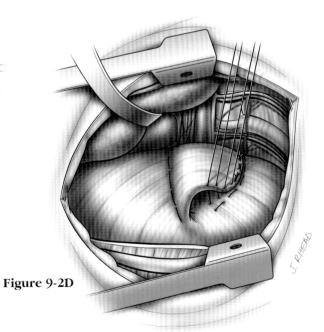

Figure 9-2D

J. R. HEAD

9-3   Giant Paraesophageal Hernia Repair

Giant paraesophageal hernias are likely the final end product of a wide spectrum of hiatal hernia disorders. Hiatal hernias are classified as Type I: sliding or axial hernia, characterized by the gastroesophageal junction being displaced into the mediastinum along the axis of the esophagus, with no portion of the stomach extending alongside of the esophagus; Type II: a hiatal hernia in which the gastroesophageal junction is in its normal intraabdominal location, and a portion of the gastric fundus is herniated through the esophageal hiatus into a paraesophageal position; Type III, which is really a combination of types I and II, in which the gastroesophageal junction is displaced into the mediastinum and a portion of the stomach is herniated through the esophageal hiatus alongside the esophagus (Fig. 9-3A); and Type IV, which is a Type III hernia in which other abdominal content, usually the colon or small bowel, is also herniated into the mediastinum. All of these hernias are classified as true hernias, in which a hernia sac contains the abnormal contents. The sac comprises endothoracic fascia, parietal pleura, and the attachment of these structures to the hiatus (termed the phrenoesophageal ligament).

Giant paraesophageal hernias are almost exclusively Type III and Type IV hernias. In these giant hernias, at least half of the stomach is displaced into the chest. The pylorus is displaced upward almost to the esophageal hiatus. The stomach frequently suffers organoaxial and mesentericoaxial volvulus, resulting in a complex endoscopic and radiographic image that is often difficult to decipher clearly (see Fig. 9-3A). The volvulus creates relative or complete obstruction, often leading to symptoms such as postprandial pain, early satiety, and regurgitation. The mass effect of the displaced organs often leads to shortness of breath and dyspnea on exertion.

When such symptoms exist in patients who are in otherwise good health, elective hernia repair is indicated. In some patients incarceration and strangulation develop, leading to the need for emergency intervention that carries substantially increased risk compared to the risk of elective surgery. In the absence of obvious symptoms related to a giant paraesophageal hiatal hernia, however, routine repair is not indicated.

Repair of a giant paraesophageal hernia may be performed through an open thoracic approach or through an open or laparoscopic abdominal approach. The choice depends on co-morbid factors affecting the patient, the possible need for an esophageal lengthening procedure, and on the surgeon's personal preferences. The objectives of the operation are similar regardless of which approach is selected. The hernia is reduced, the sac is resected, and the defect in the hiatus is repaired. Additional considerations are the need for a fundoplication wrap and provision of a mechanism for anchoring the stomach within the diaphragm to prevent recurrent herniation. If a thoracic approach is selected, the steps are very similar to those described in Section 6-6, the Belsey fundoplication. The hernia contents are reduced, the sac is resected, and additional crural stitches are placed to provide appropriate sizing of the hiatus.

This section describes an abdominal approach for repair of a giant paraesophageal hiatal hernia in which a lengthening procedure is not required. The contents of the hernia sac are reduced into the abdomen. The sac is grasped and is drawn into the abdomen (Fig. 9-3B), putting on stretch the junction between the hernia sac and the rim of the diaphragmatic hiatus. The sac is incised along this line, and blunt dissection is used to separate the sac from the underlying mediastinal structures and parietal pleura (Fig. 9-3C). The dissection is continued circumferentially, and the sac is then excised from its attachments near the esophagogastric junction, the original site of the insertion of the phrenoesophageal ligament.

Figure 9-3A

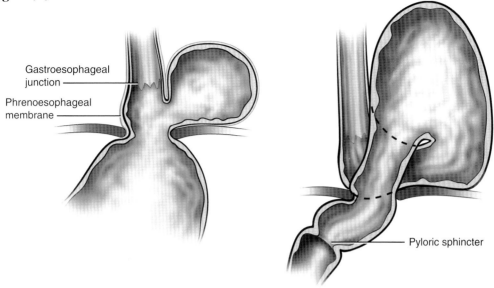

Gastroesophageal junction

Phrenoesophageal membrane

Pyloric sphincter

Figure 9-3B

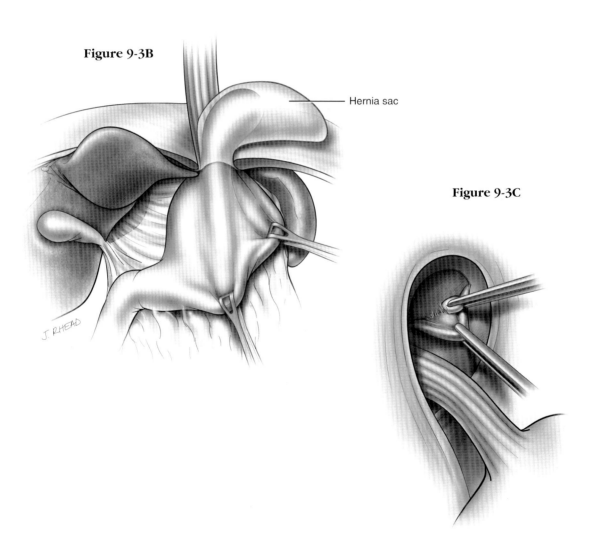

Hernia sac

J. RHEAD

Figure 9-3C

The esophagus is mobilized from the mediastinum sufficiently to provide an intraabdominal length of at least 3 to 4 cm. The hiatal closure is undertaken with heavy interrupted sutures. Assuming that the crural tissues are of adequate caliber and strength, simple sutures are sufficient to approximate the edges of the crura to obliterate the hernia (Fig. 9-3D). If the tissues are not of sufficient strength, consideration is given to repair of the hiatus with artificial material, such as a patch of Gortex or other similar substance. Even if prosthetic reconstruction is not deemed necessary, randomized trials have demonstrated that the addition of a reinforcing patch of Gortex or other material in a donut fashion can help prevent recurrent herniation. The patch is cut to an overall diameter 5 to 6 cm wider than the hiatus. A hole is cut in the middle that is larger than the esophagus, and the ring is incised radially at one point to enable its placement around the esophagus. The radial opening is oriented anteriorly to align it with the strongest portion of the hiatal ring. The patch is sewn to the diaphragm with interrupted sutures (Fig. 9-3E).

It is sometimes apparent, during hiatal closure, that there will be too much tension on the sutures to permit primary closure without subsequent breakdown of the suture line. In such instances, use of artificial material abutting the esophagus can be avoided with use of a relaxing incision. This is best performed through a thoracic approach, and is illustrated in Figure 9-3F as seen from this vantage point. An 8-to-10-cm relaxing incision is created lateral to the distribution of the phrenic nerve, permitting the crural tissues to be approximated without tension. The relaxing incision is closed with Gortex or other similar patching material. Placement of the artificial material distant from the esophagus helps to avoid complications, such as erosion of such material into the esophagus.

Figure 9-3D

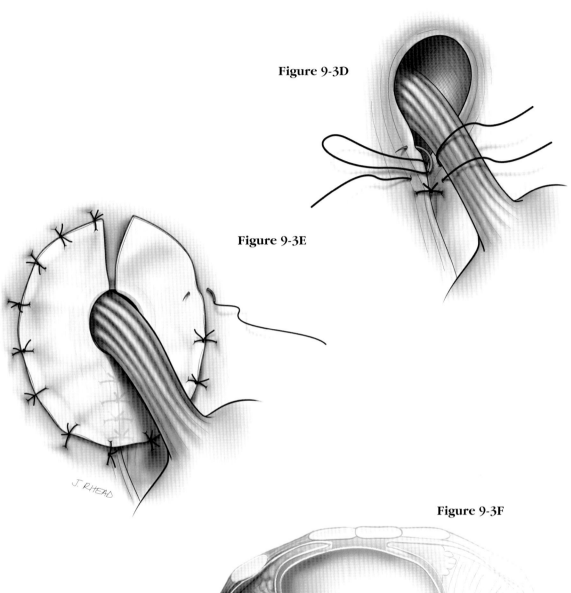

Figure 9-3E

J. RHEAD

Figure 9-3F

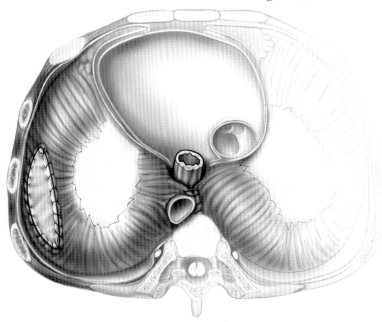

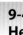

9-4 Congenital Diaphragmatic Hernia Repair

The two common types of congenital hernias are pictured in Figure 9-4A. Imaged from below, the Morgagni hernia is evident anteriorly as a defect in the diaphragm extending from the parasternal region laterally for a distance of 5 to 10 cm. The depth of the defect is of a similar size range. The hernia is easily approached from the abdomen, and laparoscopic or open techniques are equally appropriate for repair. Repair through open or minimally invasive thoracic approaches has also been described, although access to this region is more difficult than when using an abdominal approach. Small hernias in which there is sufficient tissue to permit approximation of the edges of the defect are closed with interrupted simple or figure-of-eight sutures after reduction of the hernia contents (Fig. 9-4B). The free edge of the diaphragmatic defect needs to be approximated to the anterior abdominal wall if there is no rim of diaphragmatic tissue in this region.

Most often, however, there is an insufficient amount of diaphragmatic tissue present to permit primary closure, and prosthetic repair of the defect is required. The omentum and colon are the most common tissues occupying the hernia space. The hernia contents are reduced, which may require division of adhesions within the pleural cavity. Once the edges of the defect are clearly defined, a patch of Gortex or other suitable material is brought into the abdomen and is cut to an appropriate size. The posterior margin is sutured first, followed by the lateral margins, taking care not to include any thoracic contents in the repair (Fig. 9-4C). Use of a laparoscopic technique with carbon dioxide insufflation greatly facilitates this. The anterior margin of the patch may be sutured to the free edge of any existing diaphragmatic tissue, or can be attached to the anterior chest wall using staples or screws (Fig. 9-4D).

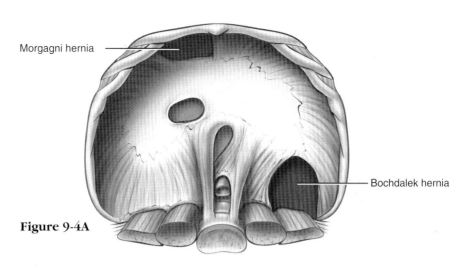

Morgagni hernia

Bochdalek hernia

Figure 9-4A

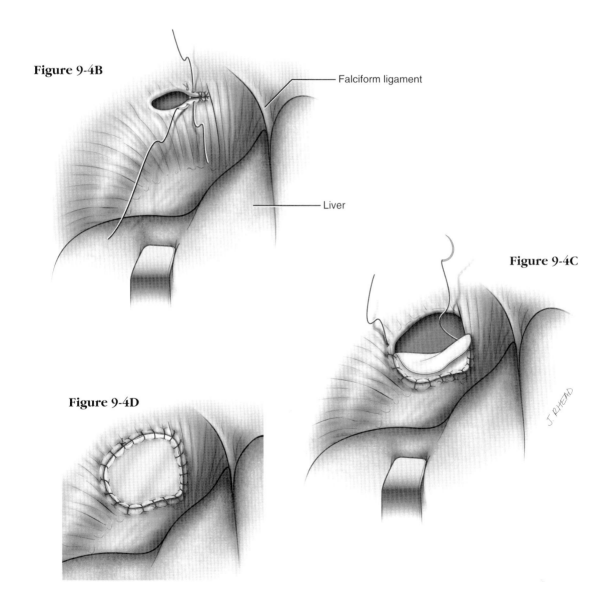

Figure 9-4B

Falciform ligament

Liver

Figure 9-4C

Figure 9-4D

J R HEAD

Bochdalek hernias occur posterolaterally and often are characterized by rather large diaphragmatic defects in neonates, accompanied by various degrees of pulmonary hypoplasia or even agenesis. It is unusual for adults to present with such findings; Bochdalek hernias in this age group are typically of moderate size with little or no lung hypoplasia (see Fig. 9-4A). Because of their location, these hernias are usually approached through the chest rather than through the abdomen. The use of minimally invasive techniques may be appropriate for pediatric patients (other than infants) who are in good general condition and for adults not previously operated on, but this approach should be considered only by surgeons with extensive experience in minimally invasive surgery of the diaphragm. In most instances an open transthoracic approach through the seventh or eighth interspace is best. The defect may be small and amenable to primary repair after reduction of the hernia contents, especially if a rim of diaphragm muscle remains on the chest wall (Fig. 9-4E).

Larger Bochdalek hernias are more challenging to repair. The abdominal contents are sometimes difficult to reduce because of positive intraabdominal pressure, the volume of abdominal contents that require reduction, and the resultant loss of domain within the abdomen. Once this is accomplished, the edges of the diaphragm are defined. It is common to have complete absence of diaphragm tissue along the chest wall side of the defect. The defect is closed with a patch of Gortex or similar material. The lung is retracted anteromedially (Fig. 9-4F). Suturing the edges of the patch to the free edge of diaphragm along the defect is straightforward. The posterolateral edge must be sutured to the chest wall (Fig. 9-4G). The use of mattress sutures, sometimes buttressed with pledgets on the outer surface of the bony chest wall, is useful to provide a secure closure.

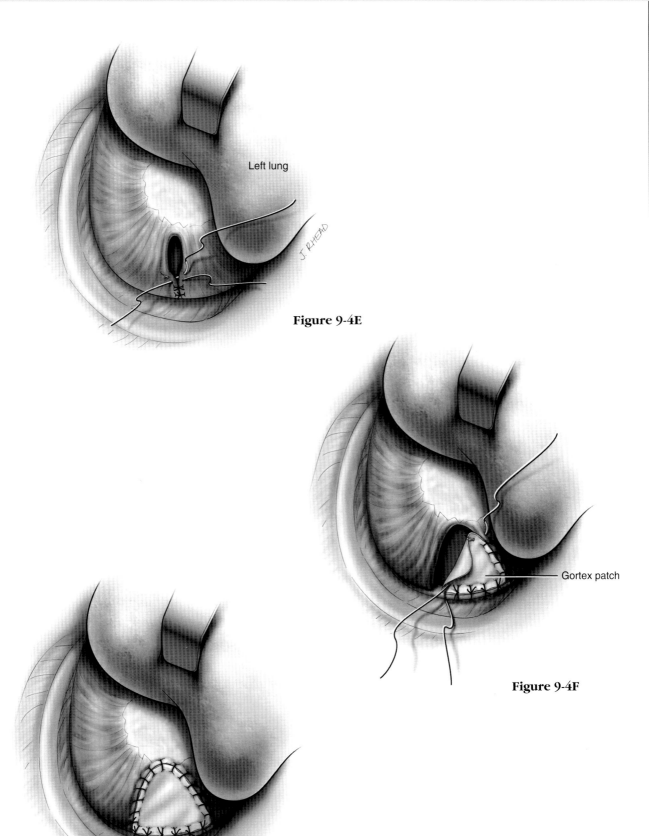

Left lung

Figure 9-4E

Gortex patch

Figure 9-4F

Figure 9-4G

9-5 Traumatic Diaphragmatic Hernia Repair

Traumatic diaphragmatic hernias occur after blunt or penetrating trauma. They present acutely or in a chronic phase, and the time from injury dictates to some extent which approach to hernia repair is optimal. Most traumatic hernias should be repaired when they are diagnosed because the natural force of intraabdominal pressure working against the negative intrathoracic pressure results in enlargement of the hernia over time. Although most traumatic diaphragmatic hernias affect the left hemidiaphragm, repair of a right diaphragmatic hernia is illustrated in this atlas because of some of the pitfalls of repairing a hernia on the right side that are not encountered on the left side. This atlas illustrates the approach to a chronic hernia rather than an acute hernia. When an acute left diaphragmatic hernia is encountered, an abdominal approach to repair is often appropriate. In contrast, chronic hernias on either side of the diaphragm are best approached using a transthoracic route. In particular, right-sided hernias are best approached in this manner because their repair through an abdominal approach is complicated by the presence of the liver.

The chest is entered through the eighth interspace laterally and the abdominal contents are usually immediately evident. On the left side, the stomach, spleen, and colon are most commonly encountered. On the right side, the liver is the most prominent organ occupying the pleural space (Fig. 9-5A). Depending on the length of time since the injury, varying degrees of adhesions between abdominal contents and the lung and chest wall must be dissected. Following this, the abdominal contents are gradually reduced through the aperture in the diaphragm. When a large segment of the liver is displaced into the thorax, the defect in the diaphragm may not be sufficiently large to permit reduction of the liver into the abdomen, and the aperture must be enlarged by cutting laterally to allow the liver segment to pass through it. As the abdominal contents are reduced, the edges of the diaphragm defect are identified and marked with Allis clamps. This serves to retract the diaphragm as adhesions are dissected and permits countertraction on the diaphragm as the abdominal contents are pushed caudad, providing ready markers for subsequent repair (Fig. 9-5B).

Although usually no diaphragm tissue is lost as a result of a traumatic hernia, especially when it results from blunt force trauma, rarely is it possible or wise to attempt to close the defect primarily unless it is very small. If a counterincision has been made in the diaphragm, it is closed primarily with heavy sutures in an interrupted figure-of-eight pattern. As the edges of the diaphragm are put on stretch, bringing them close to approximation, an estimate of the size of the defect is made. A 2-mm thick patch of Gortex or other material is cut to size, leaving a 1-to-2-cm margin larger than the defect for sewing. The medial edge of the diaphragm is attached to the patch first, beginning near the inferior vena cava (Fig. 9-5C). The sutures are placed circumferentially, keeping the diaphragm under moderate tension through judicious suture placement. As the lateral edge is approached, the sutures are left untied until all have been placed. Care is taken to leave an aperture posteromedially so that the inferior vena cava is not constricted by the patch. Once all lateral sutures have been placed, they are tied down while the patch and diaphragm are approximated by placing tension on the untied sutures, distributing tension evenly across the patch (Fig. 9-5D).

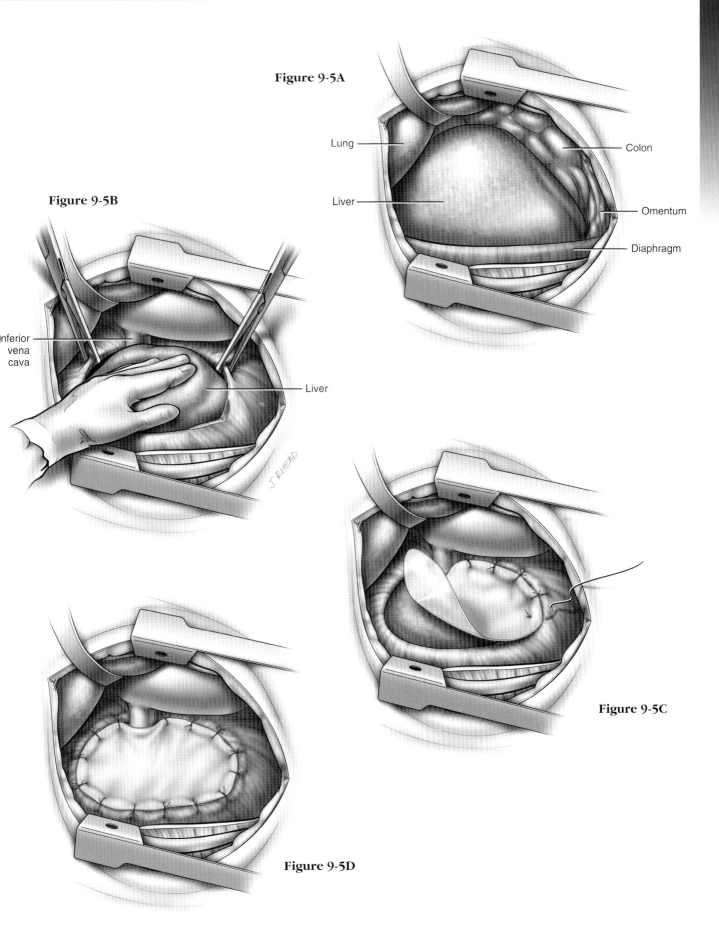

Figure 9-5A

Lung

Colon

Liver

Omentum

Diaphragm

Figure 9-5B

Inferior vena cava

Liver

Figure 9-5C

Figure 9-5D

Chapter *10*

Trachea

10-1 Anatomy

The trachea is a roughly cylindrical organ that extends from the cricoid cartilage in the neck at the level of the sixth cervical vertebra to the carina in the middle mediastinum at the upper border of the fifth thoracic vertebra (Fig. 10-1A). The trachea comprises incomplete cartilaginous rings, which wrap from anterior to lateral surfaces, and a muscular membranous portion posteriorly. It measures 10 to 11 cm in length in the average adult; the length varies according to the height of the individual. The transverse external diameter is 2 cm in males and 1.5 cm in females. There are 1 to 2 rings per centimeter of length in the adult.

The cervical trachea is related to the superficial and deep cervical fascia and to the strap muscles. The second through fourth rings are covered by the thyroid isthmus. Posteriorly the trachea is related to the esophagus, which lies between it and the vertebral column. The recurrent laryngeal nerves lie in or near the grooves between the esophagus and trachea. Laterally the lobes of the thyroid gland descend to the level of the fifth or sixth tracheal rings. The common carotid arteries and inferior thyroid arteries are also related to these tracheal surfaces.

The thoracic trachea, which constitutes half of the total length of the trachea, descends sharply away from the sternum and approaches the vertebral column near its bifurcation. The angle between the trachea and sternum increases with age; people who are older or who have kyphosis have a substantial angle between the sternum and the trachea. The trachea initially lies behind the manubrium, and passes between the left common carotid and brachiocephalic arteries on the left and right, respectively. It then passes behind the brachiocephalic vein, the brachiocephalic artery, and eventually descends posterior to the aorta (Fig. 10-1B). As in the neck, the esophagus lies between the thoracic trachea and the vertebral column. Laterally on the right the thoracic trachea is related to the right lung, brachiocephalic vein, superior vena cava (SVC), right vagus nerve, and azygos vein. On the left, the trachea is related to the aortic arch, left common carotid artery, and left subclavian artery. Just anterior to the tracheal bifurcation is the bifurcation of the main pulmonary artery.

The blood supply to the trachea arises primarily from the thyrocervical trunk via the inferior thyroid arteries (Fig. 10-1C). Most commonly the inferior thyroid artery gives off three branches to the upper trachea that anastomose to form a longitudinal vessel that gives off segmental branches. The thoracic trachea is supplied by branches of the bronchial arteries and by branches from the subclavian, innominate, and intercostal arteries. The vessels enter the trachea on its lateral aspect from a longitudinal network that feeds the spaces between the cartilaginous rings. The rings receive their blood supply from the submucosal network, indicating that persistent pressure on the mucosa can lead to ischemia and eventual necrosis of the rings, causing scarring and stenosis. The membranous trachea is supplied by secondary branches that are primarily from esophageal vessels and do not contribute significantly to the blood supply of the trachea. These facts indicate that dissection anteriorly and posteriorly is possible without seriously disturbing the tracheal circulation. The venous drainage is mostly into the inferior thyroid venous plexus. The trachea is innervated by branches of the vagus nerves, recurrent laryngeal nerves, and sympathetic trunks.

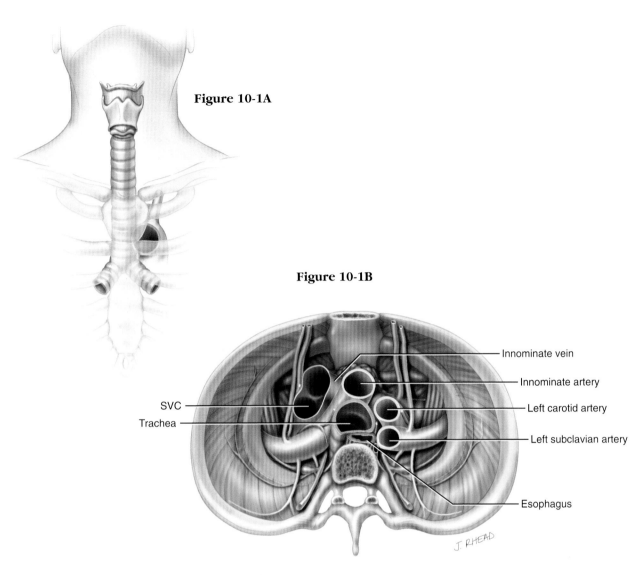

Figure 10-1A

Figure 10-1B

- Innominate vein
- Innominate artery
- SVC
- Left carotid artery
- Trachea
- Left subclavian artery
- Esophagus

J. RHEAD

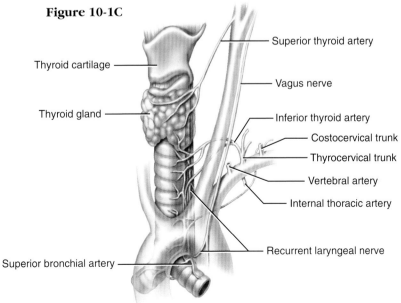

Figure 10-1C

- Superior thyroid artery
- Thyroid cartilage
- Vagus nerve
- Thyroid gland
- Inferior thyroid artery
- Costocervical trunk
- Thyrocervical trunk
- Vertebral artery
- Internal thoracic artery
- Recurrent laryngeal nerve
- Superior bronchial artery

10-2   Resection for Tracheal Stenosis

Despite decades of improvements in endotracheal tubes, tracheostomy tubes, and the balloon cuffs for these devices, tracheal stenosis for postintubation injury remains the most common indication for tracheal resection. There are a variety of types of postintubation injury, including cuff stenosis that typically occurs in the upper and mid-trachea (Fig. 10-2A), stomal stenosis related to tissue loss at the site of a tracheostomy, subglottic stenosis that results from injury to the cricoid tissues due to complications from cricothyroidostomy or an oversized endotracheal tube, and glottic stenosis that is caused by an endotracheal tube resting against the posterior vocal cords or arytenoid structures while the patient is maintained in a supine position. This section focuses on management of cuff stenosis of the upper and mid-trachea.

Cuff stenosis typically is located within 3 to 4 cm of the vocal cords, but the exact location is dependent on the location of the cuff during intubation. Cuff stenosis often does not present at the time of extubation, but takes days or weeks to develop as the result of the maturation of cicatricial tissues. The etiology of cuff stenosis, transmural ischemic injury of several adjacent tracheal rings, suggests that local therapy, such as laser resection, will not provide longstanding relief from the stenosis. However, dilation, stenting, and laser therapy may provide short-term relief from dyspnea and permit an electively planned operation for permanent relief of stenosis.

At the time of surgery, if the patient requires dilation to permit intubation, the stenosis is visualized with a rigid bronchoscope after induction of anesthesia. For stenoses that measure 5 mm or more in diameter, the initial dilation is performed with a 7-mm rigid bronchoscope and subsequently with 8- and 9-mm bronchoscopes, after which the location and extent of the stenosis is assessed. If the diameter is smaller than 5 mm, Jackson esophageal dilators are passed down the rigid scope to dilate the stenosis sufficiently to permit passage of pediatric rigid bronchoscopes and, subsequently, the adult rigid bronchoscopes. The patient is then intubated with a 6- or 7-mm diameter endotracheal tube in preparation for resection. If it is determined that the operation

for tracheal stenosis is not to be performed at the time of tracheal dilation, the patient will likely have a satisfactory airway for a period of at least a few days after dilation. If the airway must be secured for a longer period of time, a tracheostomy tube may be placed for this purpose. It should be positioned through the region of stenosis so that the subsequent resection does not require removal of an additional length of trachea necessitated by placement of the tracheostomy tube above or below the region of stenosis.

Resection of tracheal cuff stenosis can almost always be approached through a low collar incision that is sometimes combined with a partial sternotomy (Fig. 10-2B). The patient is positioned with the neck extended to bring as much of the trachea as possible out of the thorax. It is necessary that the patient be positioned so that the neck can be placed back in a neutral position as the operation is concluded. Subplatysmal flaps are raised proximal and distal and the strap muscles are separated in the midline. The thyroid isthmus is divided and the lobes are separated to the sides. Dissection is carried out on the anterior surface of the trachea proximally and distally. Circumferential dissection is limited to the region of the stenosis only, extending no more than 5 to 10 mm proximal and distal to the stenosis to avoid injury to the blood supply in the region of the planned anastomosis. The tracheal dissection is performed immediately on the wall of the trachea and the cicatricial tissues, which helps prevent injury to the recurrent laryngeal nerves. No effort is made to visualize or dissect out these nerves; the avoidance technique is used instead.

The region of the stenosis is identified by inspection or is visualized with the aid of bronchoscopy. Most lesions are proximal enough that the trachea distal to the stenotic segment is divided initially (Fig. 10-2C). Stay sutures are placed, and the distal trachea is intubated across the field with a small diameter endotracheal tube to permit ventilation while the rest of the dissection is performed. The stenotic trachea is dissected proximally until normal trachea is reached, and the damaged segment is removed (Fig. 10-2D). Inspection from within is sometimes useful to ensure that normal tissues are left at either end of the remaining trachea, which can be facilitated by opening the anterior wall of the damaged trachea to assess the appropriate point for proximal transection.

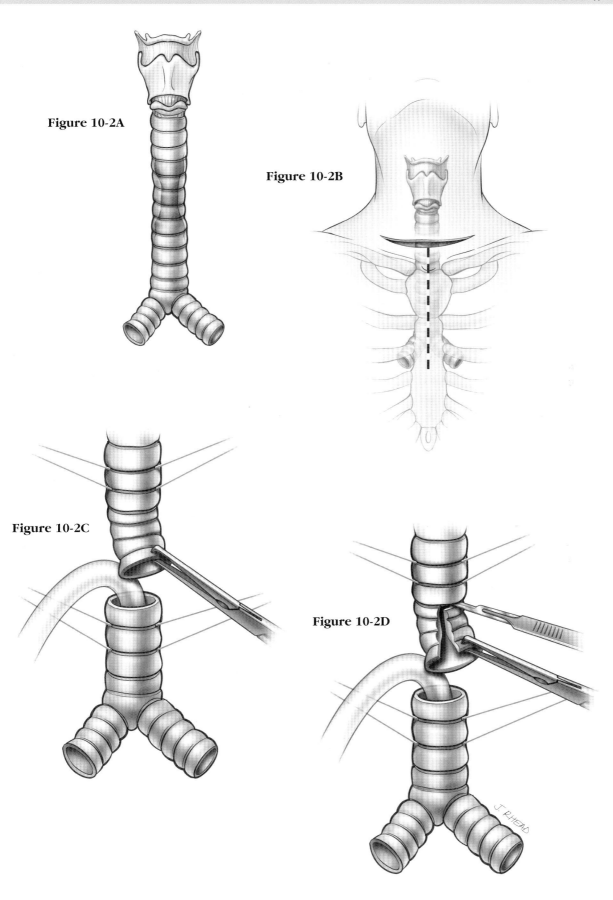

Figure 10-2A

Figure 10-2B

Figure 10-2C

Figure 10-2D

The patient's neck is flexed forward and the degree of apposition of the ends of the trachea is assessed. The amount of trachea that can be resected depends on the height, age, sex, and body habitus of the patient. Additional length can be gained by anterior and posterior dissection of the trachea proximal and distal. If necessary a laryngeal release maneuver is performed, which provides an extra 1 to 1.5 cm of length to lessen tension on the anastomosis. Posterior sutures are placed initially, beginning in the ends of the cartilaginous rings and extending across the membranous portion of the trachea (Fig. 10-2E). This segment can be approximated using a running or interrupted suture technique, employing 4-0 stitches of absorbable braided or monofilament suture. Additional sutures are placed in simple or figure-of-eight fashion to include the rest of the circumference of the trachea (Fig. 10-2F). The endotracheal tube is removed from across the field and the patient is reintubated across the impending anastomosis. The stay sutures are tied to bring the ends of the trachea together, and the anastomotic sutures are tied. The thyroid tissues are approximated over the anastomosis. Alternatively, the anastomosis may be reinforced with a segment of strap muscle that is mobilized for this purpose (Fig. 10-2G). Such a segment of strap muscle may also be interposed between the anastomosis and the innominate artery if the artery lies near the anastomosis.

The patient is extubated in the operating room and is maintained in a neck-flexed position postoperatively. In some cases it is appropriate to place a suture between the patient's chin and anterior chest wall to encourage the patient not to extend his neck.

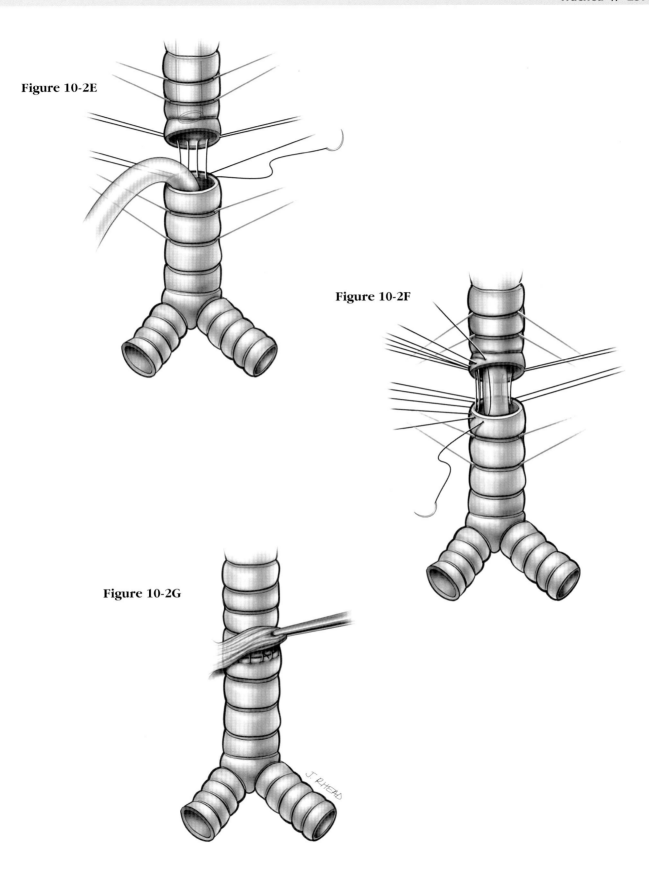

Figure 10-2E

Figure 10-2F

Figure 10-2G

10-3   Carinal Resection

Carinal resection is a technically challenging operation fraught with potential complications of a life-threatening nature. As such, careful patient selection and operative planning are necessary for optimal outcomes. The most common indication for carinal resection is a non-small cell lung cancer involving the carinal airways in the absence of obvious mediastinal nodal involvement. Other indications include primary airway tumors, such as adenoid cystic carcinoma, and other rare benign and malignant conditions. Patients undergo a careful preoperative evaluation to ensure that they have adequate pulmonary reserve to permit major lung resection, which is necessary in the majority of patients undergoing carinal resection. Contraindications to carinal resection include: (1) a history of chronic steroid use, which is the factor most strongly associated with postoperative complications; (2) the perceived need for prolonged postoperative mechanical ventilation; (3) the presence of mediastinal nodal involvement when operating for non-small cell lung cancer; (4) the need to perform a long segment tracheal resection (4 cm or more of trachea) when a trachea to the left mainstem bronchus anastomosis is planned; and (5) a possible history of prior mediastinal irradiation.

Patients with non-small cell lung cancer who are being considered for carinal resection should undergo mediastinoscopy to assess mediastinal nodal status and the status of the carinal involvement. This procedure also enables thorough anterior dissection of the trachea, and so should be performed under the same anesthetic as the carinal resection if at all possible. Performing mediastinoscopy remotely in time creates fibrosis in the plane of dissection, making the subsequent carinal resection more difficult.

Appropriate anesthetic management of the patient undergoing carinal resection is fundamental to the success of the operation. The patient must be managed with early postoperative extubation in mind. Use of a double lumen tube complicates carinal resection; instead, a small caliber, armored endotracheal tube is used. This can be passed easily down the left mainstem bronchus to provide single lung ventilation during the dissection, and is small enough to pass across the tracheobronchial anastomosis after its completion without causing injury to the anastomosis. A small caliber, single lumen endotracheal tube must be available for intubating the patient across the sterile field as the carinal resection is performed and before the anastomosis is completed. Frequent communication with the anesthesiologist, who must be skilled in single lung ventilation and be familiar with the operative steps, is vital to the outcome of the operation.

The operation is performed through a standard right posterolateral thoracotomy to provide adequate access to the trachea and carina. This is certainly the case when right lung resection is planned as part of the carinal resection. Alternative approaches include median sternotomy or a clamshell incision if an isolated carinal resection is performed, or thoracoscopic division of the pulmonary vessels supplying the left lung followed by median sternotomy for a left carinal pneumonectomy. After opening the chest, a thorough assessment of operability is performed.

Once it is ascertained that resection is appropriate, the pulmonary vessels are isolated and divided if a major lung resection is planned as part of the carinal dissection. The trachea and left mainstem bronchus are dissected only to the extent necessitated by the resection. Additional circumferential dissection beyond these limits only serves to devascularize the tissues to be included in the anastomosis. When approaching the trachea from the right side, care must be taken to ensure that no injury occurs to the left recurrent laryngeal nerve.

To limit tension on the planned anastomosis the pretracheal plane is developed bluntly to the level of the thoracic inlet. A similar dissection can be performed on the left mainstem bronchus anteriorly to provide additional length. Hilar release maneuvers provide additional length by permitting the hilum to rise several centimeters, but are not always possible to perform. For example, a right carinal pneumonectomy performed through a right posterolateral thoracotomy does not permit a left hilar release. In contrast, a right hilar release provides substantial benefits in patients in whom a carinal resection with reimplantation of the right mainstem bronchus into the trachea is planned. The hilar release is usually accomplished by creating a U-shaped incision in the pericardium inferior to the hilum with division of the attachments between the inferior pulmonary vein and the inferior vena cava. Additional length can be obtained by completely encircling the hilum with the pericardial incision. Such release maneuvers are best performed prior to division of the airways.

In the case of a right carinal pneumonectomy, the carina is divided from the trachea superiorly and from the left mainstem bronchus inferiorly, and the specimen is removed (Fig. 10-3A). The patient's left mainstem bronchus is intubated across the field. Stay sutures are placed laterally in the trachea and left mainstem bronchus (Fig. 10-3B). Interrupted absorbable sutures are placed to approximate the two structures (Fig. 10-3C). No attempt is made to tailor the orifices, although sutures are differentially spaced to make up for any size mismatch and enable complete approximation or telescoping of the anastomosis. Once the sutures have been placed the endotracheal tube passed across the field is removed and the indwelling endotracheal tube is advanced across the gap into the left mainstem bronchus (Fig. 10-3D). The stay sutures are tied to take tension off the anastomosis, and the anastomotic sutures are tied. In patients at high

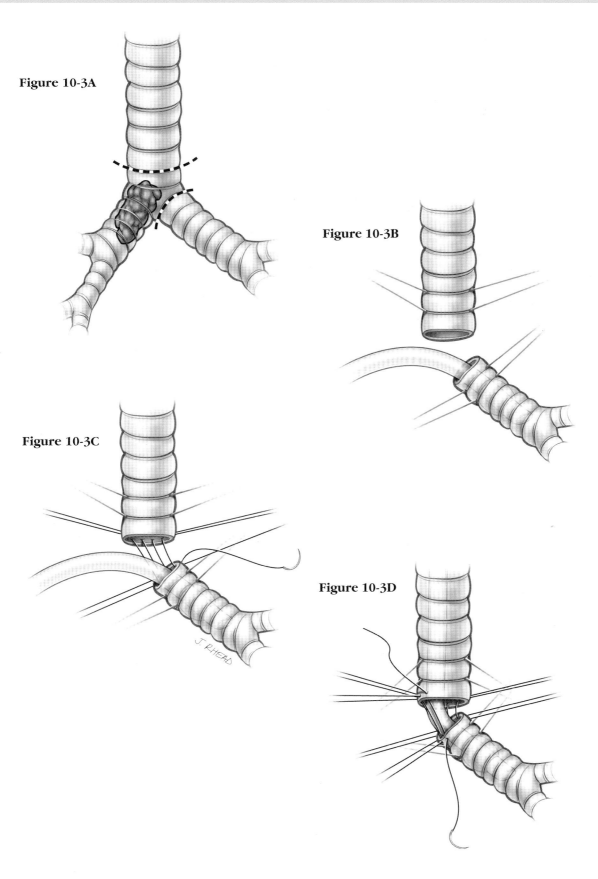

Figure 10-3A

Figure 10-3B

Figure 10-3C

Figure 10-3D

J. R. HEAD

risk for anastomotic complications, the anastomosis is wrapped with vascularized tissue such as an omental flap. The anastomosis is visualized bronchoscopically prior to concluding the operation. The patient is extubated as soon as is feasible, ideally in the operating room. Neck flexion and extension do not measurably affect the mobility of the thoracic trachea, and no fixation suture is needed to keep the patient's neck in mild flexion.

An alternative to an end-to-end anastomosis in reparative surgery of the carina is a side-to-end anastomosis between the trachea and a mainstem or lobar bronchus. A side-to-end anastomosis is created much in the same way an end-to-end anastomosis is performed, with two important caveats. First, the aperture for the anastomosis must be created by removing a small amount of tissue from the trachea to produce an ovoid opening. This aperture must be located entirely in the cartilaginous section of the trachea, avoiding the membranous portion entirely. Second, the opening needs to be located at least 1 cm from the cut end of the trachea to avoid creating ischemia in the tissues used to create the end-to-end anastomosis (Fig. 10-3E).

Other than the right carinal pneumonectomy described above, a few other options exist for reconstructing the airway after carinal resection. If the right mainstem bronchus or bronchus intermedius is preserved after carinal resection, an end-to-end anastomosis is created to the shorter of the right or left bronchus (Fig. 10-3F). The remaining bronchus is then anastomosed to the side of the trachea as described above. This high anastomosis usually requires that a complete hilar release maneuver be performed on the side of the higher anastomosis to eliminate as much tension as possible. Another option when bilateral bronchi remain after carinal resection is to create a neo-carina by anastomosing both bronchi to the trachea (Fig. 10-3G). This technique reduces the likelihood of tension on the anastomosis but introduces confluent suture lines that expose the anastomosis to an increased risk of ischemic complications at the angles where the suture lines meet.

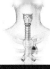

Figure 10-3E

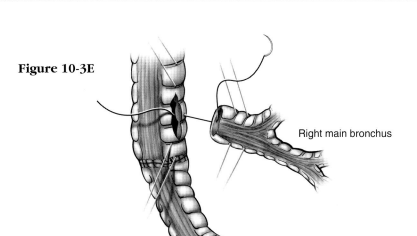

Right main bronchus

Left main bronchus

Figure 10-3F

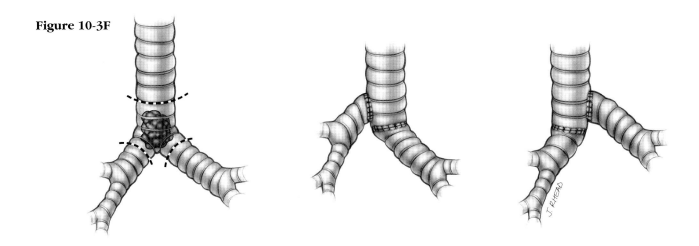

Figure 10-3G

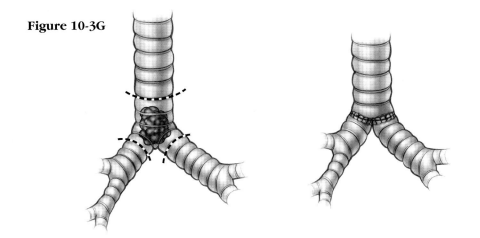

10-4 Management of Esophageal-Airway Fistula

Acquired esophageal-airway fistulae occur as a result of malignancy, trauma, iatrogenic injury, infection, stents, and intubation for purposes of ventilation. This section discusses management of intubation injuries resulting in benign, acquired esophageal-airway fistulae. Risk factors for the development of such an injury include steroid use, diabetes, infection, cuff overinflation, and excessive motion of the tube against the airway. The presence of a nasogastric tube further increases the risk of fistula formation. When fistula formation is suspected, the evaluation may include a chest radiograph or computed tomography, but the best assessment is performed endoscopically. Bronchoscopy is used to assess the presence and location of the fistula, and its relative distance from the vocal cords and the carina. The condition of the trachea is evaluated to determine whether the fistula is a small, localized process or is related to generalized destruction of the airway in the vicinity of the fistula (Fig. 10-4A); making this differentiation is important in selecting subsequent surgical therapy. Esophagoscopy may also be helpful in evaluating for the presence of a fistula but does not provide much information as to the best means for correcting the problem.

Initial management includes making the patient NPO, removing the nasogastric tube if one is present, and placing a gastrostomy tube if gastric decompression or drainage is required. Nutrition is maintained using a jejunostomy feeding tube or parenteral feedings. The patient is maintained in a head-elevated position to decrease the risks of aspiration of refluxed gastric contents. Aggressive pulmonary toilet measures are instituted. In most situations esophageal exclusion is not necessary and should be avoided, as this substantially complicates future reconstructive procedures. If pulmonary toilet is inadequate, despite the conservative measures outlined above, esophageal exclusion may be considered. Every effort is made to wean the patient from ventilatory support to optimize the outcomes from future fistula repair.

Appropriate anesthetic management of the patient undergoing repair of an esophageal airway fistula is critical to the success of the operation. Maintaining adequate ventilation in the face of such a fistula requires endotracheal intubation after anesthetic induction, positioning the balloon distal to the fistula. If division of the trachea is necessary, the patient is temporarily intubated across the field as described previously in Section 10-2. Distal fistulae create additional challenges for the anesthesiologist and the surgeon. Initial ventilatory management may require the use of high frequency ventilation, but prolonged use of this technique results in carbon dioxide accumulation resulting in acidosis. When feasible, the airway is transected distally and the mainstem bronchi are intubated across the field with individual small diameter tubes to permit adequate gas exchange. Every effort is made to end the operation with the patient breathing spontaneously and without the aid of ventilatory support.

In patients with a small fistula who have an otherwise relatively normal trachea, direct repair of the fistula from a lateral approach is appropriate. A cervical incision is performed and the trachea is mobilized from the esophagus, taking care to avoid injury to the ipsilateral recurrent laryngeal nerve. At times the nerve may be involved in the inflammatory process; if this is the case, identifying it inferior to the site of inflammation and continuing the dissection proximally into the inflamed area with the nerve accompanying the trachea can help avoid injury.

The site of the fistula is identified and the fistula is divided (Fig. 10-4B). Interrupted absorbable sutures are used to repair the membranous trachea, tying the knots on the outside of the airway. The esophagus is closed in two layers: the mucosa is closed with interrupted absorbable sutures, and the overlying muscle is closed with running or interrupted absorbable sutures (Fig. 10-4C). It is important that vascularized tissue be positioned between the two repair sites. A healthy flap of strap muscle is usually sufficient for this purpose. The muscle is interposed and is sutured circumferentially to the esophagus (Fig. 10-4D). No drain is usually necessary after this repair. The patient is extubated at the conclusion of the procedure. If a tracheostomy tube is required, an uncuffed tube is used if possible. If a cuffed tracheostomy tube is required, a tube with an extended tracheal portion is used, and the balloon is positioned distal to the site of repair.

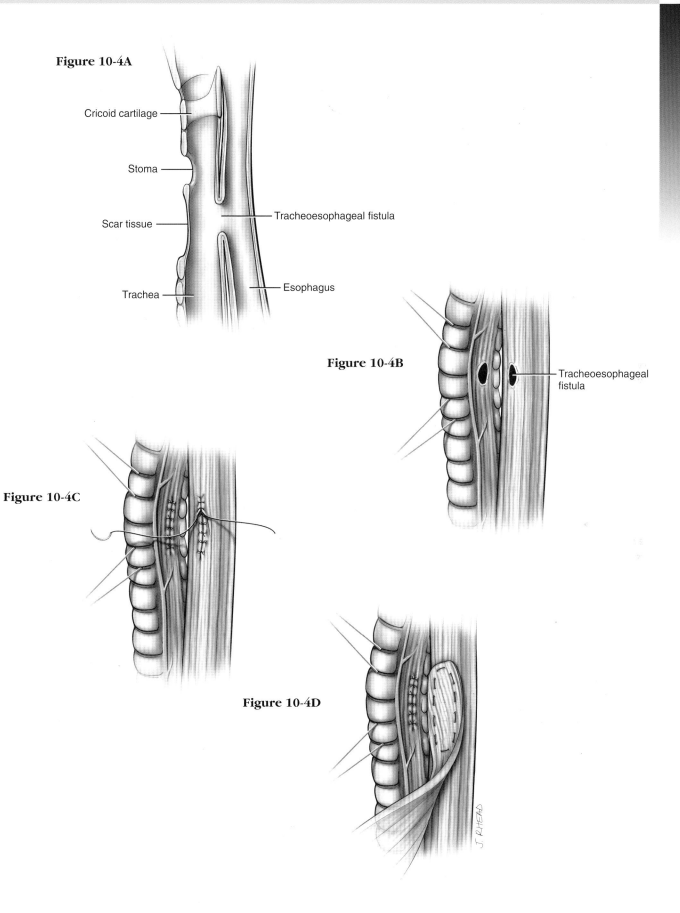

Figure 10-4A

Cricoid cartilage

Stoma

Scar tissue

Tracheoesophageal fistula

Esophagus

Trachea

Figure 10-4B

Tracheoesophageal fistula

Figure 10-4C

Figure 10-4D

Patients who have circumferential tracheal damage associated with an esophageal-airway fistula require resection of the damaged airway as part of the fistula repair process. This is performed through an anterior rather than a lateral approach, which provides much better exposure for the fistula repair. A collar incision is performed, preserving the option for a partial sternotomy should additional exposure be required. The trachea is exposed as described in Section 10-2. The dissection is carried directly on the wall of the trachea to minimize the risk of recurrent laryngeal nerve injury. Dissection proximal and distal to the circumferentially damaged portion of the trachea is limited to preserve the blood supply to the remaining trachea. The airway is divided distally and the patient is intubated across the field (Fig. 10-4E). The damaged trachea is dissected off of the underlying esophagus, and in the process the fistula is divided. The tracheal dissection is continued proximally until normal tracheal tissue is reached. In some instances the dissection may contain the tracheostomy site, in other situations the tracheostomy site needs to be preserved. The trachea is transected proximally and the damaged portion is discarded.

The edges of the esophageal defect are debrided leaving only viable tissue. The esophagus is closed in two layers using interrupted absorbable sutures for the mucosal layer and running or interrupted absorbable sutures for the muscular layer (Fig. 10-4F). A well-vascularized flap of tissue, typically a strap muscle, is mobilized and is sutured over the esophageal closure (Fig. 10-4G). The ends of the trachea are brought close to apposition using stay sutures placed laterally, and anastomotic sutures of fine, absorbable material are placed circumferentially. The endotracheal tube positioned across the field is removed and the indwelling endotracheal tube is positioned across the anastomosis. The anastomosis is completed as described in Section 10-2 (Fig. 10-4H).

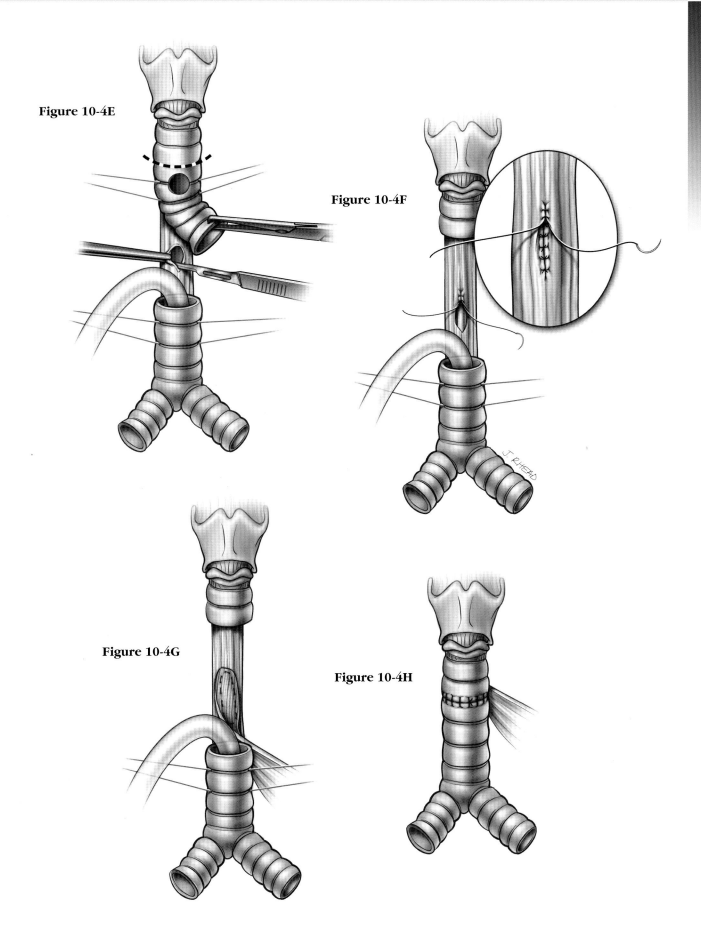

Figure 10-4E

Figure 10-4F

Figure 10-4G

Figure 10-4H

10-5 Management of Subglottic Stenosis

Subglottic stenosis is a more challenging entity to manage than stenosis of the mid-trachea. Subglottic stenosis may be associated with glottic stenosis and/or vocal cord dysfunction, and these problems must be assessed thoroughly endoscopically prior to any surgical intervention. Separate glottic or vocal cord problems must be corrected prior to any surgical approach to a subglottic stenosis. In some instances a combined approach may be necessary, including laryngotracheal fissure, which is not within the purview of this atlas.

An isolated subglottic stenosis (Fig. 10-5A), which usually results from a proximally placed tracheostomy or cricothyroidostomy, cannot be dissected circumferentially for purposes of resection because the recurrent laryngeal nerves enter the glottic mechanism in the region of the cricoid cartilage. Instead, an anterior resection is performed and scar tissue is resected from the inner surface of the posterior wall of the cricoid cartilage to restore the usual caliber of the airway. The operation is commenced as was described in Section 10-2, exposing the anterior surface of the cervical trachea to the level of the inferior margin of the thyroid cartilage. The extent of the stenotic segment is evident by inspection of the surface of the airway, but rigid bronchoscopy may aid in verifying the distal margin.

The anterior region of resection, which extends from the inferior margin of the thyroid cartilage to the inferior margin of the stenotic segment, is indicated in Figure 10-5B. Superiorly and laterally the resection margin dips to exclude the entire posterior half of the cricoid cartilage, leaving this region of cricoid cartilage and the recurrent laryngeal nerves untouched. Inferiorly, a standard extent of anterior resection is performed. A flap of membranous trachea is preserved that will line the posterior plate of the cricoid cartilage as the reconstruction is performed.

The distal end of the stenotic segment is divided, tailoring the membranous portion as described above. The patient is reintubated across the field. The superior resection is performed, tailoring the cricoid cartilage as described earlier. The true vocal cords are easily visualized during this portion of the procedure, providing good visual cues regarding the appropriate extent of resection. Scar tissue is excised from the posterior cricoid plate, restoring the normal caliber of the airway in this region. Stay sutures are placed laterally in the glottic region and in the transected trachea. Fine interrupted absorbable sutures are placed from the apex of the flap of membranous trachea to the apex of the denuded area of the cricoid plate (Fig. 10-5C). Additional sutures are placed to complete the relining of the cricoid plate. The endotracheal tube placed across the field is removed and the posterior sutures are tied after tension is placed on the stay sutures to align the two ends of the airway. Anastomotic sutures are placed in the rigid portion of the airway and are then tied, completing the anastomosis (Fig. 10-5D). Postoperative management is similar to that described in Section 10-2.

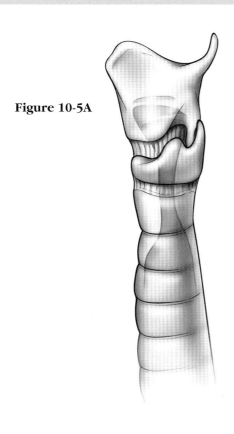

Figure 10-5A

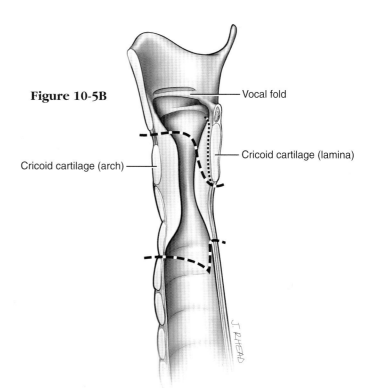

Figure 10-5B

Vocal fold

Cricoid cartilage (lamina)

Cricoid cartilage (arch)

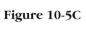**Figure 10-5C**

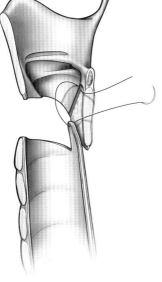

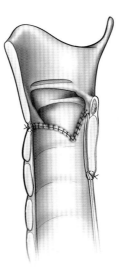

Figure 10-5D

10-6 Management of Airway Trauma

Tracheal trauma results from either blunt or penetrating injuries. Blunt trauma, including deceleration, stretching, and barogenic forces, typically causes disruption without tissue loss. Penetrating injuries from knives result in barrier disruption without tissue loss and are the easiest injuries to manage. Penetrating injuries from gunshot wounds and blast injuries cause loss of soft tissues that are a challenge to control and then surgically treat.

Acute management of airway injuries includes avoidance of blind intubation in patients who have functional airways. If intubation is necessary, it is best performed in a controlled setting in which intubation over a flexible bronchoscope is performed to avoid intubating a false passage and losing the airway entirely (Fig. 10-6A). Unstable intrathoracic injuries that cannot be intubated necessitate urgent thoracotomy for repair in the salvageable patient. If the injury is sufficiently proximal and the airway is unstable, tracheostomy may be performed through the site of injury, avoiding unnecessary trauma to the healthy airway. The patient's neck is maintained in a neutral position until verification that no injury has occurred to the cervical vertebrae or spinal cord. Airway management is performed simultaneously with control of bleeding, resuscitation, and assessment of other injuries.

If a stable airway is established, management of the airway injury itself is performed acutely or subacutely, depending on the overall condition of the patient and the status of other associated injuries. The choice of surgical approach depends on the location of the injury. Simple laceration injuries of the cervical airway are sutured. Most other cervical injuries, including disrup-

tion and blast injuries, require debridement, circumferential resection, and reanastomosis. Extensive injuries such as these are often accompanied by damage to adjacent organs. Once the airway has been controlled, repair of adjacent injuries is performed, such as esophageal repair and vascular repair (Fig. 10-6B). As for elective operations, the esophageal repair in this situation is separated from the tracheal repair by a local tissue flap (Fig. 10-6C). Cervical tracheal injuries are repaired and buttressed with local tissues because of the possibility of contamination and persistent adjacent necrotic tissue (Fig. 10-6D). Prolonged endotracheal intubation is sometimes necessary in difficult cases because of ventilatory requirements associated with neurologic injury, bilateral recurrent laryngeal nerve injury, or cardiovascular instability. In such situations the patient's endotracheal tube is positioned so that the balloon is distal to and does not impinge on the site of repair.

Intrathoracic injuries to the trachea, right mainstem bronchus, and left mainstem bronchus up to 1.5 to 2 cm distal to the carina are managed though a right posterolateral thoracotomy approach. More distal injuries to the left mainstem bronchi are managed through a left thoracotomy. Laceration injuries are sutured if there is no tissue loss. Injuries with associated tissue loss are resected and repaired through standard techniques described earlier. It is important to reinforce these repairs with local tissue flaps to help ensure adequate healing. Patients are managed such that extubation at the conclusion of the operation is possible. Situations in which early extubation is not possible subject patients to a higher risk of failed primary healing of the airway repair. Soft tissue reinforcement is most important in these patients, and periodic bronchoscopic monitoring of the airway repair is appropriate during the period of mechanical ventilation.

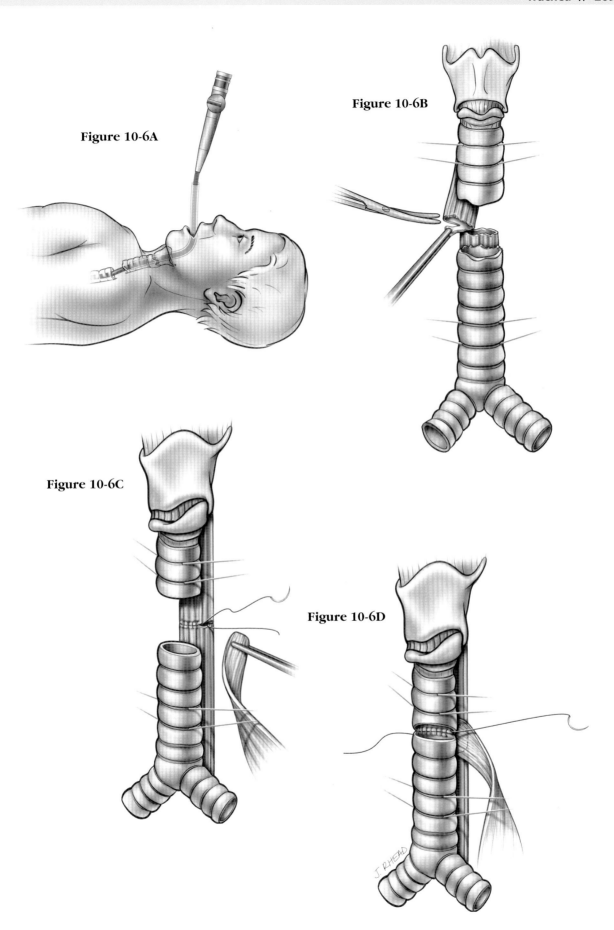

Figure 10-6A

Figure 10-6B

Figure 10-6C

Figure 10-6D

10-7 Management of Tracheoinnominate Artery Fistula

A fistula between the trachea and brachiocephalic artery is a life-threatening complication that is challenging to manage. This problem develops low in the innominate artery, within 1 to 2 cm of its takeoff from the aortic arch, and involves the posterior wall of the artery as it crosses anterior to the trachea (Fig. 10-7A). The most common etiology is erosion by the cuff or tip of a tracheostomy tube (Fig. 10-7B). Angulation of the tube, particularly if the patient is on positive pressure ventilation and the ventilator tubing is allowed to weigh upon the tracheostomy tubing, can force the cuff or the tracheostomy tip against the anterior wall of the trachea in the region of the artery. Erosion into the trachea results in surrounding inflammation, causing adhesion between the airway and the artery. As the erosion deepens, entry into the artery occurs. If the balloon is the primary site of erosion, a sentinel bleed may occur primarily through the trachea into the lungs and oropharynx. If the tip of the tracheostomy tube is the lead point of the erosion, bleeding will also occur substantially though the tracheostomy tube itself. Patients in whom a low-lying tracheostomy tube is placed or in whom the innominate artery lies very proximal are at increased risk for developing a fistula (see Fig. 10-7B inset). Other causes include trauma, tracheal stenting, iatrogenic injury in the setting of inflammation or infection, and complications of tracheal stenting.

The diagnosis of tracheoinnominate artery fistula is sometimes difficult. This entity accounts for about 10% of bleeding from tracheal stomas, other more common causes being granulation tissue, bleeding from lung parenchyma and distal airways, and postoperative bleeding from soft tissues around the tracheostomy site shortly after tracheostomy tube placement. All moderate to major bleeding, even if it stops, should be considered indicative of a possible tracheoinnominate artery fistula. Early investigation includes flexible or rigid bronchoscopy in an OR setting. After other sources of distal bleeding are excluded, the tracheostomy tube cuff is deflated, and the anterior wall of the trachea is examined for erosion or bleeding. The presence of suspicious findings is an indication for exploration. Massive bleeding is a life-threatening emergency and must be controlled immediately to stop blood loss and keep the airway free of blood. The first step is overinflation of the tracheostomy tube cuff. If this fails an endotracheal tube is passed orally as the tracheostomy tube is removed. The cuff is inflated distal to the site of erosion. A finger is passed through the tracheostomy site and the pretracheal plane is bluntly dissected, permitting the tip of the finger to compress the injured artery against the manubrium (Fig. 10-7C). Pressure is maintained until the patient can be taken to the operating room where operative control is gained.

Repair is performed through a sternotomy incision. Because of the high risk of contamination by an open tracheostomy site, a partial sternotomy traversing the sternum to the right in the third intercostal space provides access to the takeoff of the innominate artery proximally and distally without exposing the entire sternum to infectious complications. As the area of bleeding is controlled, the innominate artery is clamped proximally and distally and the area of adhesion between the artery and trachea is dissected. Under most circumstances the artery is divided proximal and distal to this site and the ends are oversewn. This is usually sufficient management as long as back bleeding is obtained from the distal end of the innominate artery (ensuring adequate flow through the right carotid artery), and the confluence of the carotid and subclavian arteries is preserved (ensuring backflow from the carotid artery into the subclavian artery). If inadequate cerebral flow is suspected intraoperatively or in the immediate postoperative period, a crossover graft is sewn in place from the contralateral carotid or subclavian artery.

The area of tracheal injury is debrided. Options for subsequent management include coverage with vascularized tissue, primary closure, or segmental resection and anastomosis. Regardless of what type of repair is selected, it is vital that vascularized tissue be interposed between the area of tracheal injury and the ends of the innominate artery (Fig. 10-7D). Available tissues include strap muscles, sternocleidomastoid, thymus, and omentum. The endotracheal tube is positioned with its cuff distal to the site of repair. If necessary, a repeat tracheostomy can be performed several weeks later if the patient is doing well.

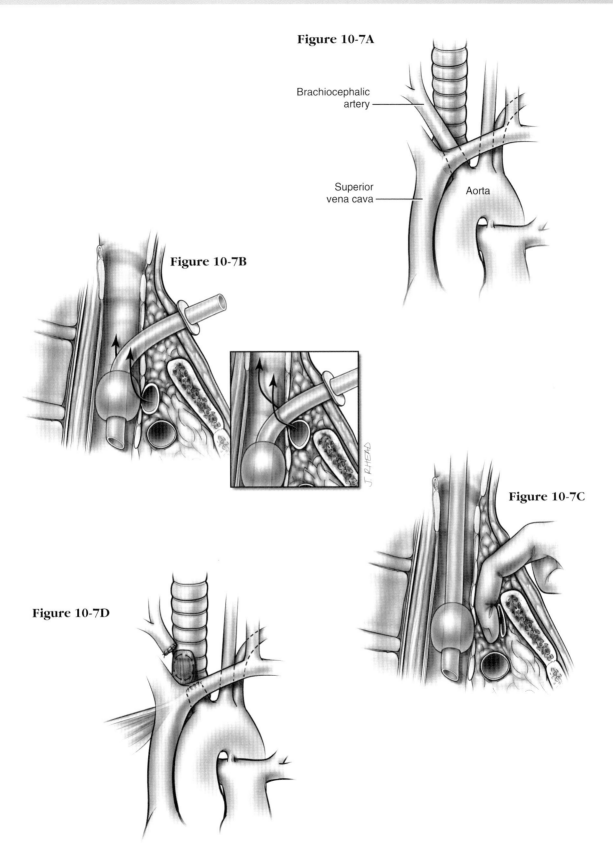

Figure 10-7A

Brachiocephalic
artery

Superior
vena cava

Aorta

Figure 10-7B

Figure 10-7C

Figure 10-7D

Chapter *11*

Pleura

▮ 11-1 Decortication

Pulmonary decortication is a common procedure used for management of a variety of inflammatory problems affecting the pleura space, ranging from pleural empyema to fibrothorax with trapped lung. In general, decortication accelerates the process of recovery from a pleural space infection compared to more conservative therapy, such as chest tube drainage combined with antibiotics and even the addition of intrapleural fibrinolytics. Exceptions to this include children with uncomplicated postpneumonic empyema, which can usually be managed with aspiration and systemic antibiotics, and adults with pleural space infections that are not fibrinous in nature and are completely evacuated with a pleural drain. Adult patients whose infectious processes evolve to the fibrinopurulent stage are best treated operatively. The choice of open versus minimally invasive surgery depends on the surgeon's experience and the degree of fibrothorax that has developed as a result of the inflammation. This chapter will illustrate general principles of open decortication that also apply to thoracoscopic decortication.

Patients are treated for any signs or symptoms of sepsis prior to being brought to the operating room. Systemic antibiotics are administered perioperatively because of the bacterial showering that occurs during decortication. The operation is performed with the patient in a straight lateral position through a muscle-sparing lateral thoracotomy (see Fig. 11-1A inset). In some instances, a standard lateral or posterolateral thoracotomy is necessary to gain adequate access to the pleural space, but preservation of the latissimus and serratus muscles is advisable whenever possible in case a space problem subsequently develops and requires man-

agement with a muscle flap. In many patients, computed tomography will direct the surgeon to the region most severely affected by the empyema. In the absence of this, a posteroanterior and lateral chest radiograph will provide sufficient information as to the affected regions. In most cases, the base of the pleural space is more involved than is the apex, and a low interspace (the sixth) is selected for pleural entry.

There are usually two distinguishable areas of pleura involvement in most empyemas. Rinds develop over the parietal and visceral pleural surfaces that enclose pockets of pus and fibrinous exudate between them. These regions of pleural involvement do not normally require pleurectomy; in fact, pleurectomy should be avoided if at all possible to reduce the risk of postoperative bleeding from the raw and very inflamed surfaces that result. After opening into the parietal pleural space, the intact surface of the parietal peel is evident (Fig. 11-1A). Using a combination of blunt and sharp dissection, this rind is separated from the parietal pleura across the entire chest wall to the point where the mediastinum and diaphragm are reached (Fig. 11-1B). After the easily visible planes are developed under direct vision, the surgeon manually extends the planes to their natural limits bluntly (Fig. 11-C).

When the parietal peel has been dissected from the chest wall, the empyema cavity is opened (see Fig. 11-1D inset). The fibrinous contents of the empyema cavity are evacuated by suctioning or, more commonly, are removed piecemeal by hand or with ring forceps (Fig. 11-D). It is important to send adequate samples of this material for culture and susceptibility to ensure that subsequent antibiotic therapy is appropriately tailored to the specific infectious organisms involved.

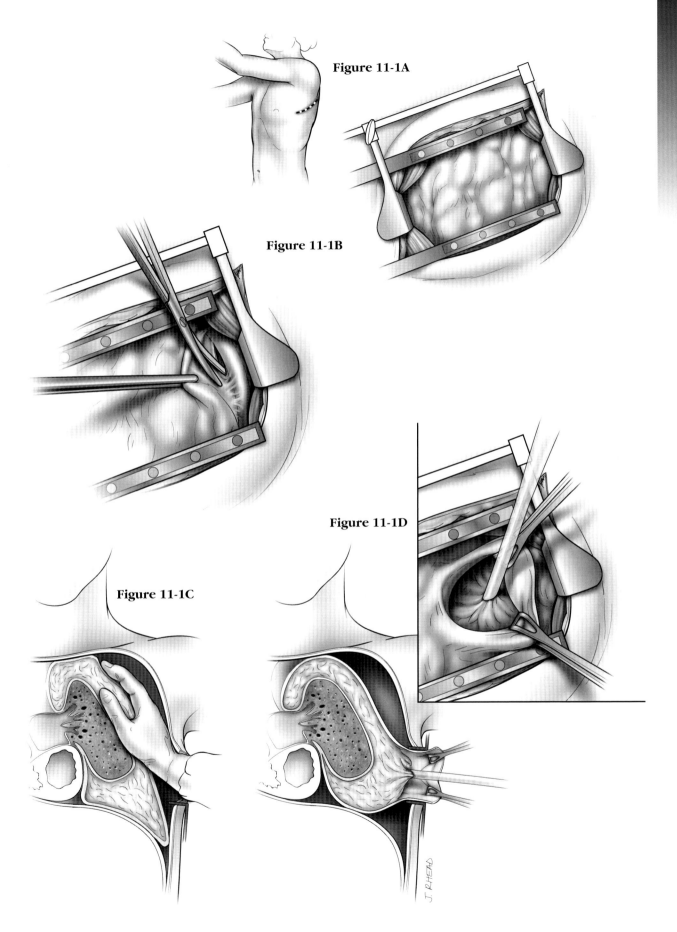

Figure 11-1A

Figure 11-1B

Figure 11-1C

Figure 11-1D

The parietal peel is then excised sharply. Frequently there are remnants adherent to the sulci, including the pericardiophrenic sulcus and the interlobar spaces, which must be carefully excised to permit complete evacuation of infected material (Fig. 11-1E). The visceral decortication is then begun. This may be very easy or can be quite challenging, depending on the phase of the empyema and how fibrinous and adherent the peel is. Often the optimal pleural plane can be opened bluntly, exposing the correct plane for dissection. More often, sharp dissection with a blade is necessary to permit identification of the pleural surface. This and subsequent visceral pleural decortication are performed with the ipsilateral lung being ventilated to optimize the ability to distinguish between lung and pleural peel. The visceral decortication proceeds with a combination of sharp and blunt dissection (Fig. 11-1F). Use of appropriate grasping instruments (blunt-tipped forceps such as Russians; Allis clamps) facilitates obtaining countertraction and avoids hand fatigue during long procedures. If parenchymal injury occurs because of adherent tissues, this area is temporarily abandoned and more fruitful areas are pursued.

The decortication is complete when the entire visceral pleural surface is clean and the lung expands com-pletely. At times it is not possible to completely clear the visceral pleural surface, leading to failure of complete lung expansion. This is usually a result of infiltration of the fibrinous process into the lung parenchyma. This situation can be managed in several different ways, including excision of the visceral pleura, creating a gridiron effect on the fibrous pleural surface by cross-hatching it with a blade, or treating the patient expec-tantly for a possible space problem by considering muscle flap rotation in the future if the space problem fails to resolve with either of the aforementioned options.

The pleural cavity is irrigated copiously with warm saline to evacuate any particles left behind during the decortication. Adequate drainage of the pleural space ensures that no pockets of infected fluid will remain after closure of the incision, creating a risk for a recurrent loculated empyema. One way to effect this is to place two large-bore tubes extending from the base of the cavity to the apex of the hemithorax, while an angled tube is placed at the base across the diaphragm (Fig. 11-1G). These tubes are maintained on suction for two to three days before converting them to underwater seal, and are not removed until the amount of drainage is very low.

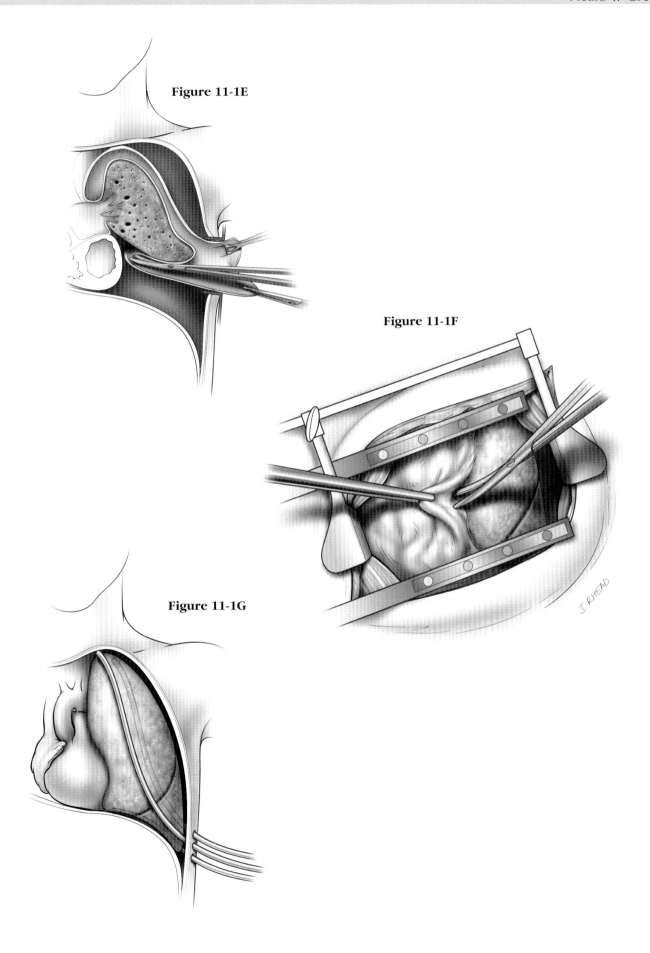

Figure 11-1E

Figure 11-1F

Figure 11-1G

J. RHEAD

11-2 Thoracoplasty

Collapse therapy for managing infected pleura space problems and chronic pulmonary infections was popularized in the late 19th and early 20th centuries. Surgical collapse therapy, including thoracoplasty, was championed by John Alexander in the era when there were no effective antituberculous agents but when anesthetic and surgical techniques had evolved to the point of permitting safe multiple rib resections. The technique remains useful today, although it has been supplanted by muscle flap transposition, which provides similar or improved outcomes without as much disfigurement as thoracoplasty (see Chapter 12). The primary current indication for thoracoplasty is the presence of an isolated space problem, ideally located apically, in a patient in whom muscle flap transposition is not feasible. Most often this occurs in patients in whom available muscles have been damaged by prior surgery or in whom muscle wasting results in inadequate muscle bulk to provide sufficient volume to fill the affected space.

The operation is performed through a generous, high, posterolateral thoracotomy incision (see Fig. 11-2A inset), which permits exposure of wide areas of the upper ribs (Fig. 11-2A). The procedure is performed in an extrapleural manner in most cases, although thoracoplasty for chronic empyema may be accompanied by the need for evacuation and drainage of the empyema space prior to collapse therapy, necessitating entry into the pleural space. Apical spaces require excision of several ribs, and the first rib must always be taken if the tissues are to collapse properly into the apical space.

The excision begins at the apex, progressively working inferiorly until the proper amount of collapse is achieved. The majority of the first rib is removed, and the entire second rib excluding the costal cartilage is removed. As the resection proceeds more inferiorly, it is not necessary to take quite as much of the ensuing ribs anteriorly. Rib resection is accomplished by scoring the periosteum with cautery and raising it from the underlying rib with a periosteal elevator (Fig. 11-2B). Preservation of the perichondrium permits regrowth of bone, ultimately reducing any paradoxical chest wall motion engendered by the thoracoplasty operation. Once the plane has been adequately established and dissected, a Doyen is used to completely free the rib to the limits of resection. The longer ribs are divided where convenient, subsequently taking the anterior and posterior parts separately.

It is important that the excision includes the transverse processes of the associated vertebral bodies, as the presence of these may prevent adequate collapse of tissues into the awaiting space. Options for accomplishing this include disarticulation of the rib heads from the vertebral bodies followed by excision of the transverse process with a rongeur, or transection of the articular mechanism with a rongeur without further dissection (Fig. 11-2C).

When used for collapse therapy for chronic pulmonary infections, thoracoplasty is performed in stages as illustrated in Figure 11-2D. For management of chronic space problems in which no functioning lung tissue is compromised, a total of three (first stage illustration) or five ribs (second stage illustration) can be performed under a single anesthetic. It is unlikely that a more extensive resection would be necessary for a chronic space problem, and the illustrated third stage thoracoplasty is not apropos of this process. In contrast, staging the extent of thoracoplasty is necessary if functioning lung tissue is to be progressively lost, as when thoracoplasty is performed for chronic lung infection. Fortunately the need for the latter procedure, in an era of improved drug therapy, is vanishingly small.

Figure 11-2A

Figure 11-2B

Figure 11-2C

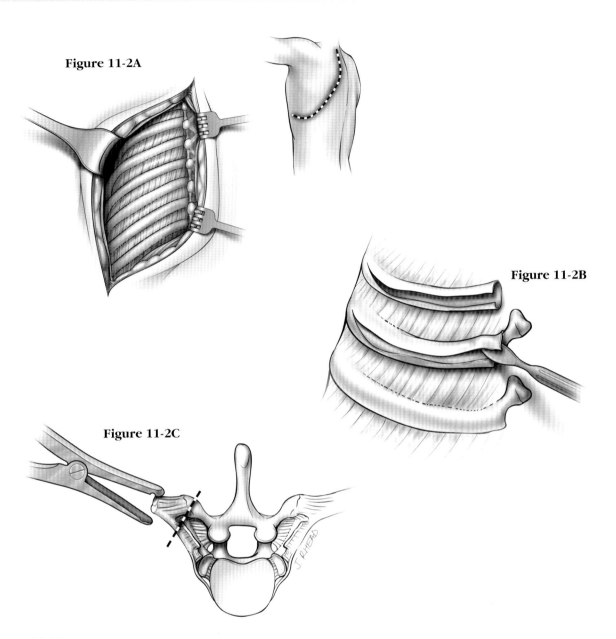

Figure 11-2D

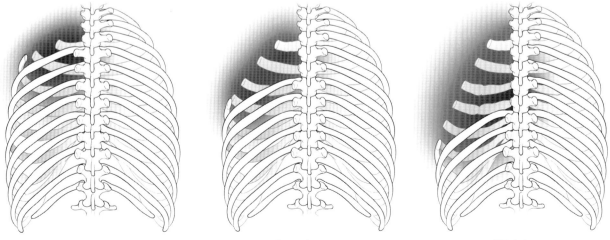

First stage

Second stage

Third stage

11-3 Eloesser Flap

Thoracoplasty, as described above, is a useful technique for managing chronic apical space problems and selected instances of chronic parenchymal infection. Basilar space problems are not usually amenable to this technique, because adequate collapse is virtually impossible given the geometry of the region. In patients with a chronic basilar space problem, often in the presence of a bronchopleural fistula, options for management include decortication, muscle flap transposition (see Chapter 12), or open drainage using an Eloesser flap technique. The latter option is reserved for patients who cannot undergo more definitive therapy because of medical contraindications or technical contraindications, such as lack of adequate soft tissue to fill the space, and in whom an adequate decortication with lung re-expansion is not possible. The Eloesser technique may be used as a temporizing measure until more definitive therapy is instituted, or can be used as destination therapy in selected patients. Even in the latter group healing sometimes is sufficient to permit closure of the flap months after it is created.

The procedure is performed with the patient in a straight lateral position (see Fig. 11-3A inset). Although the operation can be performed in selected patients under sedation and with local anesthetic, most patients will prefer a general anesthetic. Given the underlying pathophysiology of the space problem, patients are not at risk for inadequate ventilation due to lung collapse when the pleural space is opened in the absence of positive pressure ventilation, and single lung ventilation is not required. However, in patients in whom an undrained empyema is being treated, caution must be exercised in the presence of a bronchopleural fistula to ensure that infected empyema contents do not drain into the airway when the patient is positioned laterally. Usually this problem is avoided by adequately draining the space with a thoracostomy tube prior to the operation.

The aperture into the thoracic cavity must be positioned at the base of the pleural space problem to facilitate adequate dependent drainage. Under ideal circumstances the indwelling drainage tube has been placed at a level commensurate with this, and the insertion site may be used as the access point for opening into the space (see Fig. 11-3A inset). If the tube has been placed in a higher interspace, a separate access incision is performed to achieve the goal of adequate dependent drainage.

A 6-to-8-cm transverse incision is made, and the incision is extended in a "Y" fashion laterally and medially. Dermal flaps are raised in the region as outlined in Figure 11-3A. The incision is carried through the chest wall muscles to the ribs, and the pleural space is opened and digitally explored. The position of the base of the pleural space is assessed, indicating which ribs are to be resected. Six-to-8-cm lengths of two adjacent ribs are removed, including the periosteum and intervening intercostal muscles (Fig. 11-3B). This creates an open window into the pleural space. The space is debrided and irrigated, taking care not to flood the airway with irrigation fluid if a bronchopleural fistula exists.

Once the space has been adequately exposed and cleaned, the edges of the space are marsupialized, creating a continuous epithelial-lined surface, preventing closure of the space by cicatricial contracture. This is accomplished by suturing the edges of the dermal flaps to the thickened parietal pleura circumferentially using heavy absorbable sutures (Fig. 11-3C). The resultant defect permits good visualization of the space and allows dependent drainage of the space (see Fig. 11-3C inset). The space is initially packed with moist gauze until adequate hemostasis is achieved, after which it may be packed or left to drain into a dressing, depending on the amount of drainage that occurs and on the degree of bronchopleural fistula that may exist.

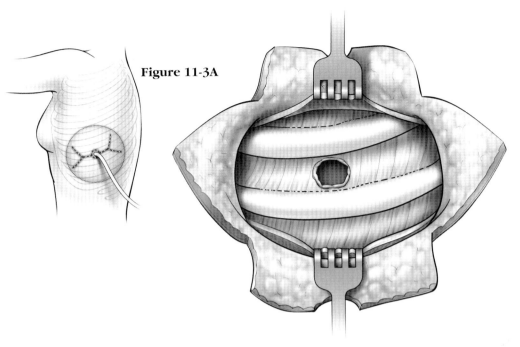

Figure 11-3A

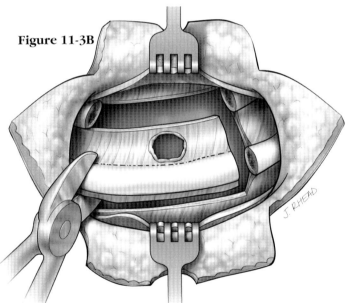

Figure 11-3B

J. RHEAD

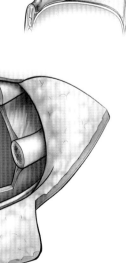

Figure 11-3C

11-4 Extrapleural Pneumonectomy for Mesothelioma

Aggressive therapy for malignant pleural mesothelioma includes pleurectomy/decortication for palliation of symptoms; when all gross disease is removed using this technique, it is an important adjunct to potentially curative therapy, including chemotherapy and radiation therapy. Many patients with pleural mesothelioma, because of the local extent of disease, are not candidates for pleurectomy/decortication, and aggressive surgical therapy must then consist of extrapleural pneumonectomy (EPP) to optimize local control of disease. Indications for this operation include epithelial histology, absence of mediastinal nodal involvement, no evidence for peritoneal space involvement, the ability to encompass all disease with EPP, and the patient's ability to tolerate pneumonectomy.

The operation is performed with the patient in a full lateral position (Fig. 11-4A). Lung isolation is achieved with a double lumen endotracheal tube. A right-sided resection is described. The elements are similar to those necessary for a left EPP. The incision extends along the sixth rib from 2 cm lateral to the costovertebral junction to the costochondral junction. The sixth rib is excised, and the chest is entered through the bed of the periosteum. The extrapleural dissection is initiated first by sharply developing the plane between the pleura and chest wall. If extensive chest wall involvement beyond the pleura is encountered, the EPP is aborted and decortication/pleurectomy is performed instead. Most of the extrapleural plane can be developed bluntly, beginning anteriorly and then working superiorly. Care is taken to avoid injury to the subclavian artery and vein, the superior vena cava, the azygos vein, and the internal mammary vessels (Fig. 11-4B). The posterior dissection is performed, ensuring that there is no esophageal involvement (Fig. 11-4C). This phase of the dissection is complete when the mainstem bronchus is identified. The pericardium is opened anteriorly and palpation is performed to ensure the absence of invasion of the pericardial space.

If, at this point, a complete resection appears feasible, the diaphragm is resected. The blunt dissection is carried to the level of the costophrenic sulcus laterally and posteriorly. The diaphragm muscle is divided anteriorly to the level of the peritoneum, and this incision is carried laterally and then posteriorly. The edges of the diaphragm muscle are elevated with Allis clamps and the plane between the diaphragm muscle and peritoneum is developed bluntly (Fig. 11-4D). The pericardium is opened further anteriorly to visualize the inferior vena cava (IVC), helping to avoid injury to the IVC as the diaphragm resection continues lateral to it. A 2-cm rim of diaphragm muscle is left attached in the region of the esophagus for use in anchoring the reconstruction.

Figure 11-4A

Figure 11-4B

Internal thoracic
artery and vein

Trachea

Superior
vena cava

J. RHEAD

Figure 11-4C

Figure 11-4D

Peritoneum

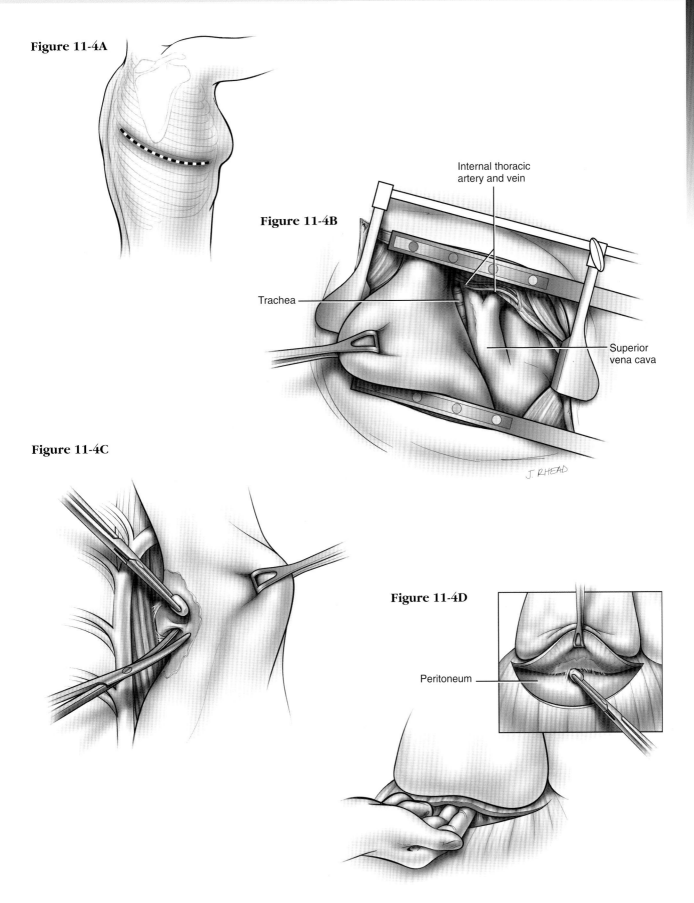

The specimen is retracted posteriorly and the pericardium is incised anteriorly to the apex of the hilum. The pulmonary artery and superior and inferior pulmonary veins are divided intrapericardially. The specimen is retracted anteriorly, and the posterior pericardium is divided. The mainstem bronchus is dissected, closed with a stapler, and divided. The specimen is removed (Fig. 11-4E). A pericardial fat pad flap is dissected and is sutured over the bronchial stump to separate it from the pulmonary artery stump. Hemostasis is obtained.

Reconstruction of the diaphragmatic surface is accomplished with a 2-mm patch of Gortex. A relatively loose patch avoids unnecessary tension on the closure, which can lead to breakdown of the sutures lines and herniation of abdominal contents. Another option is to use a "dynamic" patch, which is constructed from two sheets of Gortex that overlap by 5 cm. The sheets are stapled laterally, leaving the central part of the overlapping portions free to slide over each other, accommodating changes in intraabdominal pressures. The patch is sutured anteriorly, laterally, and posteriorly by bringing mattress sutures through the patch, through the chest wall, and through a button prior to tying them over the outer chest wall. Anteromedially the patch is sutured to the cut edge of pericardium/diaphragm, and posteriorly it is sutured to the diaphragmatic rim that was left adjacent to the esophagus (Fig. 11-4F).

The pericardium is reconstructed to prevent herniation of the heart into the empty hemithorax. Reconstruction is accomplished with a 1-mm patch of Gortex by suturing it to the divided edges of pericardium posteriorly and anteriorly and to the diaphragm patch inferiorly. As the posterior and anterior edge closures approach the apex, a gap is left for egress of the pericardial fat pad that is covering the bronchial stump (Fig. 11-4G). The patch is fenestrated to avoid postoperative tamponade (Fig. 11-4H). Hemostasis is achieved. A small drainage catheter is placed to permit medialization of the mediastinum postoperatively. The incision is closed in an airtight manner.

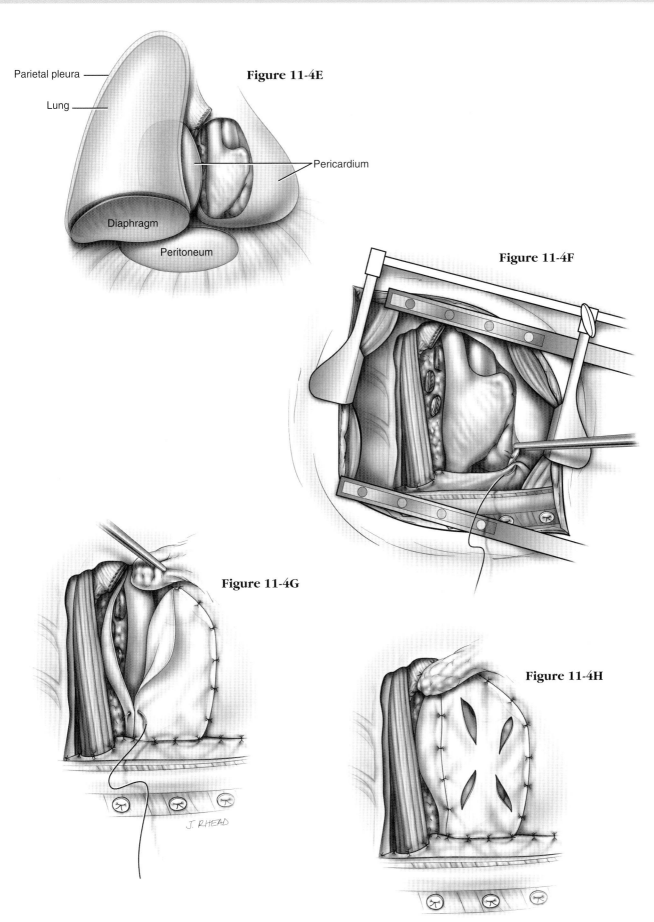

Parietal pleura

Lung

Figure 11-4E

Pericardium

Diaphragm

Peritoneum

Figure 11-4F

Figure 11-4G

Figure 11-4H

J. RHEAD

Chapter 12

Soft Tissue Flaps

12-1 Applications

Reconstruction of soft tissue defects of the chest wall, myoplasty or omentoplasty for management of intrathoracic space problems, and reinforcement of vital structures of the mediastinum all require pedicled flaps. A detailed knowledge of the availability and application of such flaps is vital to the successful management of complex thoracic surgical problems. Reconstruction of the bony chest wall is detailed in Chapter 4 and will not be addressed further here. In addition to the flaps described in this chapter, a variety of other methods of soft tissue coverage are available, including musculocutaneous flaps, fasciocutaneous flaps, and osteomyocutaneous flaps, either as pedicled flaps or as free flaps. They are not discussed in detail in this chapter.

Most soft tissue defects of the chest wall that require reconstruction occur anteriorly or laterally; it is uncommon to require soft tissue reconstruction for posterior defects. Defects of the anterior chest wall occur after sternectomy for tumors or infection, chest wall resection for invasive breast cancer or primary chest wall tumors, management of radionecrosis, and trauma. The blue- and orange-shaded areas in Figure 12-1A depict the range of anterior soft tissue defects that result after upper and lower partial sternectomy and adjacent tissue resections. They are optimally managed with local tissues, such as pectoralis major flaps based laterally on the thoracoacromial artery (used as advancement flaps) or based medially on perforators arising from the internal mammary vessels (used as turnover flaps) (Fig. 12-1B). The latter option often is not available after sternectomy. Other alternative tissues for managing such anterior defects include rectus abdominus flaps based on the superior epigastric vessels and omental flaps based on the right gastroepiploic artery.

Anterolateral chest wall soft tissue defects result from tumor resection, radionecrosis, and trauma, and are depicted in pink and purple (see Fig. 12-1A). They typically involve loss of portions of the pectoralis muscles and/or serratus anterior muscles. Small defects are reconstructed with rectus abdominus or serratus anterior flaps, whereas larger defects are ideally managed with latissimus dorsi flaps based on the thoracodorsal artery. Use of free flaps with microvascular anastomoses may be considered in the absence of available local pedicled flaps.

Large pleural space problems for which myoplasty or omentoplasty is considered for obliteration require a substantial amount of tissue bulk to achieve this objective. Tissues available for this task include latissimus dorsi, omentum, and possibly pectoralis major. Sometimes more than one flap is necessary to adequately obliterate a space. Smaller spaces are successfully managed with serratus anterior based on the lateral thoracic artery or pectoralis major flaps. Entry into the pleural space is facilitated by removal of a portion of one or two ribs underlying the narrowest portion of the pedicle, creating sufficient space to prevent impingement on the blood supply to the flap.

Intrathoracic situations that require soft tissue for coverage include high-risk esophageal anastomoses, vascular repair in the presence of infection, and major lung resection after induction chemoradiotherapy, to name just a few. Flaps for these purposes must have long pedicles to enable them to reach the mediastinum without tension (see Fig. 12-1A, green shaded portion). Bulk is not usually an important issue for such reinforcement/coverage flaps; in fact, thin, pliable tissue flaps are often more effective for these purposes than are bulky flaps. Local intrathoracic flaps that are useful for reinforcing mediastinal structures include intercostal muscle and pericardial fat pad. The best external flaps that reach to the mediastinum without creating excessive bulk include serratus anterior and omentum.

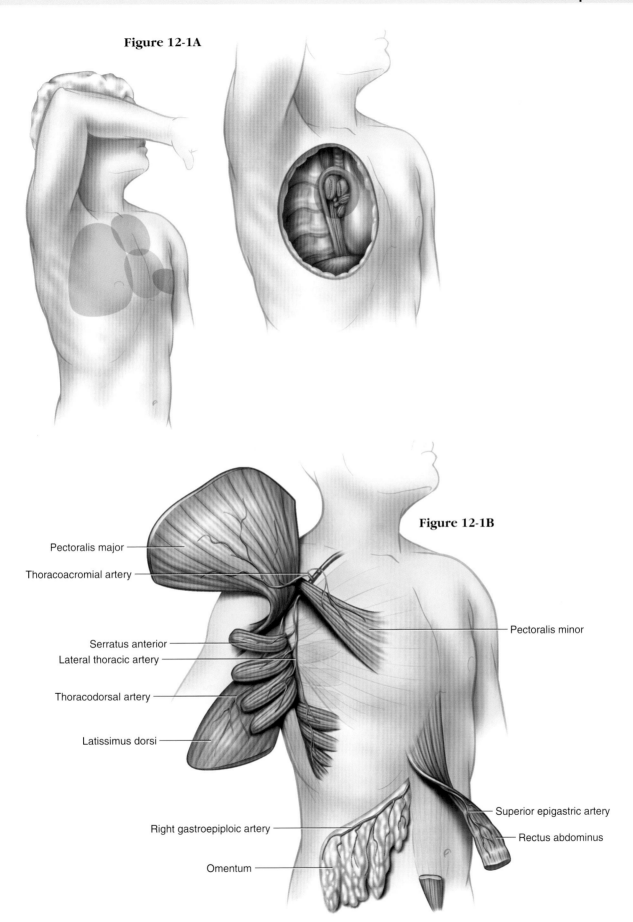

Figure 12-1A

Figure 12-1B

Pectoralis major

Thoracoacromial artery

Pectoralis minor

Serratus anterior

Lateral thoracic artery

Thoracodorsal artery

Latissimus dorsi

Superior epigastric artery

Right gastroepiploic artery

Rectus abdominus

Omentum

12-2 Latissimus Dorsi and Serratus Anterior Flaps

The workhorse of chest wall reconstruction is the latissimus dorsi (LD) flap. The most common drawback to its use is that it is often cut during performance of a standard lateral or posterolateral thoracotomy. The LD can be used as a free flap, and has a large arc of rotation when used as a pedicled flap. It may be fashioned as a muscle or myocutaneous flap. Its origin is broad-based, and includes the spine of the lower six thoracic vertebrae, sacral vertebrae, and posterior iliac crest. The superior and lateral borders of the muscle are relatively free. The muscle fibers converge in a spiral pattern into a tendon that inserts onto the intertubercular groove of the humerus. The dominant vascular supply is the thoracodorsal artery, a branch of the subscapular artery, which enters the deep surface of the muscle about 10 cm inferior to the muscle insertion onto the humerus (Fig. 12-2A). The motor nerve supply is the thoracodorsal nerve, which arises from the C6 to C8 nerve roots. Although this muscle functions to adduct, extend, and medially rotate the humerus, similar functions are provided by other shoulder girdle muscles.

To prepare this muscle for myoplasty, the borders of the LD muscle are marked with the help of external landmarks: the superior extent lies at the tip of the scapula, and the anterior margin is evident as the posterior axillary line; the posterior extent corresponds to the posterior vertebral column, and the muscle extends inferiorly to the posterior iliac crest. Flap elevation is performed with the patient prone or in a lateral position. Prepping the ipsilateral upper extremity into the field permits shoulder abduction that facilitates flap mobilization.

Dissection is performed through a 10-to-20-cm incision, which originates in the posterior axilla and extends inferiorly on the surface of the muscle (Fig. 12-2B). The muscle is divided from the tip of the scapula and is separated from the interdigitations with the inferior fibers of the trapezius. The surface of the muscle is freed with the aid of exposure, using a headlight or lighted retractor. Dissection is carried inferiorly until the origin of the muscle can be divided from the vertebral bodies and from the lumbosacral fascia 5 to 7 cm cephalad from the posterior iliac crest. Mobilization then proceeds proximally. Minor vascular pedicles from the lumbar and posterior intercostal arteries are identified and controlled. Adhesions between the anterior margin of the LD and the serratus anterior are divided, moving proximally until the crossing branch from the thoracodorsal artery to the serratus anterior artery is identified. The flap is elevated superiorly and the site of entry of the dominant vessels into the posterior surface of the muscle is found. These vessels are carefully identified and preserved. Adhesions between the LD and teres major are divided. If a relatively small arc of rotation is all that is needed, the LD insertion may be left intact. If more length and greater arc are necessary, the insertion ligament/muscles are divided proximal to the dominant vessels and the dissection proceeds distally toward the vessels. Additional vascular pedicle length may be gained by dividing the vascular branch to the serratus anterior.

The LD muscle reaches anteriorly through a subcutaneous tunnel on the surface of the serratus anterior muscle, or can be brought either superficial or deep to the pectoralis major muscle. Superior mediastinal coverage is facilitated by excising segments of the second and third ribs in the midaxillary line. Inferior mediastinal coverage is accomplished by creating a similar defect in the fifth or sixth interspace. The donor site is closed primarily unless a large skin pedicle has been taken with the flap, which may then require grafting.

The serratus anterior (SA) flap is a broad, thin flap, which can be used to reconstruct relatively small surface defects or can reach into the pleural space for myoplasty. It is generally raised as a muscle flap, and its use as a myocutaneous flap is rare. The SA origin is the outer surface of the upper eight or nine ribs anterolaterally, and the insertion is on the ventral surface of the medial border of the scapula. There are two dominant blood supplies, one from the lateral thoracic artery and the other being lateral branches of the thoracodorsal artery (Fig. 12-2C). The motor nerve supply is the long thoracic nerve, which arises from the C5 to C7 nerve roots. The SA muscle functions to pull the medial border of the scapula anteriorly, and its complete loss results in winging of the scapula.

The muscle is harvested with the patient in a standard lateral position. The anterior edge of the latissimus dorsi and the posterior edge of the pectoralis major are marked; the SA lies between these landmarks and extends deep to the LD. A diagonal incision is made across the axilla and is carried inferiorly for 8 to 10 cm. Either the upper few slips are harvested, based on the lateral thoracic pedicle, or the lower three to five slips are harvested, based on the thoracodorsal pedicle; use of the latter is most common. The slips are divided anteriorly at their origin on the ribs (Fig. 12-2D). The dissection proceeds from anterior to posterior, where the muscles are divided from their insertions and are elevated off the chest wall. The lateral thoracic nerve, which supplies motor function to the muscle, is identified on the outer surface of the muscle and preserved. It joins the thoracodorsal vessels at the level of the sixth rib. The vessels are dissected in a cephalad direction; if necessary, branches to the LD are divided to provide an adequate arc of rotation for the SA muscle flap. Intrathoracic transposition is accomplished through a thoracotomy incision or through a window created by resection of portions of two ribs near the vascular pedicle. The donor site is closed primarily.

Figure 12-2A

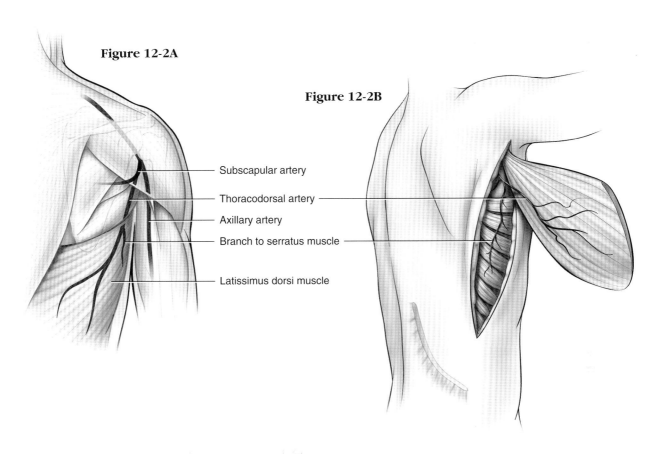

Figure 12-2B

- Subscapular artery
- Thoracodorsal artery
- Axillary artery
- Branch to serratus muscle
- Latissimus dorsi muscle

Figure 12-2C

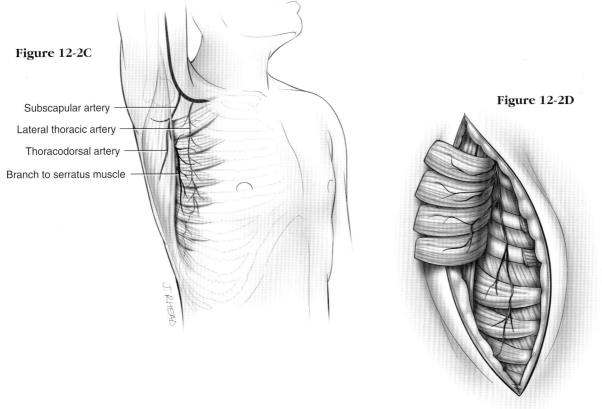

Figure 12-2D

- Subscapular artery
- Lateral thoracic artery
- Thoracodorsal artery
- Branch to serratus muscle

12-3 Rectus Abdominus and Pectoralis Major Flaps

The rectus abdominus (RA) muscle flap is typically used for reconstruction of the anterior chest wall. It is somewhat more technically demanding to prepare, and the incidence of hernia in the flap donor site is an ongoing topic of concern when selecting among reconstructive options. In addition, prior injury to the ipsilateral internal thoracic vessels often precludes use of the rectus abdominus muscle, and a prior ipsilateral subcostal incision is an absolute contraindication to use of the RA muscle.

The rectus abdominus muscle extends from the costal margin to the pubis, having tendinous intersections at the level of the xiphoid process, midway to the umbilicus, and at the level of the umbilicus. The origin is from the symphysis pubis and the crest of the pubis, and the insertion is on the cartilages of the fifth through seventh ribs (Fig. 12-3A). For purposes of thoracic reconstructive surgery, the dominant pedicle is the superior epigastric artery and vein. The motor nerve supply is from the seventh through twelfth intercostal nerves. The function of the rectus abdominus is to flex the vertebral column forward and to stiffen the abdominal wall. Loss of the muscle leads to substantial cosmetic deformity and some limitation of truncal flexion.

The muscle is prepared through a paramedian or a midline incision with the patient in a supine position. The anterior rectus sheath is divided and dissected from the surface of the muscle. Portions of the anterior rectus sheath may be left attached to the muscle flap at the level of the tendinous junctions. The lateral and medial margins of the RA muscle are mobilized. The posterior aspect of the flap is freed from the posterior rectus sheath and the distal muscle is divided. The inferior epigastric vessels are divided at the lateral margin of the muscle to complete the dissection. The muscle is generally tunneled under a flap of skin crossing the costal margin to permit it to pass to the anterior chest wall for use in reconstruction. The tunnel must be made wide enough to avoid constriction of the blood supply to the flap. The flap is turned over the costal margin and is laid in place (Fig. 12-3B).

The donor site is closed in a manner that avoids herniation and avoids compression on the vascular pedicle of the graft. The medial and lateral edges of the anterior sheath are sutured together; if weakness in this closure is of concern, reinforcement with synthetic mesh is appropriate.

The pectoralis major (PM) muscle flap is a very useful tissue flap for use in reconstructive surgery of the sternal region and upper chest in general. It can be fashioned as a muscle, myocutaneous, or osseomusculocuta-neous flap. Its origin is the medial half of the clavicle, the anterior surface of the sternum, the cartilaginous portion of ribs 1 to 7, and the fascia of the external oblique muscle. The PM fibers converge into a tendon that inserts onto the humerus. The dominant vascular supply is the pectoral branch of the thoracoacromial artery, which enters the deep surface of the muscle at the midpoint of the clavicle (Fig. 12-3C). Minor pedicles include the pectoral branch of the lateral thoracic artery, and the perforating arterial branches arising through the intercostal spaces medially, primarily from the internal mammary vessels and the lower intercostal vessels. Motor function is supplied by the lateral or superior pectoral nerve for the clavicular and sternal heads, whereas the medial and inferior pectoral nerves supply the lateral and posterior segments of the muscle. The function of the pectoralis major is to adduct and medially rotate the arm. Use of this muscle in reconstructive surgery results in cosmetic deformity (loss of the anterior axillary fold) and functional loss.

Preparation of the PM flap can often be performed through an incision that exists as part of the need for reconstructive surgery; in most cases, this is a median sternotomy incision. Alternatively, an incision is made parallel and inferior to the clavicle for purposes of preparing a PM muscle flap. To create a standard flap that is based laterally on the dominant vascular pedicle, the muscle is dissected from the overlying skin, carefully preserving its fascial covering. The muscle origins are divided from the sternal region, costal cartilages, and clavicle. The flap is rotated superiorly, enabling visualization of the vascular pedicle on the deep surface of the muscle. The dissection is completed up to the clavicle, and the muscle fibers are divided lateral to the pedicle. The flap may be rotated and advanced to cover the upper two thirds of the sternum (see Fig. 12-3D inset).

A turnover, or reverse, flap is based on medial perforating vessels, and is very useful in reconstructing sternal defects when the ipsilateral internal thoracic vessels remain intact. The anterior muscle surface is exposed as outlined above. The lateral border of the muscle is freed, and the fibers are divided at the junction of the lateral third and the medial two thirds of the muscle. The clavicular attachments are divided medial to the thoracoacromial pedicle. The flap is dissected lateral to medial, preserving the medial 2 to 3 cm of attachments to the chest wall. The perforating vessels in this region provide segmental supply to the flap, indicating that the flap can be divided into two or three separate slips as needed for reconstructive purposes. The PM flap is turned over into the sternal defect and is sutured (Fig. 12-3D). The lateral portion of the muscle that was left intact is sutured under tension to the pectoralis minor muscle to preserve the anterior axillary fold.

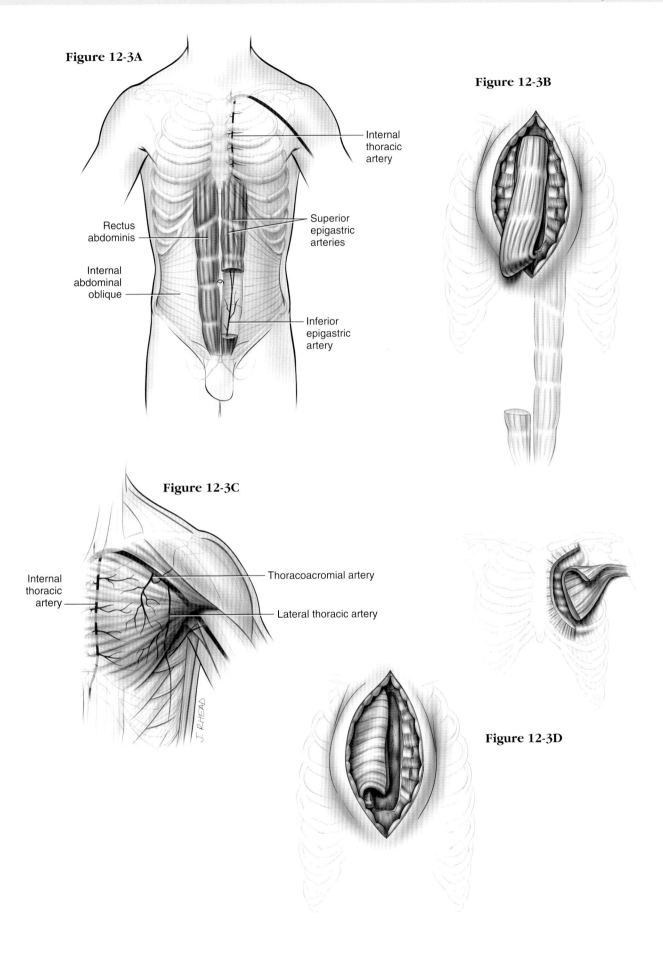

Figure 12-3A

Internal thoracic artery

Rectus abdominis

Superior epigastric arteries

Internal abdominal oblique

Inferior epigastric artery

Figure 12-3B

Figure 12-3C

Internal thoracic artery

Thoracoacromial artery

Lateral thoracic artery

Figure 12-3D

12-4   Omentum and Intercostal Muscle Flaps

The omentum is a useful flap for reinforcing anastomoses and for providing bulk to fill space defects. Its use is restricted to patients who have maintained an adequate level of nutrition such that the omentum is a fatty apron of tissue rather than a thin translucent sheet. There are two dominant blood supplies, the right and left gastroepiploic vessels. A minor pedicle is formed by a secondary vessel, which courses inferiorly in the omental apron that connects the two dominant blood supplies (Fig. 12-4A).

There are a wide variety of ways that the omentum can be fashioned for reconstruction. It may be dissected from the transverse colon, taking care to preserve the middle colic vessels, and turned over to be brought superiorly to reach the anterior abdominal wall without further dissection. The omentum can be divided vertically such that only half of the apron is turned over onto the anterior chest wall in a similar fashion, based on the gastroepiploic vessels without requiring further dissection. Most often, however, the omentum is dissected from the transverse colon and from the stomach by dividing the short branches between the gastroepiploic vessels directly on the gastric wall. In this way it is used as a pedicled flap. The flap is based either on the origin of the right gastroepiploic artery or of the left gastroepiploic artery, depending on where the flap is to be transposed. If there is a need to preserve the vascular supply to the stomach, the omental flap may be based on the minor pedicle distally in the apron by separating the gastroepiploic vessels from the omentum, leaving them intact on the stomach, to the point where the communicating branch inferior in the apron anastomoses with the gastroepiploic vessels, and this branch is carefully preserved (Fig. 12-4B). The pedicled flap thus prepared is tunneled over the costal margin to reach anterior chest wall or mediastinal defects.

Intercostal muscle flaps are used primarily for reinforcing intrathoracic repairs, such as closure of esophageal perforation, divided hilar structures in the presence of infection or prior radiation therapy, and high risk enteric organ or vascular anastomoses. Flaps can be created from intercostal tissues from ribs 3 to 11; the blood supply for ribs 1 and 2 is not based on intercostal vessels and is unreliable, while the twelfth rib is too short to provide meaningful reconstructive tissues. The dominant blood supply is the posterior intercostal artery, and the motor nerve supply is from the intercostal nerves. The external and internal intercostal muscles are accessory muscles of respiration; there is considerable redundancy in the system because of the multiplicity of such muscles.

The intercostal flap is best prepared prior to completing any planned thoracotomy. Use of intercostal muscle lying in the thoracotomy incision after completion of the thoracotomy may not be optimal if the intercostal retractor has placed pressure on the intercostal bundle, adversely affecting the viability of the flap. After exposure of the chest wall, the latissimus dorsi is reflected posteriorly and the interspace to be used for the thoracotomy is identified. There are at least two ways to prepare the intercostal muscle flap at this point. To create a flap with the most reliable blood supply, the rib at the superior aspect of the planned intercostal incision is excised subperiosteally. The intercostal muscle is divided from the inferior rib, and the deep periosteum of the resected rib is incised. The muscle flap is transected anteriorly at the desired limit of the length of the flap, and the dissection is carried posteriorly to near the origin of the intercostal vessel. This technique has the advantage of avoiding dissection near the intercostal bundle. However, leaving the periosteum intact may lead to new bone formation in the future that may be undesirable.

Alternatively, the muscle is divided at the lower boundary of the selected intercostal space, and the muscle is dissected from the superior rib with a periosteal elevator. This is best accomplished by taking the external intercostal muscles from anterior to posterior, and then taking the internal intercostal muscles from posterior to anterior. The relative orientation of the muscle fibers permits their easy separation from the underlying rib. As dissection of the internal intercostal muscles proceeds, care is taken to follow the undersurface of the rib to avoid injury to the intercostal bundle (see Fig. 12-4C inset). The flap is dissected posteriorly until the origin of the intercostal artery is reached, defining the posterior extent of the flap (Fig. 12-4C). The flap is then turned over into the pleural space, permitting coverage of the desired tissues (Fig. 12-4D).

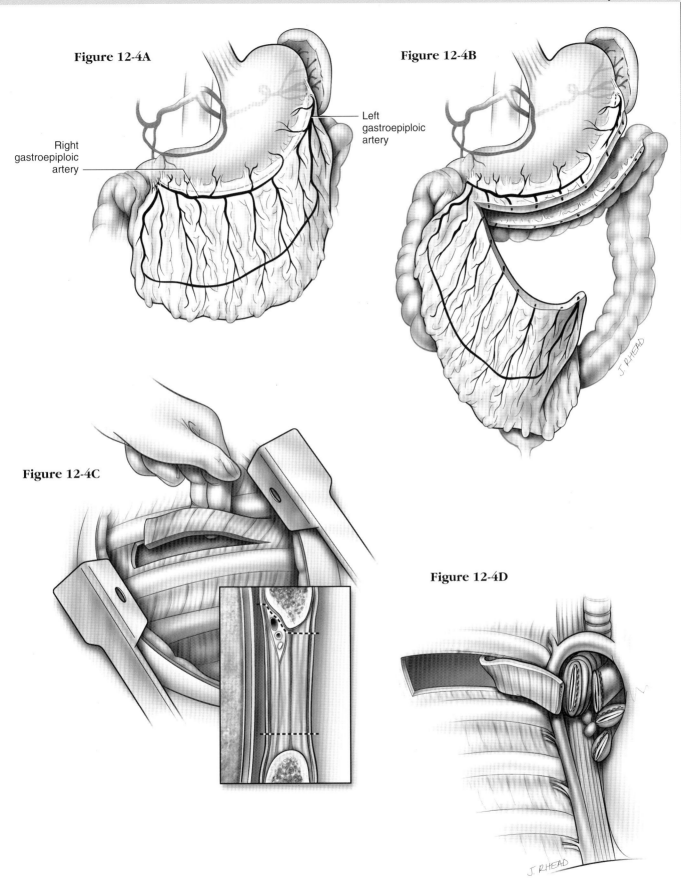

Figure 12-4A

Right gastroepiploic artery

Left gastroepiploic artery

Figure 12-4B

Figure 12-4C

Figure 12-4D

Index

Note: Page numbers followed by f indicate figures; those followed by t indicate tables.